AṢṬADAḶA YOGAMĀLĀ

AṢṬADAḶA YOGAMĀLĀ

(COLLECTED WORKS)

B.K.S. IYENGAR

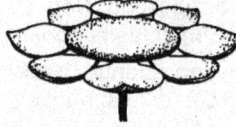

Volume 8

Questions and Answers, Interviews
Articles & Comprehensive Index
for all Volumes (1 to 8)

Allied Publishers Private Limited
New Delhi • Mumbai • Kolkata • Lucknow • Chennai
Nagpur • Bangalore • Hyderabad • Ahmedabad

ALLIED PUBLISHERS PRIVATE LIMITED
Regd. Off. : 15 J.N. Heredia Marg, Ballard Estate, **Mumbai**–400001
Ph.: 022-42126969 • E-mail: mumbai.books@alliedpublishers.com
47/9 Prag Narain Road, Near Kalyan Bhawan, **Lucknow**–226001
Ph.: 0522-2209942 • E-mail: lko.books@alliedpublishers.com
F-1 Sun House (First Floor), C.G. Road, Navrangpura,
Ellisbridge P.O., **Ahmedabad**–380006
Ph.: 079-26465916 • E-mail: ahmbd.books@alliedpublishers.com
3-2-844/6 & 7 Kachiguda Station Road, **Hyderabad**–500027
Ph.: 040-24619079 • E-mail: hyd.books@alliedpublishers.com
5th Main Road, Gandhinagar, **Bangalore**–560009
Ph.: 080-22262081 • E-mail: bngl.books@alliedpublishers.com
1/13-14 Asaf Ali Road, **New Delhi**–110002
Ph.: 011-23239001 • E-mail: delhi.books@alliedpublishers.com
17 Chittaranjan Avenue, **Kolkata**–700072
Ph.: 033-22129618 • E-mail: cal.books@alliedpublishers.com
60 Shiv Sunder Apartments (Ground Floor), Central Bazar Road,
Bajaj Nagar, **Nagpur**–440010
Ph.: 0712-2234210 • E-mail: ngp.books@alliedpublishers.com
751 Anna Salai, **Chennai**–600002
Ph.: 044-28523938 • E-mail: chennai.books@alliedpublishers.com

Website: www.alliedpublishers.com

First Published 2008

Reprinted 2010, 2012

ISBN : 978-81-8424-391-8

Front cover design : The Author
Artwork : S.M. Waugh
Back Cover Photograph : © Michael O'Neill, N.Y.

Published by Sunil Sachdev and printed by Ravi Sachdev at Allied Publishers Pvt. Ltd., Printing Division, A-104 Mayapuri Phase II, New Delhi - 110064

Invocatory Prayers

ॐ

Yogena cittasya padena vācāṁ
Malaṁ śarīrasyaca vaidyakena
Yopākarottaṁ pravaraṁ munīnāṁ
Patañjaliṁ prāñjalirānato'smi
Ābāhu puruṣākāraṁ
Śaṅkha cakrāsi dhāriṇaṁ
Sahasra śirasaṁ śvetaṁ
Praṇamāmi Patañjaliṁ

I bow before the noblest of sages Patañjali, who gave yoga for serenity and sanctity of mind, grammar for clarity and purity of speech and medicine for pure, perfect health.

I prostrate before Patañjali who is crowned with a thousand headed cobra, an incarnation of Ādiśeṣa (Anañta) whose upper body has a human form, holding the conch in one arm, disk in the second, a sword of wisdom to vanquish nescience in the third and blessing humanity from the fourth arm, while his lower body is like a coiled snake.

Yastyaktvā rūpamādyaṁ prabhavati jagato'nekadhānugrahāya
Prakṣīṇakleśarāśirviṣamaviṣadharo'nekavaktrāḥ subhogī
Sarvajñānaprasūtirbhujagaparikaraḥ prītaye yasya nityaṁ
Devohīṣaḥ savovyātsitavimalatanuryogado yogayuktaḥ

I prostrate before Lord Ādiśeṣa, who manifested himself on Earth as Patañjali to grace the human race in health and harmony,

I salute Lord Ādiśeṣa of the myriad serpent heads and mouths carrying noxious poisons, discarding which he came to Earth as a single headed Patañjali in order to eradicate ignorance and vanquish sorrow.

I pay my obeisance to him, repository of all knowledge, amidst his attendant retinue.

I pray to the Lord whose primordial form shines with peace and white effulgence, pristine in body, a master of yoga, who bestows on all his yogic light to enable mankind to rest in the house of the immortal Soul.

BY THE AUTHOR

This volume of *Aṣṭadaḷa Yogamālā* published by Allied Publishers, Delhi, is the eighth volume of the "Collected Works" of Yogācārya B.K.S. Iyengar. The Collected Works are comprised from Articles, Interviews and Questions and Answers given by the Yogācārya throughout is extensive life of practice, teaching and imparting yoga.

Also by the Same Author

Light on Yoga
Light on Prāṇāyāma
Concise Light on Yoga
Art of Yoga
Tree of Yoga
Light on the Yoga Sūtras of Patañjali
The Illustrated Light on Yoga
Yoga Dipika (Marathi)
Yoga Ek Kalpataru (Marathi)
Ārogyayoga (Marathi)
Light on Aṣṭāṇga Yoga
Aṣṭadaḷa Yogamālā (Vols 1 to 7)
Yoga: The Path To Holistic Health
Yoga Sarvānasāṭhi (Marathi)
Basic Guidelines for Teachers of Yoga (co-authored with G.S. Iyengar)
Yogacandan (Marathi)
Light on Life

Also on Iyengar Yoga

Body the Shrine, Yoga Thy Light
70 Glorious Years
Iyengar His Life and Work
Yogapushpanjali
Yogadhārā

TABLE OF CONTENTS

PLATES

TABLES

ACKNOWLEDGEMENTS

It is a great joy for me to express my sense of gratitude to all those who from the very first day of undertaking this voluminous work, assisting immensely by participating with involvement in both the intellectual head as well as the emotional feelings. Hence, this acknowledgement to those who helped is not a formal one, but is filled with love and affection from the very source of my own life.

Geeta S. Iyengar – For going through the scattered materials which were difficult to present and in dissarray, for assisting me with her valuable suggestions and corrections to the subject matter which made it comfortable for me to braid with ease.

Faeq Biria – Who with dedication to the subject and to me, came to India every year specifically to help me, lending his unimagineable memory power which was a great help for me to re-build the subject from his constructive thoughts which guided me to remove those repetitions that non-deliberately appeared in the volumes. With his memory power, he has made the readers free from boredom

Patxi Lizardi – Who also with love and devotion travelled every year to India, printing the same manuscript umpteen times, pointing out how the words were not balancing with the subject matter and taking notes to bring not only harmony in the subject, but also a smoothness in reading.

John J. Evans – Who graciously looked into the volume bringing a cohesive English throughout.

Stephanie Quirk – Editing assistance, book layout and preparation of the plates.

Uma Dhavale – For editing assistance.

Raya Uma-Datta – Assisting with tables and plates.

Montserrat Gonzalez and Emilio Hidalgo for their help in the preparation of the indexes.

Mr Kokate – For artwork of the front and back covers.

Surojit Banerjee – Overseeing editorial work for Allied Publishers (Delhi).

The various subjects depicted in the plates who willingly allowed themselves to be photographed for this volume in order to express with clarity so that the readers adopt with ease to follow in their practices.

FOREWORD

One night in 1949, an extraordinary and momentous event occurred in my life. It was to become a turning point of my personal fortunes and it dictated the direction my life was to take.

With it, there came to a close what had been my most severely testing period, grim years lasting from 1940 to 1949 and which had followed the termination of my job at the Deccan Gymkhana Club. I had served there from 1937 to 1940. Indeed it was for this position that, at the request of Dr. V.B.Ghokale, I had moved away from the familiar language and society of my own upbringing. Dr. Ghokhale was a surgeon who had retired to Poona (Pune) at the end of his service to the government of the Bombay Presidency.

Even with the Deccan job, my situation had remained exposed, lonely and unstable but at least it had provided me with a livelihood and place to live, learn and grow. Each of us needs some vital base from which to participate in society and when mine was abruptly terminated, it fell on me as a catastrophic blow.

Yet some mysterious force kept me on my feet. It made me hold on to the one thing I had: Yoga.

I persisted and persevered in practice, and by dint of willingness to teach whosoever approached me, just kept our heads financially above water. I say "our" as I had recently married my wife, Ramamani, who along with yoga turned out to be both the rock and blessing of my life. And she participated equally with me in the singular event which took place on a night in 1946.

Simultaneously, we both had a dream.....

Our family deity, Lord Venkateṣvara (Balaji), came to me in my dream and gave me a handful of rice with these words, "Now devote your time to yoga and the rest will be taken care of". That same night the Lord's consort, Mahalaksmi, appeared to my wife, telling her, "I had borrowed 25 paisa from your husband and am now returning the same to you".

These remarkable dreams marked a new dawn in our lives. Fear, worry and anxiety began gradually to fade out. Although I had been initiated into the practice of yoga at an early age, there had never before appeared any sort of divine injunction that yoga should be my path. I again started practising with increased vigour, rigour and confidence. The doubt which had constantly sapped my morale gave way to renewed enthusiasm and aspiration. By the grace of Balaji and Mahalaksmi, my *sādhanā* began bearing fruit, not only economically but also in the writing and publication of what become standard books on the subject; *Light on Yoga, Light on Pranayama, Tree of Yoga, Art of Yoga, Light on the Yoga Sutras of Patanjali, Yoga: The Path to Holistic Health, Light on Astanga Yoga, Light on Life* and now the *eight volumes of Aṣṭadaḷa Yogamālā.*

It has been a long journey and the way ahead has not always been clear. It is only now, in the fulfilment of this major undertaking to gather and organise, as one collected work, the entire fruit of my experience and distilled reflections that I find I can look back and recognise how, hour after hour, one book at a time, the discipline of authorship has refined, honed and crafted my thought.

Our dreams of long ago have been realised, their double visitation guiding towards the divine source of inspiration. At the conclusion of this final volume, I prostrate before Lord Shri Venkatesvara as I have now fulfilled his summons to yoga. My lifelong work is an offering to the Lord in gratitude for his benediction. My devotion to Him has transformed a life that could easily have lacked worth or meaning into a useful life of service and significance.

It has been an honour to present, through Allied Publishers, these volumes on India's most valuable heritage. In the hope that these books will become a source of reference and research for the seeker of today and of tomorrow, I have included a comprehensive index for the entire series, from volume 1 to 8. In the event that these works serve as a foundation to aspirants of yoga, then both credit and merit must be shared not only between the publisher and myself, but with those innumerable students without whom, whether directly or indirectly, the formulation and execution of this immense work would not have been possible.

For millennia yogi have practised yoga as paths of karma, jnana and bhakti. These volumes of teachings are the karma, or the result, of my dedicated sadhana. Any Master on a particular path who has attained a level of exalted, yet subjective, knowledge, finds himself in a situation analogous to that of the newly enlightened Buddha, seated under the peepul tree. He realised that he had to find his followers, wherever they were, return to them and try to help them also to "See what he had Seen". In that insightful decision, he became a Teacher.

As regards the path of *jñāna*, in the process of writing, I have had endlessly to sift my thoughts and reflections so as to clarify and bring lucidity to the deepest ramifications of my felt experience. It has been necessary to search the knowledge base of several languages to find suitable expression so that you may read my words and hopefully hear their message. Fortified by knowledge, you too will, I hope, dive into the great depth and richness that yoga-sadhana offers.

As concerns *bhākti*, following Lord Venkatesvara's behest I pray to continue in yoga and provide a "sheltering monastery" for all who seek its cool shade. To this end I surrender to you the best that I can do.

B.K.S. Iyengar

Pune, India

INTRODUCTORY MESSAGE*

First of all, I'm touched by my pupils who have done this wonderful decoration work with the expression of my *Naṭarājāsana* as I salute the Lord with that *āsana*. At the same time I hope God will pardon and forgive my students who have shown my foot to the Lord; though there is no difference for them between foot and hand.

As soul exists everywhere, God too exists everywhere.

In my early days birthday celebrations were not at all performed. Today I am happy that the love and affection you all shower upon me, shows that even though people call me a wild person, that 'wild' nature has brought so many of you close to me. If I was really soft, I don't know how many I would have drawn to my side. I was just sitting in the corner and wondering what to say; because birthdays have become ritualistic; just say hello, cut the cake, eat and go. On such occasions to speak on a dry and serious subject is going to be boring as it is a hard subject to grasp. To make this hard and dry subject moist and pleasant requires tremendous effort. As some people mentioned here today that they are in the *bahiraṅga sādhanā* state, others say they are in the *antaraṅga sādhanā* state while some say they are in the *antarātma sādhanā*. Note the word *sādhanā* that is present in all the three states.

To be very honest, even today I do not know why I am practising and what makes me practise. Concerning teaching I had to do it because I had to survive, I had to live and I have done this for years. Of course now I do not teach but I guide whenever students go wrong, or fail to get the correct position. But the moment I begin my practice, I become very inquisitive yet remaining innocent. With this innocence and inquisitiveness I enjoy things that surface in my practices. While practising my mind remains watchful and completely quiet, but my body acts dynamically with alertness. Of course you have seen the fire-brand character while I am teaching, but not while practising. It may surprise you how soft I remain while practising. The inner 'I' becomes even softer than the petals. If I am hard in body and mind, probably the elegance and

---

* This Message was given on the occasion of the author's 79th Birthday celebrations, 14th December 1997, at the Ramāmaṇi Iyengar Memorial Yoga Institute, Pune, India.

beauty of the *āsana* would not have surfaced in me. For many the body fibres and the intelligence would become hard in their practices. Fortunately I keep them softer than the petals, so that the knowledge that flashes out is received by the fibres of the body with care and comfort. Our bodies, according to our yogic science, are like lots of petals with various designs. Unless and until these petals are kept in a right shape, knowledge will not bloom at all. Hence, I am happy that I keep my mind innocent and open in my practice. When I keep my mind in such a state and practise, unthought of things flash like lightning. Whatever new things strike me I share with you all. I do not know if what I share is accepted or rejected or taken with indifference by you. As an honest student of yoga, I at once pass what I am experiencing and the thoughts that strike me on to all of you, in order to make you finer and finer in your practices. I filter and re-filter the same experiences over and over untill it is well established before sharing them with you all. Each time by re-doing my practices I reach a seasoned state of understanding, which registers all changes in my head and heart. Just one experience cannot give a matured or seasoned understanding, the same has to be re-done, re-filtered and re-felt to bring the best out of it, so that the essence of the experience is brought out without bringing in the past memories. I do not practise with the past memories though they are registered within. Yet I keep my brain and mind afresh the moment I begin my practice. I am neither in the future nor in the past, I follow the whole body while journeying in it in each *āsana*. I follow living in moments without allowing them to roll into movements. I accept whatever comes and if the feeling is bad, I work out at once how to change the bad actions and feelings into good actions and feelings.

Today my interest is to tell you about my subject and its *sādhanā*. You know about the kites that children play with. There are different shapes of kites, each having a different form, design, thread and person to play. As one observes children's kite games, the yogi learns by using his body as a kite. We have got hundreds of muscles and joints, thousands of fibres, millions and billions of cells and hence this body can be compared to a kite. The Self which is hidden inside plays the kite; if the wind is not there the kite cannot fly. As such children move and pull the thread to make the kite fly by pulling and pushing the thread forwards or backwards until the kite catches the wind to soar up. Similarly I use the intelligence as a thread to act on the muscles to work properly and move evenly with rhythm. In our body, the calf or thigh muscles or hinges or ankles or heels, are like different kites. To control these various muscles and structures that are like different kites, the thread of intelligence is made to be held by the holder – the Self *(sūtradhāra)* – to make the fibres, tissues, joints and muscles move with control.

If the anatomical/physiological body is the kite, its thread is the intelligence and the Self is the holder of the thread. In order to adjust each muscle, joint and fibre, the Self has to hold the thread and pull the intelligence in such a manner that all the various parts of the body are brought to a single state of stability like the kite that remains stable though soaring high in the sky.

While practising the *āsana* one has to grip these various deformities in the performance of the *āsana* and remove them, resulting in the state where the intelligence as thread grips the various parts of the body (the kite), so that the holder (the Self) feels the oneness with the intelligence (thread), as if the kite, the thread and the Self are one.

Like the kite with the thread and its holder, there is no difference between *antaraṅga*, *bahiraṅga* and *antarātma sādhanā*; it is only for the sake of convenience that these differences are created to facilitate understanding of the difference and oneness. When the child is playing with the kite, for him the thread, the kite and himself is one. If the thread is cut the kite is lost, similarly these divisions are shown so that we penetrate from the periphery (the body), to the inner core (the Self), through the power of the intelligence so that the inner core is one with the outer body. This is the 'dual avenue' to study the movement of the intelligence, consciousness and conscience so that the soul moves freely everywhere with the help of all these vehicles.

Practice of *āsana* is like kite-flying wherein different designs and shapes are struck. In the same way the human body assumes so many different shapes and forms in the *āsana* which need attention to reach perfection. If somebody says that it is 'physical yoga', then I say that that person does not know anything about the subject. Such a person is an impostor and not an honest *sādhaka* at all.

Let me give another example. A potter makes different types and shapes of pots: it may be oval, round, longish and so forth. But when the pot or the jar is filled with water, whatever shape the jar is the content takes that shape and touches the vessel evenly everywhere. If the vessel is crooked, the content also takes that crooked shape and similarly makes contact. There is no gap or space left, no air bubbles present. This is what you have to learn when you are practising the *āsana*. These *āsana* are like different vessels or containers but the content – the *ātman* covers the body whether one part is contracting or another part is expanding. As you are sitting now you are aware of the frame of the body. Similarly in various positions, one has to feel the content (the soul), touching the container or the body, both inside and outside, without any deviation or air gaps.

Take *Śīrṣāsana* or *Tāḍāsana*. You might not know how many empty spaces remain unattended while you are practising. If the inner core – the Self – comes in contact with the entire container which is five to six feet long and two to two and a half feet broad, then one can see that the divided two feet have to be made as if it is one in practice. If there is a gap the divisions become apparent. These divisions come only to those who are empty in their intellect. Those who know and seek to bring totally the container and the content in contact are the true practitioners. This is what yoga has taught me on account of my attentive observation in my practices. It is this innocence or freshness in approach which gave me wisdom towards precision in my presentations. It is my consciousness *(citta)* or the conscience *(antaḥkaraṇa)* and my *ātmā* or the Self, which questions the emptiness or fullness of the intellect and I immediately pull my intelligence of the heart (the thread) to pierce, to reach that empty area so that the kite (body) feels that there is a contact of my body through the thread of intelligence to myself. I want you all to practise yoga with this analogy of the kite flying.

You have to learn when practising these *āsana* that you have to fill the container of the body with the Self without leaving any space in between. The moment you experience this, then that period of time is a divine time. Divinity does not bring division. To understand this union in division is very subtle. Hence observe carefully while practising. I repeat again my words: "Consciousness is the needle, the eye of the needle is the intelligence, the mind is the head of the thread which you sharpen in the beginning to push into the eye of the needle". With this insertion into the intelligence the mind connects the *bahiraṅga* (outer body), with the *antaraṅga* (inner body) and both disappear from the scene for the Self to act directly.

If you take the five elements of nature: *pṛthvī, āp, tej, vāyu* and *ākāśa, tejas* is in the middle of all elements. As *tejas* is connected to the mind *(manomaya kośa),* it connects the first two gross elements, *pṛthvī* (physical body) and *āp* (vital body), with the later subtle elements *vāyu* (intellectual body) and *ākāśa* (the space i.e. the core). After the *tejas* (mind) does its job it is the *sūkṣmendriya* in our body, the intelligence that has to sew the nerves, fibres with the entire systems of the body. Then as a *sādhaka* you understand that the divisions disappear. You are one with yourself not only at one point but at every point. This is what *āsana* teaches.

Know the way. Knowledge comes as the senses of perception are the gateways of knowledge. Though one may say that one must control them, yet without these knowledge cannot come. Unfortunately these gates of knowledge run with the external world. But the same gates of knowledge are to be introverted in the practice of *āsana* to derive the knowledge of the inner world, our inner body where the *ātmā* exists. These senses of perception are connected with *jñāna* of the *prakṛti* which has to come in contact with the *jñāna* of the *puruṣa,* giving rise to *ojas-śakti. Ojas-śakti* or *puruṣa śakti* merges the *prakṛti* in its *śakti.* For this one has to use all the five sheaths of the body to know the Self which has no sheath at all.

Finally, all the five sheaths are to be connected through the needle (the consciousness), using the eye of the needle (the intelligence), to weave the entire body from the skin to the self and vice versa into a fine muslin cloth. It should be even finer than the muslin cloth because the intelligence is a refined instrument in all of you and very sensitive so that it can even feel the thickness (darkness) or the thinness (light of action) of your inner body.

Right method of *āsana* practice makes this thick coating in the body to become transparent. Actually this is the beauty of each *āsana*. Hence it is not done just as physical exercise but it is used to make this inner coating of the body transparent and sensitive so that the intelligence, consciousness and the soul can pass through these veils of the self. In short *āsana* are done by the body for the mind, intelligence and consciousness to sensitise them. This sensitive inter-penetration or the opening of the inner layer of the skin, makes it even finer than the muslin cloth so that the soul can move everywhere as it likes while practising *āsana*, *prāṇāyāma* or *dhyāna*.

An analogy can be made with the river water that is collected in the reservoir and allowed to seep through the sluices so that the soil of the earth is nourished gradually. Similarly these *āsana* should be practised. Don't just take it as physical yoga. If you are real 'Iyengar' practitioners then you must know that we are merely using this body as an agent to trim the intelligence and make the intelligence seep into the system. The mind as an agent works to make the thread (intelligence) sharp and thin. These vehicles as agents have to touch the Self, then made to dissolve or act as secondary instrument of support. Instead of having indirect connections through *pṛthvī*, *āp*, *tej*, *vāyu*, *ākāśa*, as well as the *buddhi*, *citta* and *antaḥkaraṇa*, the *ātman* directly contacts these to guide you for good and auspicious practices. The *piṇḍāṇḍa* (microcosm) and the *brahmāṇḍa* (macrocosm) have to become one in our practice. It means the outer world comes directly in to contact with the inner world as if they are one. The coarse cloth (body) becomes a fine cloth which makes the coarse body to become as fine as the Self.

These gates of knowledge, namely; the organs of action and senses of perception are looked on as outside organs, they enable you to develop what *Haṭhayoga Pradīpika* calls as *antar-lakṣya* and *bahirdṛṣṭi*. It means that even though the physical eyes *(darśana jñāna)* may be looking out, the intellectual eye *(jñānacakṣu)* as the third eye will be looking inside. Hence all the five senses are connected to the intelligence as a single thread which takes you closer to the Self, so that from the *jñānendriya* you are able to reach the inner core of the being through your mind, intelligence and consciousness. This is what *āsana* teaches.

Patañjali says, *vitarka vicāra ānanda asmitārūpa anugamāt saṁprajñātaḥ* (*Y.S.*, I.17) – practice and detachment develop four types of *samādhi:* self-analysis, synthesis, bliss and the experience of pure being.

Though he has used the word *samprajñāta samādhi* I say they are various types of awareness. These are *vitarka*-awareness, *vicāra*-awareness, *ānanda*-awareness, *asmitā*-awareness. What you have to learn while doing the *āsana* is this: *Vitarka* is the biological frontal brain and *vicāra* is in the back portion, called the old oriental brain or the *saṁskārita* brain or the store-house of impressions. This frontal brain of analysis and the back brain of latent imprints of past experiences have to commune and finally unite with each other. When both these brains are made to function unitedly, one will not be able to differentiate at that moment whether the action is physical or mental or spiritual. When these two commune and unite with each other there is a joy that sprouts from within and at that time one just smiles. This smile is from the heart, the *ānanda*. It is this smile, this *ānanda* that further takes you to trace the source of that *ānanda* which is neither in the biological head nor in the old brain, but sprouts from a different place altogether. That place is the core of the being, *asmitā*. While practising *āsana*, one studies from *vitarka-vicāra*. This is the gross part of the intellect that kindles the subtle intelligence of the heart to sprout with bliss, *ānanda* or *muditā* (gladness). This memory of *ānanda* makes one search from where it sprouts. This is what *āsana* gives us, not just physical health. Just to say that my liver is fine or my haemoglobin content is high is not the real effect of *asana* but their by-products.

From now on practise *āsana* using *vitarka-vicāra* (head) to trace the cause of *ānanda*. It is interesting to note that the process reverses in *prāṇāyāma* practice, as one begins with *asmitā*, then comes to *ānanda* and from *ānanda* one moves to *vicāra* and *vitarka*. This is a beautiful way in studying the *sūtra*. This *ānanda* cannot be explained theoretically. Can anyone inhale from the head? If done that is hypertension. Any person who inhales from the head will soon become a cardiac patient. He will have high blood pressure and hypertension. Without the use of the head can you inhale or exhale? That is how to know the differences in *vitarka*, *vicāra*, *ānanda* and *asmitā*.

We theoretically explain the four states of *prajñā* (awareness). But in which position, in which part of yoga do these four surface? Which works in *āsana* and which in *prāṇāyāma*, has to be noted, is it not? All these have to be learnt under the guidance of an able teacher or a master. We understand in totality the various *prajñā*, the various awarenesses which have been given to us which psychologists can explain better than me. The four awarenesses (*vitarka*, *vicāra*, *ānanda* and *asmitā*), correspond to the four lobes of the brain, as *maitrī*, *karuṇā*, *muditā* and *upekṣā* correspond to the heart which also has four lobes (sections). It is only through Patañjali that these words became clear and we learn to connect the *prajñā* of the head to the *prajñāna* of the heart and vice versa, and to experience how yoga helps in maintaining serenity in the brain and the heart.

It is only when we practise these things through yogic *āsana* that we understand this depth and not just by standing on one's head. One cannot do *Śīrṣāsana* without using the head and one cannot do *Setu Bandha Sarvāṅgāsana* without using the heart. Each *āsana* has its own characteristic and as such we have to observe and study from where to where the source of action takes place. What happens when one loses the attention? For example, if one loses attention for a fraction of a second in *Śīrṣāsana* he loses his balance and falls down. In *Setu Bandha Sarvāṅgāsana* and *Halāsana* the brain remains silent but the seat of the heart remains attentive, while in *Śīrṣāsana* the brain is attentive while the seat of the heart remains pensive. This way *sādhaka* like you and me have to find out the biological, physical, chemical and mental changes that take place in each *āsana*, between the head and the heart. This way of study awakens awareness of the intelligence in various stages.

Let the medical professionals study the value of yoga and do research as Patañjali has done by changing the biological divisions of intellectual seats of the head and the emotional intelligence of the seats of the heart into one intelligent component. If you all work with a searching mind then I am sure that it would help to connect the modern technology with the wisdom of the ancients. With this combination it may be possible to understand various *prajñā* (intelligent attention and awareness) and how they work. To a great extent *āsana* can guide the medical professionals to present the value of yoga without favour or prejudice.

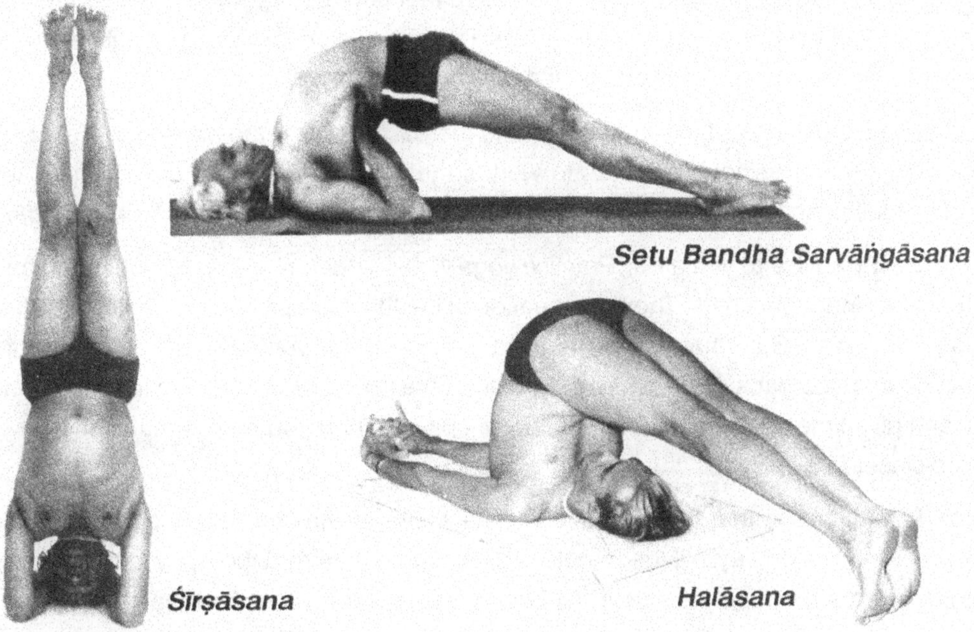

Plate n. 1 – *Āsana* which transform changes in head and heart

The *sādhaka* is graded according to his internal states. He may be *mṛdu, madhyama, adhimātra* and *tīvra*. It means the *sādhaka* may be feeble, average, keen and intense. In each *āsana* the pupil has to observe how the intelligence of the heart and the intellect of the head work, at what time it is *mṛdu*, at what time it is *madhyama, adhimātra* and *tīvra*. Each *āsana* has the potential to tell the *sādhaka* his quality and states of mind. We speak of four types of *sādhaka*, but we fail to observe at what time which part of the body is *mṛdu*. If the intuitive heart is active, the brain is *mṛdu;* if the intuitive heart is *adhimātra*, the brain is *mṛdu*, if the brain is *adhimātra*, then the heart is completely *mṛdu*, so one has to learn to understand and balance these. If there is *mṛdu* in the head there should be *mṛdu* in the heart as well as *mṛdu* in the body. Hence each one has to counter with the higher quality of the head and heart. For this the rigour of the body and the vigour of the mind have to go together.

The body does not say that it has no strength, it is the mind that says so. However for a good practitioner, the body sends the message that it cannot take it anymore. Here comes analysis to rectify with reason. Then one can recover either from the fatigue of the body or the mind in a few minutes. One has to think and act to get a right balance between the body, mind, nerves, energy and intellectual wisdom in practice.

Take my example. Many of you have seen me staying twenty to thirty minutes in the most difficult *āsana*. But you do not know why I stay. I stay to study the state of my body cells, the state of mind and intelligence. I learn to keep that original freshness throughout that time. I watch when that freshness disappears and find means to work out to bring that freshness back throughout my stay in the *āsana* without changing the position.

Mind is the one which makes or mars the *sādhanā* and the *sādhaka*. The intelligence or the eye of the consciousness has to work so that the mind does not vacillate. I keep the thread of intelligence firm and mind as subordinate to it in my practice of *āsana* or *prāṇāyāma*.

So my advice to you all is, "Practise yoga with an open mind. Keep your mind and heart like that of an innocent child." Then the creation of the things happening in the body will surface for you to cognise. But what you do is to rationalize when you practise. Instead of this see everything from the back of the brain and not from the front of the brain. Act from the front of the brain and give time for the back of the brain to absorb. Then you realise that whatever you do, you are closer to divinity.

Patañjali says that the goal is closer to a *tīvra saṁvegin* because in that person the intelligence is clear, the eye of the needle is clear, the needle and the eye are close to the soul. Whereas we have to use the thread to become firmer and finer. And that's why we have to struggle in the beginning, so that the effort becomes natural and as practises go on, it ceases to become a struggle or an effort.

Practise with an innocent mind and not with a heedless mind or with a slow-witted or dull head. There is a difference between innocence and ignorance. A child is intelligent but innocent. If the child is slow-witted or dull you think that there is something wrong with the child, and take the child to a child specialist to find out if the child is retarded or not. We are not retarded, but are neglectful and indifferent. We have to convert this indifference to make a difference. That's why these *āsana* are meant to be practised to remove indifference and for harmony to set in. When harmony sets in then you start understanding the various *prajñā*. Please do in this manner. God will bless you.

QUESTIONS AND ANSWERS

SECTION I

ON HEALTH AND THERAPEUTICS

SECTION I – ON HEALTH AND THERAPEUTICS

I.1. – The positive aspect of disease

When the modern medicines failed on certain diseased persons, they were recommended to try yoga. I tried to help such people either in controlling or curing their illness which spread from mouth to mouth like fire for yoga to gain popularity.

Aches, pains or sufferings are stepping-stones to knowledge. This philosophy of pain and the science of healing came into existence at the time of the churning of the ocean *(samudra maṁthana),* when Lord Dhanvaṁtari sprang from the ocean with a pot of medicines in his hands.[1]

Fear of disease and death brings awareness to think of health and survival. Hence, I feel that pains and diseases act as boons to maintain health and Self-knowledge.

Gautama Buddha saw a diseased person, an aged person and a funeral. He also saw a wandering mendicant. He was struck to see these sufferings in life and determined to search for the eternal truth. With this vision, he decided at once to be free from these bondages and reached *nirvāṇa* – liberation.

Diseases, suffering, aches and pains have made man discover remedies through medicines or other alternative healing acts like yoga. We have to be grateful to those savants who traced various types of remedies for the good of health and happiness.

The three demonic brothers Rāvaṇa, Kuṁbhakarṇa and Vibhiṣaṇa were masters of meditation. Yet Rāvaṇa was full of *rajas,* Kuṁbhakarṇa full of *tamas* and Vibhiṣaṇa full of *sattva.*[2] All three had excellent will power. Lord Rāma killed Rāvaṇa, Hanumān killed Kuṁbhakarṇa, while Vibhiṣaṇa became a devotee of Rāma and surrendered himself to Rāma who was an incarnation of Vishnu.

---

[1] See *Aṣṭadala Yogamālā,* vol. 2, pp. 107-108, and *The Tree of Yoga,* p. 115.

[2] See *Aṣṭadala Yogamālā,* vol. 2, pp. 239.

The fights between the gods and the demons from time unknown exist even to this day. The fight between Rāma and Rāvaṇa,[1] Lord Narasiṁha and Hiraṇyakaśyapu,[2] Krishna and Kaṁsa,[3] Indra and Vṛtrāsura[4] are very significant. These stories are the expressions of the triumph of divine qualities over demonic ones. Here, the demon represents disease and Gods represent health.

Man has been gifted to help himself. He has the capacity to handle physical, physiological and mental diseases like lust, anger and greed, and torpid diseases like doubt, laziness, dullness, heedlessness and sleep. Man can gain health freeing himself from desires and ambitions, which in turn bring pain, sorrow and disease. From this angle I say that diseases are blessings which discipline man to uncover the strength of vibrancy to work out not only in discarding the afflictions but to rise above them and to proceed towards liberation and emancipation.

The diseases, sufferings and sorrows awakened me and my intelligence through yoga and lifted me to this level of health, knowledge and wisdom. Through sufferings, I realised the value of yoga and I carried on giving relief to millions.

Patañjali explains the cause of disease in *sūtra* II.15.[5] Sorrow, pain, disease, thought and action are hidden in pleasures and enjoyments and the wise man is careful not to be caught in the net of pleasures or pains. Pleasure follows sorrow and sorrow follows pleasure.[6] These *sūtra* are an eye opener for us who are caught in disease, pain and sorrow and struggle to come out from these clutches. These things act as a mother of invention for us to search for eternal spiritual bliss.

We as human beings have the capacity to think of pain and sorrow and analyse them by discriminative knowledge. From such discriminative knowledge came medical science and other healing methods. Patañjali uses the word *bādhanā* for pain and *bhāvanā* for feeling.[7] *Bhāvanā* is a feeling to be felt by all of us. The sense of feeling is *vidyā* and the absence in

---

[1] See *Aṣṭadaḷa Yogamālā*, vol. 2, p. 239, and vol. 3, p. 191.

[2] See *Aṣṭadaḷa Yogamālā*, vol. 7, p. 71.

[3] See *Bhāgavata Purāṇa* (*skandha* 10).

[4] See *Aṣṭadaḷa Yogamālā*, vol. 2, p. 172, *Padma Purāṇa, Bhūmikhaṇḍa,* 23-24, *Ṛg-Veda,* I.16.80 and *Mahābhārata, Ādi-Parva.*

[5] *Pariṇāma tāpa saṁskāra duḥkaiḥ guṇavṛtti virodhāt ca duḥkham eva sarvaṁ vivekinaḥ* (*Y.S.*, II.15) – The wise man knows that owing to the fluctuations, the qualities of nature, and subliminal impressions, even pleasant experiences are tinged with sorrow; and he keeps aloof from them.

[6] *Sukha anuśayī rāgaḥ* (*Y.S.*, II.7) – Pleasure leads to desire and emotional attachment. *Duḥkha anuśayī dveṣaḥ* (*Y.S.*, II.8) – Unhappiness leads to malice and hatred.

[7] *Vitarka bādhane pratipkṣa bhāvanam* (*Y.S.*, II.33) – When one is affected by wrong, illogical thoughts, it has to be countered with the knowledge of discrimination. To think of contrary or contradictory thoughts which are against the principles of *yama* and *niyama* are known as *vitarka bādhana* or *bādhanam.*

feeling is nescience *(avidyā)*. *Bādhanā* means pain and sorrow. They tap and awaken sensitivity in the sufferer. It is called *pratipakṣa bhāvanam*. It is a thought used as an antidote or as a remedial approach towards obstacles. The *bhāvanā* attitude has to be developed to fight the *bādhanā*.

Bhāvana means feeling, which arises from the faculty of emotional intelligence. It has two sides: *pakṣa bhāvanam* (feeling and moving with the current) and *pratipakṣa bhāvanam* (feeling and moving against the current). Both will be acting simultaneously. Due to want of understanding they get mixed up. To go with pains, diseases and pleasant thoughts is a natural flow, but to think, act and find a remedy to fight against them is *pratipakṣa bhāvanam*.

Nature can be favourable if the practitioner happens to pursue yoga with efforts. It is said that nature helps those who help themselves. In a way nature tests us and the remedy of nature's onslaught is yoga.

As death is certain many feel, "Let me not do wrong but good, before I die". That is why the *Veda* say, *mṛtyor māmṛtaṁ gamaya* – Take me from death to immortality (eternity).[1] As fear of death and acceptance of death is there, one likes to do virtuous things. There are those who think, "Death is certain, let me enjoy as I want": then they are caught sooner or later in the chain of pains and sorrows. If there was no death, virtue would never occur to man. Awareness of death takes one towards the path of spirituality. One thinks of doing something good before one dies.

When a person does wrong, he thinks and repents that he shouldn't have done that. Repentance is virtue. Similarly, pain is also a virtue. If there is no pain then one grows arrogant. Pain helps one to be humble. If one has no sorrows and pains, one acts like a demon as if one is free from the jaws of death. The pain acts as a *guru* and teaches us to be humble.

The moment there is a slight numbness, you worry about it and think ways of removing it. Is it not a step towards transformation for the good or right action? Here the right sense of action has set in at this point of time. This is because we have been bestowed with the discriminating power *(jñāna)*. With this discriminative power, one not only reaches perfect health but also realises the truth that Self is eternal and likes to move towards it.

Hence learn to accept disease gracefully, wage a war against it through *yoga sādhanā*. Then the light of wisdom on the Self dawns.

---

1 *Bṛhad-āraṇyaka Upaniṣad*, I.3.28.

I.2. – *Āsana*-therapy

Āsana is one of the aspects of *aṣṭāṅga yoga.* It has a tremendous bearing in providing the *sādhaka* with health and harmony.

Āsana are said to be as many as the species in the vegetable and animal kingdoms. When an afflicted person adopts *āsana,* he pours out his energy to get into *āsana* and feels enlivened in proportion to his involvement. His physical, psychological and mental frames rejuvenate and transform him with a sense of gladness.

Man is made of five elements *(pañcabhūta),* namely earth, water, fire, air and ether, which correspond to the five sheaths of the body. These are structural, physiological, mental, intellectual and spiritual. These are supported by *pañcavāyu,* namely *prāṇa, apāna, vyāna, samāna* and *udāna.* This biochemical structure or the body machine *(yantra)*[1] is represented by *tridoṣa, saptadhātu* and *trimala.* The *tridoṣa (vāta, pitta* and *śleṣma)* are the humours of the body. They are formed mainly by three elements, air, fire and water. The *sapta-dhātu* have seven ingredients: chyle *(rasa)* is water *(āp),* blood *(rakta)* is water, fire and air *(āp, tej, vāyu),* flesh *(māṁsa)* is air, water and earth *(vāyu, āp, pṛthvī),* fat *(meda)* is water and earth *(āp, pṛthvī),* bones *(asthi)* is earth and air *(pṛthvī, vāyu),* bone marrow *(majjā)* is water and fire *(āp, tej)* and semen *(śukra)* is water *(āp).* The *trimala* are the three waste matters: faeces *(purīṣa)* is earth and fire *(pṛthvī, tej),* urine *(mūtra)* is water and fire *(āp, tej),* and sweat *(sveda)* like urine is water and fire *(āp, tej).* The element air (*vāyu)* is supported and made to function by five vital energy-forces. In addition to these *trimala,* the female body has two *mala* namely menstrual blood *(ārtava)* of fire and water and breast milk *(stanya)* is water.

While performing the *āsana,* the structure of the *āsana* is well placed or well designed to fit into the body so that the practitioner absorbs them properly unto himself/herself. The body is considered a machine (*yantra)* as each *āsana* comes under various techniques; it is a *tantra* as it has a methodology. When one performs an *āsana* with accuracy there occur the subtle adjustments of all the above ingredients within him bringing the required balance in all these systems.

Man imbibes the three qualities of nature namely, illumination, vibrancy and inertia *(sattva, rajas* and *tamas).* These qualities are activated and dynamised in *āsana* through their motion and action so that the body, mind and self are kept in a stable state. When rhythm and comfort set in, turmoil ends, nullifying the opposing forces. If going into the *āsana* is a *mantra* or

---

1 See *Śri yoga vidyā yantra. Mahābhārata* and *kāvya* literatures have used *yantra* for machines and engines. It is in this sense, the author uses the body machine as a *yantra.*

a *japa*, rhythmic presentation is the *artha* (means) and its deliverance and freedom, the felt feeling *(bhāvana)*.

The *sādhaka* has to put in place the skeleto-muscular structure, the earth element (*pṛthvī-tattva*) of the body. This accuracy in *āsana* helps the organic body to remain in a healthy state palpating vibrancy. The energy of the water element *(āp-tattva)* flows smoothly and throws out the waste matter. The energy of the fire element *(tejas-tattva)* burns and throws out the toxins. The air element *(vāyu-tattva)* circulates and purifies each cell of the body. The space element *(ākāśa-tattva)* maintains the required intracellular space.

Different *āsana* having different degrees of interpenetrative actions work effectively on the body and bring the required changes in the healing process. Each *āsana* has a peculiar character of its own to work effectively on the body. So selecting of different *āsana*, sequencing them correctly to fit into the structure of the body helps the afflicted areas to undergo the required biochemical changes for healing or curing a disease.

In each *āsana* several actions are involved regarding the position, reposition, extension, expansion, elongation, sustenance, suspension, retraction, traction, suction, compression, fixation, contraction, rotation, relaxation, tension, stretching, pulling, pushing, rinsing, softening and hardening. A right kind of balance and timely adjustments are involved in the performance of the *āsana* so that one establishes oneself in the *āsana* energising and enlivening one's body as well as resurrecting the mind.

The body-mind or bio-mental machine is educated and trained unitedly to function uniquely and consciously. If one practices *āsana* and *prāṇāyāma* with correct interpenetration weaving the biophysical and bio-chemical bodies with *pañcavāyu* and *pañcatanmātra*, these transform the infrastructure of the practitioner.

In case the diseased body does not indicate the improvement or is unable to perform or sustain and maintain the position of the body in *āsana*, then the external support is taken with the help of props. When the body is supported with the external props, one gets courage to perform and vitalise one's body. When one cannot walk by balancing on the legs, then one uses a stick or a walker as a support.

The *sāṁkhya darśana* says that *prakṛti* is blind and *puruṣa* is lame. Therefore the lame sits on the shoulders of the blind and guides the blind to move in right direction. The props do that. With the support of props, one stabilises the body in *āsana* and gets enlivened and charges one's body for further development. The mind opens with ease and gets illumined. The props teach one in the course of time to become independent, though at the start dependence is essential.

The practice of *āsana* and *prāṇāyāma* changes and transforms the ratio-wise balance of *sattva*, *rajas* and *tamas*. The *tamas* is lessened and *rajas* is increased. The *mūḍha* and *kṣipta* states of mind are conquered.[1] The mind enters the state of *vikṣipta*. Then, if the *sādhanā* is pursued, the *vikṣipta* mind (which vibrates and oscillates) leads towards the state of *ekāgra*. Up to this state, the props are required. Then the practitioner adjusts and readjusts in *āsana* subjectively, intently, actively, sensitively, intelligently and consciously. If one follows step by step, even the so called incurable diseases are arrested by maintaining equi-metabolism. The ascending diseases are controlled. The patient is rehabilitated and re-educated to endure the pain and sustain his life by eliminating further regression. All these help to improve the patient to come out from the diseased body and mind to be in an at-ease state.

Then one is free from all impediments. From then on *āsana* becomes the self and self, the *āsana*.

I.3. – Cardiovascular training through yoga

In 1984, When I was in San Francisco for the first International Iyengar Yoga Convention some doctors insisted I undergo a test to study my lungs since I had a history of tuberculosis. They wanted to see the chemical changes taking place in my body on account of regular practice of *āsana* and *prāṇāyāma*. I was told that they had a number of instruments and devices which carry out such tests. I underwent the test as I was curious to know scientifically how my lungs were. All the needed instruments were fixed on me and recording took place for more that an hour. I jocularly asked them, "Please let me know how long I stay on this Earth planet. I told them that I have seen life sufficiently well and I think I should say, enough". The doctors after studying the graphs were surprised and solemnly said, "Sir, we are sorry to tell you that you are going to live long", and further added, "Our study has shown that your lungs are like that of a twenty-four to twenty-five year old athlete; so when you have such good lungs, you have a long life in front of you." I was already sixty-six at that time. This gave me the satisfaction that I who had tuberculosis and bouts of other diseases had kept my lungs young through *āsana* and *prāṇāyāma* practices.

[1] The consciousness *(citta)* of a man functions on five levels namely *mūḍha* – dull, *kṣipta* – active, *vikṣipta* oscillating, *ekāgra* – one-pointed, *niruddha* – restrained. *Mūḍha* has *tamas*, *kṣipta* has *tamas* and *rajas*, *vikṣipta* has more of *rajas*, *ekāgra* is of *rajas* and *sattva* and *niruddha* is beyond *guṇa*.

The important gates of man's life are the respiratory and circulatory systems. If something goes wrong in these two gates, then diseases set into the system and the person does realise what health means. The main attention in the whole of *yogic sādhanā* is on the respiratory and circulatory systems.

When we start breathing, our defensive strength is stored on the sides of our lungs. If you look at the lungs of a person who is depressed and dejected, they cave in and appear narrow. The physical manifestation of emotional disturbances is that the sufferers cannot inhale with ease but gasp for breath. In such cases, whatever energy is stored, it is thrown out. In people who are emotionally disturbed the dissipation of energy is more predominant than in one who is strong.

In the practice of *āsana* reactions have to be studied and readjustments have to be done accordingly. Have any of you noticed the state of your mind when you look at the rising or the setting sun in a blue sky? You are in delight without the feel of I or ME. At that time, you do not notice how the chest opens out. This expansion of the chest gives an indication of the location of the storehouse of energy. The sides of the chest near the armpits are the areas where the energy gets stored. The moment one expresses the bountiful beauty of the rising or setting sun we lose that divine state but come back to the I or You or ME.

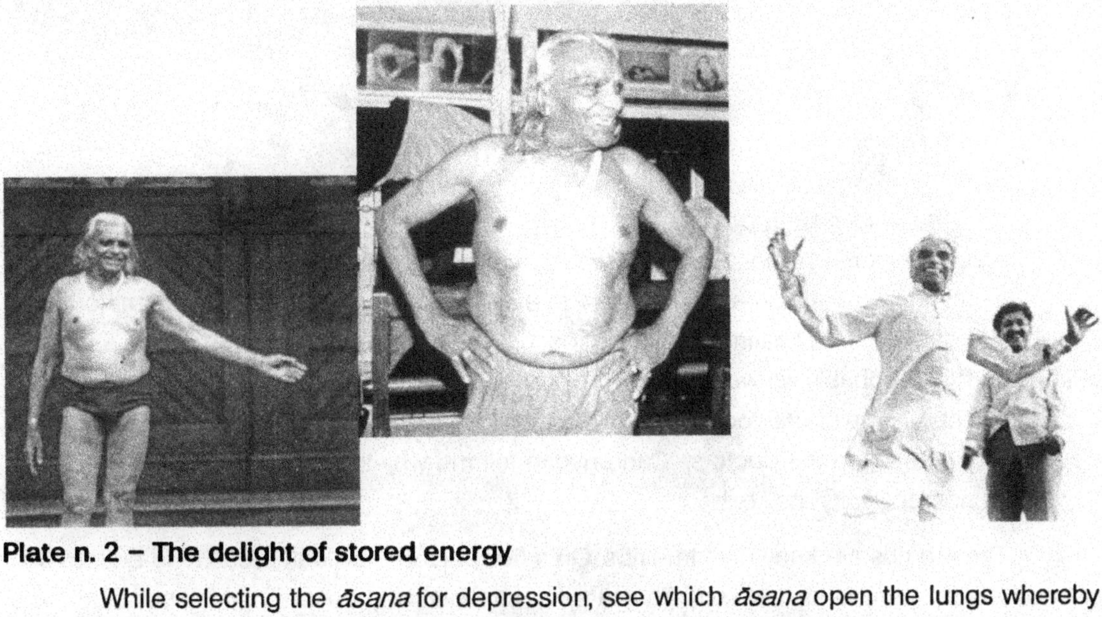

Plate n. 2 – The delight of stored energy

While selecting the *āsana* for depression, see which *āsana* open the lungs whereby the energy is stored and conserved for utilisation. I make such *āsana* for the dorsal chest, armpits and navel to open so that space is created. The moment the space is created, the air occupies the place and blood current is made to circulate well generating copious energy in the nervous system. The nerves become strong and the person gains hope and confidence in performing these *āsana* The patient begins to live positively.

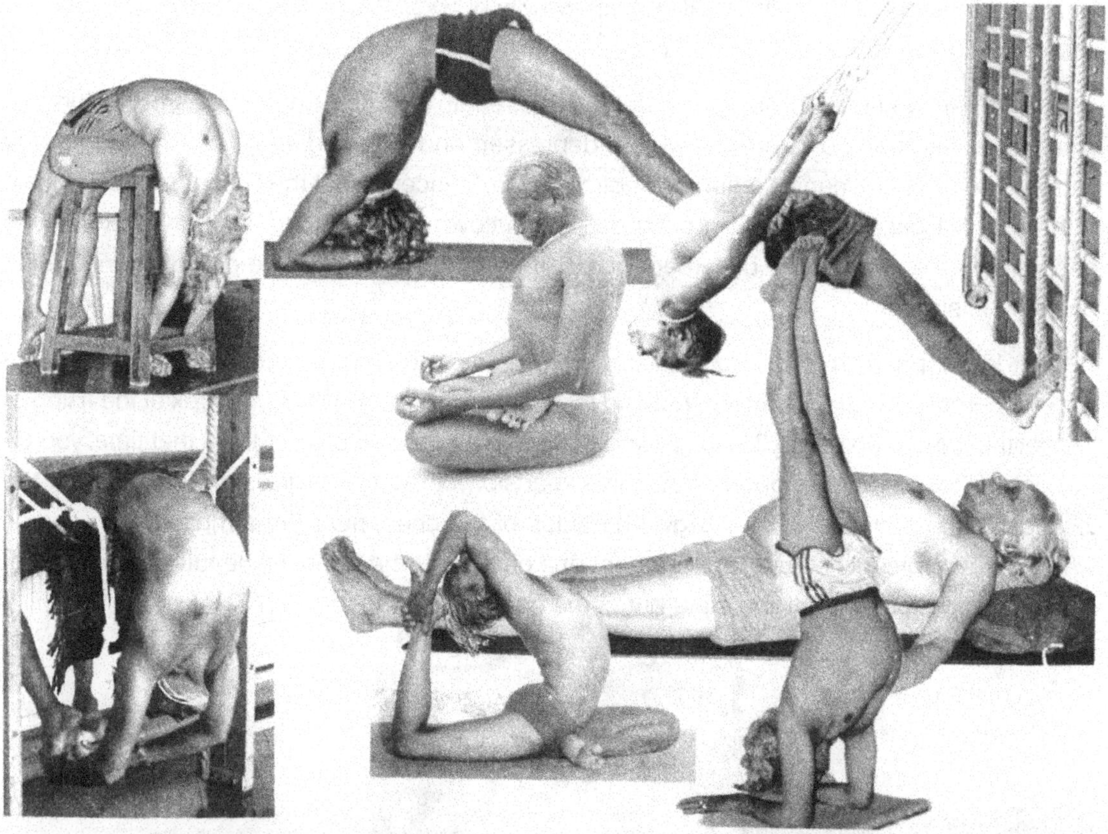

Plate n. 3 - *Āsana* to gain a positive life

Also in performing the *āsana,* the diaphragm gets expanded. I do not want to use the term 'contraction' in inhalation and 'dilatation' in exhalation which are technical terminologies. The Creator has given us floating ribs. If the floating ribs were not there and if all the ribs were united and fixed, probably we would not have been able to breathe at all. So the construction of the rib cage should be understood, wherein the two floating ribs have the power to expand and open out, I once asked the doctors, "Can anyone tell me why they exist as floating ribs?" But they could not reply why they exist.

The top ribs are known as true ribs. On a live person they look broad. The bottom ribs of the chest are termed as false ribs. They are not attached and appear narrow. If we look at a skeleton – the top chest appears narrow and the middle broad. It is interesting to note how in old age these get atrophied at the top to form a narrow top chest and a broad chest at the bottom.

In the living anatomy it is not so. When we inhale, these floating ribs have the power to expand and open sideways and in that opening they help to absorb energy from the bottom of the chest to the top. As they open out, they help expand the intercostal muscles from the bottom to the top filling the lungs. When the intake of breath is long and soft, it is like the water seen on a lake or on a beach with no tides. If the tide is not strong but weak, then the waves of the sea move gradually and wet the sand quicker and deeper. If the tide is strong, it goes back fast carrying sand along with it; when it is not strong, the waves penetrate the sand and do not take the sand back while receding.

Like the slow waves of the calm sea, inhalation and exhalation have to be done gradually for the breath to touch the banks of the lungs. In the process of the inhalation, the breath has to move gradually from the unknown inner body, then to the mind and finally through the intercostal muscles to touch its frontier – the skin. In this slow movement of the breath, the bronchioles extend and expand from the bronchi allowing the air cells to absorb the energy from the drawn-in breath and store it. Since the breath is not made to hit hard but to seep in gradually (like the sand wetted by the wave), the lungs, as storehouse of energy store and help the blood to be purer.

Also in the art of exhalation, one has to gradually release the breath from the periphery so that the magnet of the breath which is still in contact with the lungs is not blown or thrown out. The air is to be released slowly so that the drawn in energy is not thrown out at once but the unwanted air is released. This is actually the *prāṇāyāmic* method of breathing.

When we inhale, our inhalation is like pouring water into a vessel; the water first touches the bottom, spreads to the sides to find its own level and then comes to the top; this is how the breath moves. If we suddenly make the vessel topsy-turvy to empty it, the water does not flow smoothly. It gushes out with a heavy sound. If we slant the vessel and let out the water, it flows gradually and smoothly without making sounds. The exhalation has to be done this way. Though we do not tilt the torso here, the exhalation should be such that we are emptying the tank by slightly opening the lower tap – the lower torso. While inhaling the breath touches the lower torso first and fills to the top. While exhaling the breath releases from the top of the torso so that it is emptied rib after rib to reach the bottom area of the chest.

I think this mechanism of *prāṇāyāmic* breathing helps the practitioners to know the difference between deep breathing and *prāṇāyāmic* breathing. With this type of inhalation, the air touches the central part of the vessel and then spreads to the two sides of the lungs fully before starting exhalation. The breath is made to move on to either side of the lungs with the help of the intercostal muscles. During inhalation, the breath is moved to both sides of the chest However in the process of exhalation, though the breath is released from the top, the inhaled breath that is still in the lungs is made to be absorbed by the system in this slow process of exhalation. During exhalation, the breath should not be expelled but released. If the spine and the chest box are held steadily, then the breath is released with controlled action moving from the periphery towards the inner torso vertically as well as horizontally from end to end.

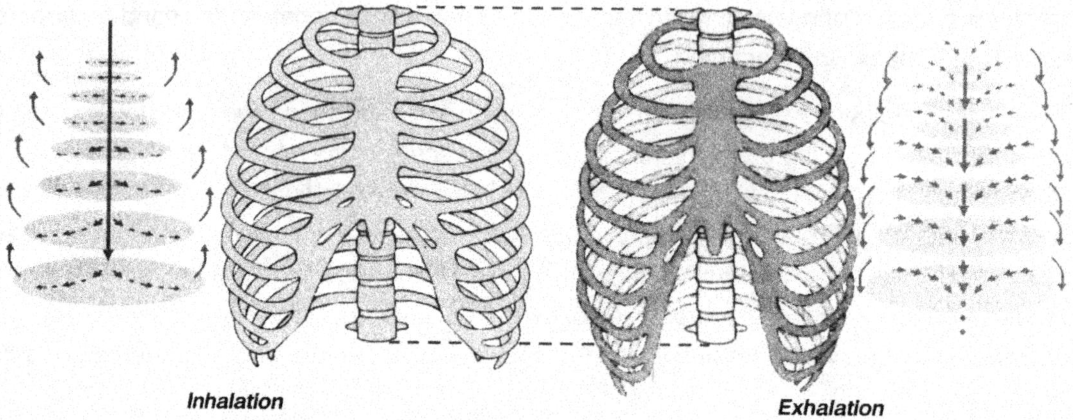

Plate n. 4 – The movement of inhalation and exhalation

As the spokes of the wheel move from the bottom to the top and from the top to the bottom, inhalation and exhalation move this way. By this slow flow of breath, absorption of energy is bound to be definitely more in the yogic method of respiration than in ordinary deep breathing. In ordinary deep breathing we use only a part of the lungs, but in *prāṇāyāmic* breathing we use the whole of the lungs.

In the beginning these facts are difficult to understand but one can learn. The actions in *prāṇāyāmic* breathing are subtle and take time to absorb.

Please remember that as one empties water gradually from a vessel, empty the chest gradually in exhalation. No force should be used during exhalation. By right method of *prāṇāyāmic* practice, one does not become a victim of environmental disturbances and emotional upheavals. In prāṇāyāmic breathing the amount of energy stored and conserved in the body makes one to withstand the onslaught of environmental circumstances and forces. The effect of *prāṇāyāma* is that it gives a great amount of energy to be stored and to be used only when necessary.

What is this stored energy? While we are driving a car, we see a person driving down the opposite side who loses control over the steering and our instincts immediately react wherein the hidden energy surfaces at once to protect from a possible accident and we say, "Thank God, we escaped". At that time, we use the energy which had been stored and after that we return to our mechanical way of driving, saying, "Thank God, we are safe". In the same way, the yogi does not allow the energy to dissipate but transforms it into dynamic power every second so that he draws in softly and fully the energy from the universal atmospheric air to make full use of it. This way of practice is known as *prāṇāyāmic* method and in this method; there is no strain on the heart. However when the sac of the heart is moved to the left, then heart diseases set in.

In yogic practices certain direct and indirect muscles play a definite role. During an earthquake, the earth trembles, shaking the whole area for miles and miles, but it does not end there. The tremors continue thereafter. Similarly, there are tremors of the heart. We get shocks physically, intellectually or emotionally and they affect the heart muscles. The heart experiences tremors for a long time. That is similar to the earthquake. You may say, "Thank God, I am saved". Though you know that you have escaped from an accident or massacre or catastrophe, the heart continues to palpitate similar to an earthquake. I call this as tremors of heart. These tremors of heart continue until the heart muscles, energy and emotions of mind find their level to settle down. In fact the tremors of the heart stop when the protective muscles of the heart are released from such spasms. The indirect muscles become hard along with the direct muscles of the heart. The direct muscles cannot release from the stress easily, and the tremor of the heart continues until spasms of the protective muscles are brought to normalcy.

So in yoga there are certain *āsana* such as *Setu Bandha Sarvāṅgāsana*, *Viparīta Karaṇi*, *Ardha Halāsana*, *Viparīta Daṇḍāsana*, where the protective muscles of the heart that are connected to the cardiac region of the spine are relaxed and released faster. When they are made to relax, then the direct muscles of the heart get relaxed. If one has to invigorate the cardio-vascular system in any other type of exercises, one needs to create tremendous movement in the body like jogging or running. This way one creates tremors made by vigorous movement whereas in yogic *āsana*, one brings a good amount of blood circulation to heart muscles without irritating or making the heart to pump fast. On this basis, I discovered the *āsana* called *Śarapañjarāsana* or *Bhīṣmācāryāsana* for the cardiac patients who find great relief.[1]

---

1 At the time of the war between the Kauravas and Pandavas, Bhīṣma was injured in the battlefield, he could not breathe with ease or turn on his sides. Bhīṣma asked Arjuna to make a bed of arrows for him to rest. As he was thirsty but could not turn or sit, he asked for water. Arjuna hit the earth with an arrow, so the water flowed into his mouth. These symptoms of Bhīṣma are similar to today's cardiac attack. The bed of arrows gave me a thought, that the bed of arrows help the ventricles of the heart to supply blood to the other chambers for a harmonious function. I designed a bed like the bed of arrows (see plate n. 6b, page 60) and named it after him as *Bhīṣmacharyāsana* or *Śarapañjarāsana (śara* = arrows, *pañjara* = a cage, net, dove-cot, aviary).

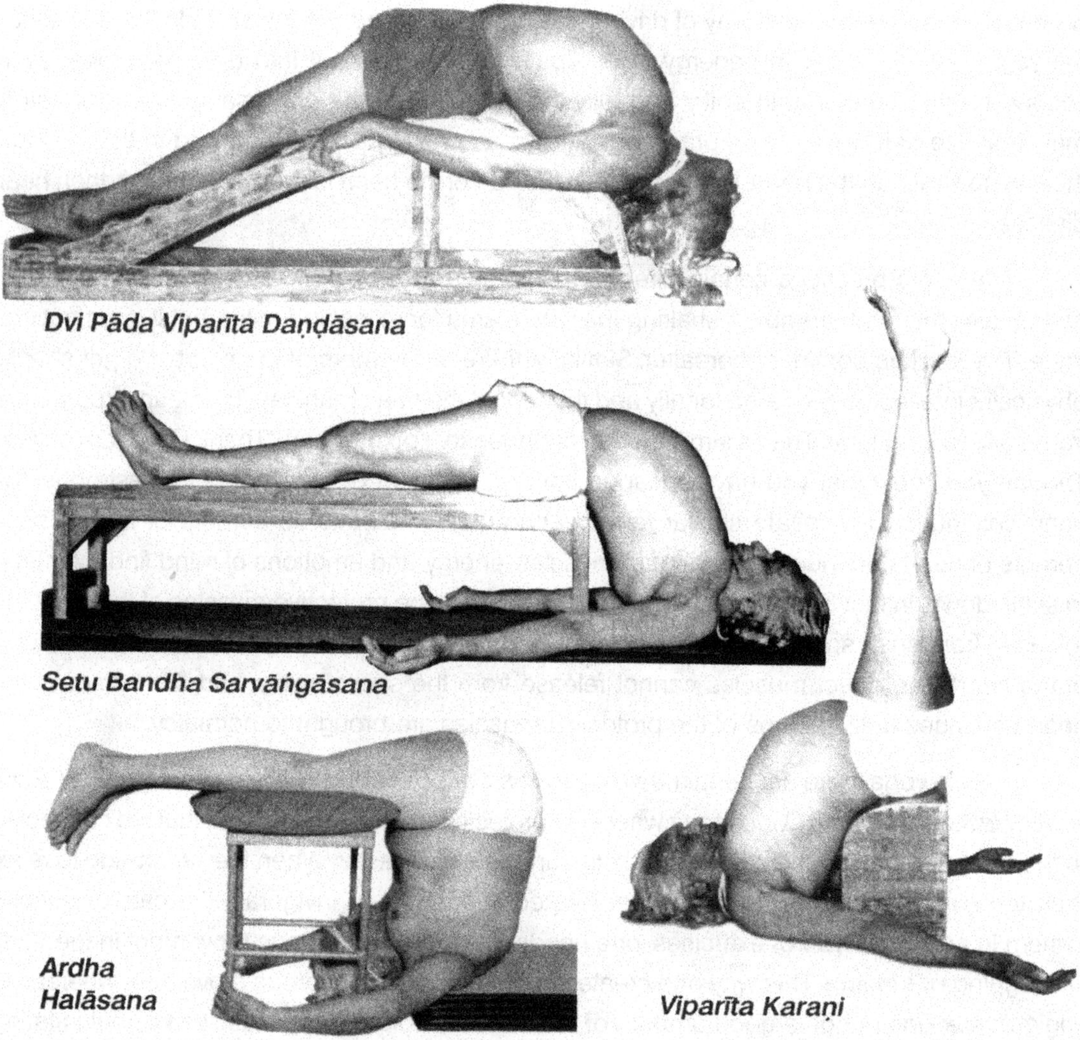

Plate n. 5 – *Āsana* that rejuvenate the heart muscles

This way, the stimulation in the yogic method takes place and life is prolonged. That is how the yogi keep their heart strong. They do not allow the heart muscles to move away from its position. All *āsana* are taught in such a way for the heart to remain in a healthy state.

SECTION II

ON DIET AND NUTRITION

SECTION II – ON DIET AND NUTRITION

II.1. – The importance of diet in yoga

I do not like to talk on diet for the simple reason that I was undernourished throughout my childhood and youth.

There is a story from the *Mahābhārata* which I would like to bring to your attention. Aśvatthāmā was the son of the great teacher Droṇācārya, the *guru* of the Kauravas and Pāṇḍavas. Due to poverty he could not afford to give milk to his son Aśvatthāmā. Aśvatthāmā's mother used to mix rice flour in water with sugar and make her son drink, saying that it was milk. This was how Aśvatthāmā was nourished on "rice flour-milk". Later he became a commander-in-chief of the Kaurava army.

In poverty I too ate for survival without any idea of nourishment in mind. The food nourishes the body on its own which is a physical need. It was so not only at the time of studentship but also even after I began teaching. Stick to yoga, it guides the diet.

Plenty of literature is available on food and diet for yogic practice. For them food comes first and then yoga. For me, it is yoga first, then food. Practice of yoga is important to me and I live on whatever suits my *sādhanā*.

Lord Krishna says in the *Bhagavad Gītā* that the suitable food for *sāttvic* growth is that which is delicious, soft, sweet, substantial, agreeable and promotes long life, vitality, energy, health, happiness and cheerfulness. *Tāmasic* food is that which has no taste and flavour, but stinky, unclean, remnants and leftover. In my childhood, I did not know what is *sāttvic* or *rājasic* or *tāmasic* food. Whatever food the circumstances were providing me, I ate for survival. But my yogic practices nourished me and kept me healthy and alive with the stale and tasteless food.

My diet depends upon what type of practice I plan to do. I avoid that food which affects my practice. In case I need to attend family problems the next day, I may perform the *āsana* of tomorrow or the day after or the day before and adjust my diet in such a manner that the practice won't suffer the next day. My system cannot take hot, savoury, spicy food. Even among the so-called good food, I choose what is congenial to my system and my practices.

If one remains on light food or on a diet and one type of food each day, this may make one feel weak. *Āsana* practice guides one in having sensitivity for eating what the body needs each day. Sometimes the system demands liquid food and sometimes sweet or salty food which all comes from the dictates of the body's needs.

My food is what an average Indian eats. I am a vegetarian. My main food is a bit of rice, one vegetable and yoghurt with honey in the day and milk with chapatti and vegetable at night. But as far as solid food is concerned I don't think my system needs much. It is the discipline of yoga which has disciplined my food. That is why I am not fussy regarding food.

There cannot be a single type of food congenial to yogic practice. *Haṭhayoga Pradīpikā* says avoid too much food *(atyāhāra)*. Eat only when hungry, or when saliva oozes from the mouth as one sees the food. Only eat what the system demands. Some say that the moment they smell something good, their mouths begin to water. But this cannot happen to one who is practising yoga. One can experiment oneself. Regular, disciplined and genuine practice of *āsana* and *prāṇāyāma* for some months makes one indifferent to one's favourite dishes even if they are placed in front of him. Stop practice for eight days, then indiscipline sets in and old habits return. When practised regularly, the digestive system gets stimulated and one eats less than what one normally consumes. After yoga, the system needs less fuel. Even the metabolism turns into *sāttvic* quality in yoga *sādhanā*. By yogic practice, one enjoys food but does not indulge in it. When one breaks the discipline of yoga, then indulgence in food returns.

Speaking on *prāṇāyāma*, Svātmārāma in the second chapter of *Haṭhayoga Pradīpikā* indicates that one should have *kśīrajya bhojanam* – rice cooked in milk and ghee. At the time of learning *prāṇāyāma* his advice is to have rice cooked in milk and ghee. This food not only comes under the category of *sāttvic* food but it is congenial to the system. The practice of *āsana* creates heat in the body and *prāṇāyāma* causes dryness. This heat and dryness is balanced with food such as milk and ghee (clarified butter) which not only lubricates the system, but also acts as fuel to the practice.

Svātmārāma in the first chapter on *āsana* says: among the discipline of *yama*, the most important is *mitāhāra* – moderate food. *Mitāhāra* means balanced food which is explained as *susnigdha madhura āhāraḥ* – sweet and lubricating.

If one feels like vomiting or there is pain in the stomach while practising back-bending know that either the food is not digested or the food that has been taken on the previous night was not congenial to back-bends. Then one is forced to avoid that food if one wants to stick to yogic practices.

If we feel pain or stiffness, we restrict our movements. Similarly, if the organic body restricts the movements, know that we have overeaten or the food that is consumed is not digested. This way we learn to take what is right food.

If one feels like vomiting one stops practice. If one feels a burning sensation in the stomach or the heart, one needs to do *āsana* which stops the burning or the vomiting sensation. But one never tries to trace the root cause of these problems. Chillies irritate one in backbends. This makes one to sacrifice that day's practice. Switch to do supine *āsana* in order to minimise the burning sensation though it should not be considered as an alternative practice. This is just adjustment for that condition and state only. A genuine and disciplined practice brings a change in food habits, then it is a yogic food. A heavy food makes the brain dull whereas yoga demands a sharp brain to watch and absorb the changes.

Chāndogya Upaniṣad says that the mind is formed by the food, *annamayam hi saumya manaḥ*. The *Upaniṣad* says that the food that is taken gets divided into three parts. The grossest part becomes faeces, the middle part becomes flesh which gets converted into ingredients (*sapta dhātu*) of the body and the subtlest part of food forms into mind. This quote from the *Upaniṣad* is enough to know that the mind is made up of food. If one wants to have sharpness and alertness while practising yoga, then one has to change his food habits.

Man has been graced with a thinking faculty. Mind, brain, intellect is a thinking faculty. Thinking process reaps thoughts. It is easy to change the food habits. I have heard that even Hitler was a vegetarian. Mahātmā Gandhi too was a vegetarian. Why did Hitler being a vegetarian have a violent attitude while Mahātma Gandhi had a non-violent approach for everything? How is it that the vegetarian food did not change Hitler's mind?

Vegetarian food is good as far as health is concerned. It is certainly cleaner than non-vegetarian food. The *Upaniṣad* is right when it says, first see that the faeces are formed correctly, because according to *Āyurveda*, those who are constipated invite diseases. Constipation is the cause of many diseases. First, if the bowel movements are correct, half the health is gained. Secondly, eat such food which nourishes the seven constituents *(sapta dhātu)* of the body namely; chile, blood, flesh, fat, bones, bone marrow and semen. The third is that the subtlest part of food is meant to build up the intellectual faculty. Hence, you have to learn to balance food that is congenial to the practice.

Modem science speaks about proteins, calcium, carbohydrates and so on. Nobody can explain how much protein the system needs. If protein is not digested but accumulated in the system, then it can cause diseases. In India, too much intake of fatty food and carbohydrates causes obesity, diabetes and so forth.

As a practitioner of yoga, see which food is congenial to practice by studying and watching the reaction on the body through your *sādhanā*.

The food we take should give that strength to develop the mind to reach towards the higher goals in life. Varying food habits brings variation in mind thoughts. Different tastes of food not only make the tongue indisciplined but also effect the mind to indulge in tastes.

As long as the physical health is concerned, one can have varieties with limitation but the moment one likes to go towards spiritual aspects then one has to check not only the stomach but also the taste. The thinking process should not get hampered. One should not keep on changing the food day in and day out. Eat not for the sake of taste but for the sake of sustenance.

Prashant told you the story the other day. Vyāsa was standing on the bank of the river Yamunā. Some of the milkmaids carrying milk-pots were eager to cross the river, but river was flooded, therefore they had to wait. Vyāsa saw the pots which were full of milk. Being hungry, he asked them for milk. The milkmaids gave him the milk and were surprised to see him emptying the pots one after the other. Then Vyāsa loudly said: "If the milk that I have taken is to satisfy the Nārāyaṇa[1] within, the Yamunā will make a path for these milkmaids to cross". Surprisingly at once the river divided into two and made a path for the milkmaids to cross over to the other side. Then they realised that he was no other than Vyāsa. Vyāsa was really hungry and consumed all the milk that was available and was sure that it is Nārāyaṇa, the very Lord within who was demanding this milk. It was a genuine hunger and not greed. Lord Krishna says in *Bhagavad Gītā: ahaṁ vaiśvānaro bhūtvā prāṇinām dehamāśritāḥ* - I am the fire *Vaiśvānara* existing in everyone's stomach.

The *Haṭhayoga Pradīpikā* also defines *mitāhāra* (moderate food) as; *bhujyate śivasaṁprītyai mitāhāraḥ sa ucyate* - One should eat thinking that the eater is Shiva, the Lord within, and not himself.

Therefore, as practitioners of yoga, discipline yourselves. Eat only when hungry and eat only as much as is essential for sustenance.

---

[1] Nārāyaṇa is the name of Lord Vishnu who dwells in the heart of everyone as *antaryāmin*.

That is how I live. Otherwise food for the diseased and the healthy has to be prescribed. Food may depend upon economic and geographic conditions. It may depend upon one's constitution. It may depend upon one's requirement, age and power of digestion. It may depend upon one's mental calibre. As a practitioner of yoga, begin to watch the subtle changes that occur within. Then learn what to eat and what to practise in order to be energetic and not lethargic.

II.2. – Yoga and vegetarianism

Many of you do not know about my early life. When young, I suffered from tuberculosis and I practised yoga. When I grew up, there was a time when I couldn't get a meal for three or four days at a stretch. When I could not get a meal each day, how could I dream of fruits and milk? This is the reason why I do not deal with diet. As I began practising yoga undernourished, who am I to talk about nutrition? Today God has given me everything but I have not forgotten my early life. I stick to what is available and eat without making choice from my head or tongue. Is yoga meant only for the well off, or is it also for the under developed? In my youth I was undernourished, yet I practised a great deal. Probably if I say that the major part of my life was dedicated to yoga, you may not believe me. The only advice I can render is that if the salivary glands do not respond to the food that is in front of you, do not eat. When you see a piece of dry bread and if it stimulates saliva, then take that and get nourished as it was for me in my early days.

Coming to vegetarianism, remember the adage that 'as you sow, so shall you reap'. 'As you eat so you grow'. The growth of mind depends on the food you eat. Regarding animal food, the instinct in animals creates the fear of death at the time of slaughtering and their cells discharge fear which many of us can recognise through their eyes. You eat that food of the animal filled with its instinctive fear and nervous breakdown. This affects the system with that complexity. Although there is life in vegetables, you do the least harm by eating them and if you do not use them they go rotten. Consuming them soothes the system. Today of course the vegetarian food is so much commercialised that there is tremendous rapaciousness in growing vegetables for money.

Non-vegetarian food was prohibited for *yoga sādhaka* since it has the element of hidden violent forces. It was an accepted norm that consuming non-vegetarian food is opposed to the principles of *yama*. I do not have to propagate it.

People were unaware of yoga in the early period of the last century and my interest was to recharge yoga and bring it to the notice of the people. Those who practise yoga with a religious frame of mind; their systems cannot take in flesh. As yoga enters into their system, the non-vegetarian food is disliked by the system. Neither the body permits nor the conscience permits. This transformation occurs as one practises with religiosity. Obviously he gives up the *hiṁsātmaka* food. All I would say is, first enhance the intensity of practice. If there is no saliva when you eat, then that food is bound to effect your health.

I will not talk about diet because I have lived on water for days. So you have to choose food that refines and keeps your mind lighter and makes you happier. If you do not feel heavy in your alimentary system one hour after eating, then that is good food. You must judge for yourself even with vegetarian food as to what is soothing to the practice.

I am for vegetarianism but first you have to embrace yoga so that it embraces you.

II.3. – A healthy diet

Why make a big fuss about food? Is it such a big issue to do *sādhanā*? When you feel thirsty you ask for water. Can this thirst for water be quenched by anything else? Does alcohol quench the thirst? When you are thirsty, if your friends offer orange juice instead of water you say you prefer water and nothing else. At that time orange juice is not the right food. Water alone is the right food.

Do not fill the stomach when it does not want. The amount of food one takes should not disturb the digestive system and metabolism. It should be digested in a period of six hours. If it does not get digested, it means one has over eaten.

Do not make a choice from the head for food. Suppose one is hungry, if anything is put on the table, what do you do? You pick it up at once and start eating it. Food is digested by the stomach and assimilated by the body and not by the choice of the brain. Assimilation is important. See the food that you eat is assimilated.

I don't recommend dieticians' books, because the authors have experimented according to their system. Just calculating food value and calories does not work. Each body may be different. People call me fiery, a man of anger. *(Laughter).* What food should I take to keep that fire down in my diet? Suppose a person is cool and soft, it means the water element predominates in that body. Diet books cannot tell this. Each one has to judge himself according to his temperament and composition of elements in the body. For example, ether element contracts and expands. When some people eat, their stomach bloats immediately as the proportion of ether is great. They have to find out food that does not create this bloating sensation. This is how one has to study the dieting system that nourishes and triggers the energy according to one's needs.

The beauty of practising *āsana* is that as one goes on practising, the system itself distinguishes between foods which are not wanted and that which is required. The system develops the sensitivity to accept the food and discard the unwanted food. Food which is wanted will be well assimilated. When the system gets properly nourished, the elements in the body balance proportionately. Often the stomach refuses to accept certain food. A feeling of repulsion comes which means that the food is not what the stomach needs. As the learning process of yoga is subjective, consumption of food is also subjective. Hence one has to think of food on the subjective level only. For example, the technique of *āsana* or *prāṇāyāma* is objective but their transmission becomes subjective and it is the same with food. As a guideline I would say eat a little less than the stomach can take, whatever the food is.

If the stomach can take a kilo of food, for example, can anybody eat a kilo of food? In that case, take half a kilo of solid food, a quarter of liquid and keep the last quarter empty. This is the healthy way of eating food according to all yoga texts.

Eat only when hungry and not from temptations. There are so many who don't even get a slice of bread. It is easy to speak on food when affluent people have plenty of everything. I came from a poor family. I know the value of food. Instead of pondering over food, eat only when hungry and whatever is available without making fuss. It is the mind, which creates fuss. Body is more honest than the mind. The body refuses the food when it does not want. One vomits or gets diarrhoea. Avoid such food which does not suit the system. When one is allergic to certain food, avoid it. Stop over eating. And don't eat what is not palatable. The brain and mind like to have the choice of tasty food, but let the stomach judge whether it can take, digest and assimilate.

For example, milk is considered to be a very *sāttvic* – good food –, which gives energy. But for some milk gives diarrhoea.

Basically everyone wants physical health and mental peace. Along with yoga if I introduce diet then how do I know whether yoga has done good or the diet? I trust yoga and yoga adjusts my food. After coming to yoga, have you all changed your eating habits or not? Tell me.

- Changed. -

What more do you want? If you are honest in your practice, then the food essentially acts as a fuel to the system. The physical body knows exactly what food it needs; the choice does not come from the brain. I don't think that by eating rich food alone one can do yoga. A real practitioner of yoga needs very little food. For him, yoga itself is a food because *prāṇa* – energy – nourishes him. Nourishing food alone is not the key to health but the assimilation of it is important. Assimilation is the golden key that unlocks the gates of good health and clear intelligence.

II.4. - Controlling appetite

Do *Śīrṣāsana* and cycle for fifteen to twenty minutes and *Sarvāṅgāsana* and cycle for twenty to twenty-five minutes regularly. These inversions controll the appetite.

If one has overeaten, then do *Supta Vīrāsana* immediately after food as long as one can stay as it takes off the load that is felt in the stomach. Be careful not to fill the stomach after feeling lightness in the stomach. One's appetite is controlled through *Ujjāyī* and *Viloma prāṇāyāma.* This feeds the body with the *prāṇic* energy and hunger fades.

II.5. - On fasting

The practitioners of yoga do not overeat. As they are all under-eaters, it is as good as partial fasting. One must have heard that Buddha fasted and came down to a single grain of rice. When he did that, he said that, "I made a mistake", and advised his disciples not to make the same mistake. So fasting is as bad as overeating. When people overeat, they are put on nature-cure or naturopathy programmes of fasting and cleansing and naturally the toxins that are formed in the system are removed. Afterwards are these people given any guidance on how they have to follow what to eat? Yogic practices teach this without outside guidance. *Āsana* and *prāṇāyāma* are meant to maintain the harmony of the five elements of nature according to their proportions. Hence the practitioners of yoga have a balanced body, a balanced mind, a healthy body and a healthy mind with a matured intelligence.

Know well that one cannot recommend fasting for one and all. One cannot stipulate the type or amount of food as the constitution of everyone is not the same. True, I do not recommend fasting but I demand practice of yoga regularly and religiously. Here the need is to understand the reality. Those who practise regularly, religiously and accurately find the change occurring in their system. Though they feel hungry the body does not take more than what it requires. Those who were taking non-vegetarian and spicy food before yoga left off on their own as the system refused to accept it. Regular practice brings regulation in food habits. Yoga practices make one to eat less. Hence, the food that is saved (indirectly) goes to the needy.

Therefore, it is the *sādhanā* that helps to know and recognise impediments and guides one to regulate food habits. Know that we are not Christ or Buddha.

Lord Krishna says that practitioners of yoga should be moderate in food, exertion, inaction and sleep as well as in wakefulness so that the purpose of destroying pain is served.

Do not go to the extremes as practitioners. Be moderate. Do not over-eat and do not under-eat. Do not make food as a "whole and sole" programme of life. We eat to live and not live to eat.These inversions controls the appetite.

SECTION III

ON SPORTS AND PHYSICAL EXERCISES

SECTION III – ON SPORTS AND PHYSICAL EXERCISES

III.1. – Yoga, superior to sports and physical exercises

First of all one should understand what yoga is. Yoga is a practical science that teaches the art of living. The art of living covers the well-being of man physically, morally, mentally, intellectually and socially. Secondly, the life of a human being is meant to know the purpose of living and the goal of life. Yoga is meant to guide the practitioner to know not only these but it is also meant to realise the Self. *Āsana* is part and parcel of yoga. As the body is the capital on which the life is projected, *āsana* acts as a foundation for health and strength to maintain the life force that keeps one to survive and live.

Āsana, unlike aerobics, jogging, weight lifting is a wholistic exercise as it attends not only to the body but integrates the mind to the life force – the Self. It is wholistic *sādhanā (sarvāṅga sādhanā),* and not working as exercises on certain parts *(aṅgabhāga sādhanā)* of the body.

In áll other exercises or sports the mind is outwardly stretched. For instance in weight lifting, the mind needs attention on the action of lifting but not the total involvement of attentive mind and awareness of intelligence and consciousness. *Āsana* acts as a base for all other systems of exercises as it works simultaneously on the respiratory, circulatory, digestive, nervous, glandular and excretory systems along with the total involvement of mind and intelligence.

It is possible to introduce *āsana* and *prāṇāyāma* as they will be supportive and complementary to other forms of exercise. It is better if done separately.

Āsana is not a physical exercise, but an organic or physiological exercise. It helps to bring a proper disposition on the physiological sheath of the body. *Āsana* creates space and extension in the body and cleanses the nervous system whereas other types of exercise create contraction in the muscles and tension in the body. Hence I advise that they should be done separately with an interval of a few hours to have a good effect on the body and mind.

Āsana act as a wonderful tool that brings focal attention on the needed part and develops power of strength and growth in those parts which are needed for various types of sports. Many of my students who are professional sports-persons and athletes have published books; for instance *Yoga for Runners, Yoga for Athletes*, and a book on yoga for cricketers is in the offing.

If a person has to make a choice because of available time, then my advice is that he should choose yoga in preference to any other exercises as *āsana* are invigorating and rejuvenating.

As *āsana* and *prāṇāyāma* develop the person from the skin to the intelligence, it definitely helps a sportsperson to become a better sportsman, a better athlete and so forth. When the practice of yoga makes an average man a better person, why not sports people? As yoga works in concord and harmony, it makes one a better human being by energising his body and mind.

I would say essentially that if yoga is done by all, one can improve all round at all levels.

III.2. – Relaxation and meditation for athletes

In the Mexico Olympics, our Indian hockey team was beaten. I was told by an authoritative person in hockey that before the match began they were asked to do *Śavāsana*. Obviously, they couldn't even run on the field after *Śavāsana*. Is yoga to be blamed for this? Those who claim to be teachers must know the norms of yoga to fit into sports.

The idea of meditation is to direct their minds and thoughts towards single attention. Practice of *āsana* spreads the flow of energy in the body and keeps it warm and mind cool. This flow of energy and warmth in body and coolness in brain rejuvenates the system with a positive effect on the body, brain and mind. For an untrained mind meditation creates a void and makes it slow in action. That was what happened to our hockey players in Mexico.

When I was in New Zealand I heard from my own students that when our cricket team went to New Zealand, our players were asked to run on the ground to keep themselves fit and warm, whereas New Zealand team were taking yoga from my students before the match. They were getting warm, fresh and agile to play as if with a fresh body and a fresh mind.

No dancer, musician or actor does *Śavāsana* before their performance. If they relax they can't dance or play or act. So meditation and *Śavāsana* are futile in competitive sports.

I am proud to say that I have taught yoga to leading cricket players, wizards in music, and dancers who swear that their success is due to yoga.

Before any competition, it is true that one needs mental peace. But there is a world of difference between relaxation needed for activity and relaxation for passivity. If this is not understood it will spell doom on players. When you have to play you need a stimulated body. The *āsana* stimulate and atomise the body and brain and at the same time keep one mentally alert. The nerves also get rejuvenated to endure the strain of the day. The *āsana* like standing postures, lateral twists, back bends help to shed out the lethargy and bring lightness and agility in body and mind.

For games, you require exhilarating action and active mind and not a passive mind. In *dhyāna* and *Śavāsana*, the energy recedes and makes one's mind passive and body cold. When the brain and mind become silent and soft, how can one expect to play with vigour? Undoubtedly *dhyāna* and *Śavāsana* are good after the day's play. Relaxation does not stimulate the body and mind at once. It is good to do so after the game. The key-note for sports is active action with a non-stressed brain which can be earned in abundance in certain *āsana*. *Āsana* practice is nothing but active and dynamic *dhyāna* or meditation. *Śavāsana* does not bring co-ordination at once between the body movements and alertness of the mind.

I stress that the cells have their own psychology, intelligence and memory. If you don't observe these through body language then you are bound to be a failure in your games or sports.

If you run to warm up before the game, you end up with fatigue whereas practice of *yogāsana* stimulates and makes you active and helps you gather mental energy for attention without tiring. Other exercises throw the mind out of gear while *yogāsana* integrate the cells of the body with the cells of the brain which makes one remain composed and attentively alert to face confrontation.

No doubt one relaxes in *dhyāna* or *Śavāsana* but it takes time for body, brain and mind to be alert and active for quick movements. Coaches have only an idea that meditation improves concentration. Meditation comes after concentration. When the intelligence of the body acts and reacts without any bodily obstacles, concentration comes on its own.

Those sports people who have undergone training with me have understood the difference. If they are warmed up without strain and kept ready to act with precision, how can they face defeat?

III.3. - Yoga or jogging - strengthening the heart

First of all the idea is illusory: these two are quite different types of exercises. One is stimulative while the other is irritative. What a paradox to understand that jogging stimulates the heart! Jogging does not help to take deep breaths. Only short breaths are possible. In jogging, only the upper lungs are used and hence the pumping of the heart increases and this makes one believe that faster the heart beat, the congested arteries get flushed but at what cost and strain? In yogic *prāṇāyāma* called *Bhastrikā*, it does the same without strain. Only one has to know whether the affected person is capable of performing this vigorous *prāṇāyāma*.

This increase in heart rate helps the blood vessels to pump and flush the blocked area but does it stimulate the heart? It is hard to say for a patient who is suffering from cardiac problems. Stimulation and irritation are of opposite poles. So it is for the heart patient to decide and not to consider the advice from those who have no heart problems. I am sure that cardiologists will be careful in advising their patients.

People are made to think that jogging increases the pumping of the heart and therefore it gets stimulated. On the contrary the heart gets irritated as improper breath movements disturb the diaphragm which create laboured breathing.

Please do not get carried away with the false idea that jogging stimulates and invigorates the heart. Jogging may invigorate the brain but not the heart. Jogging tires and exhausts the jogger as he pants for breath and feels thirsty making him to drink, perhaps a soft drink.

In running and jogging the diaphragm becomes tight and hard. Due to the un-rhythmic diaphragmatic action breathing becomes hard and fast and the heart beats fast but it does not mean that the heart has flushed out the blockages.

The aorta is bifurcated: one part takes blood towards the brain and the other towards the trunk. Running produces heat in the brain as well as in the legs and so one thinks that the circulation has increased. What about the effect on the brain cells? What about the effect of heavy laboured breathing? So I am definitely sure that jogging and running are not good for cardiac patients. What is invigorating is stimulating and what is non-invigorating is non-stimulating but irritating. If you can understand this, then you judge for yourself whether jogging is good or bad.

Unfortunately, medical science as well as the common man does not know the value of yoga. If one has to improve the circulation and cleanse the heart, one needs to know the *āsana* which stimulate the heart but do not irritate. You may not perspire heavily in *āsana* as happens in jogging. Let me tell you that the backward extensions and inverted *āsana* given here stimulate the heart. One has to choose what fits one in this list and practise or approach a teacher. After attending to these *āsana*, do *Śavāsana* with *Viloma prāṇāyāma* for total relaxation.

I have shown the re-actions of actions between yoga and jogging and now I leave this for you to decide whether you prefer the physical movements like jogging or whether you like to do the psycho-physiological exercises which are provided in the above list of *āsana*.

For me the experimental period is over. I have handled hundreds of cases and I am sure of the benefits. But it is for you to compose and judge and not me.

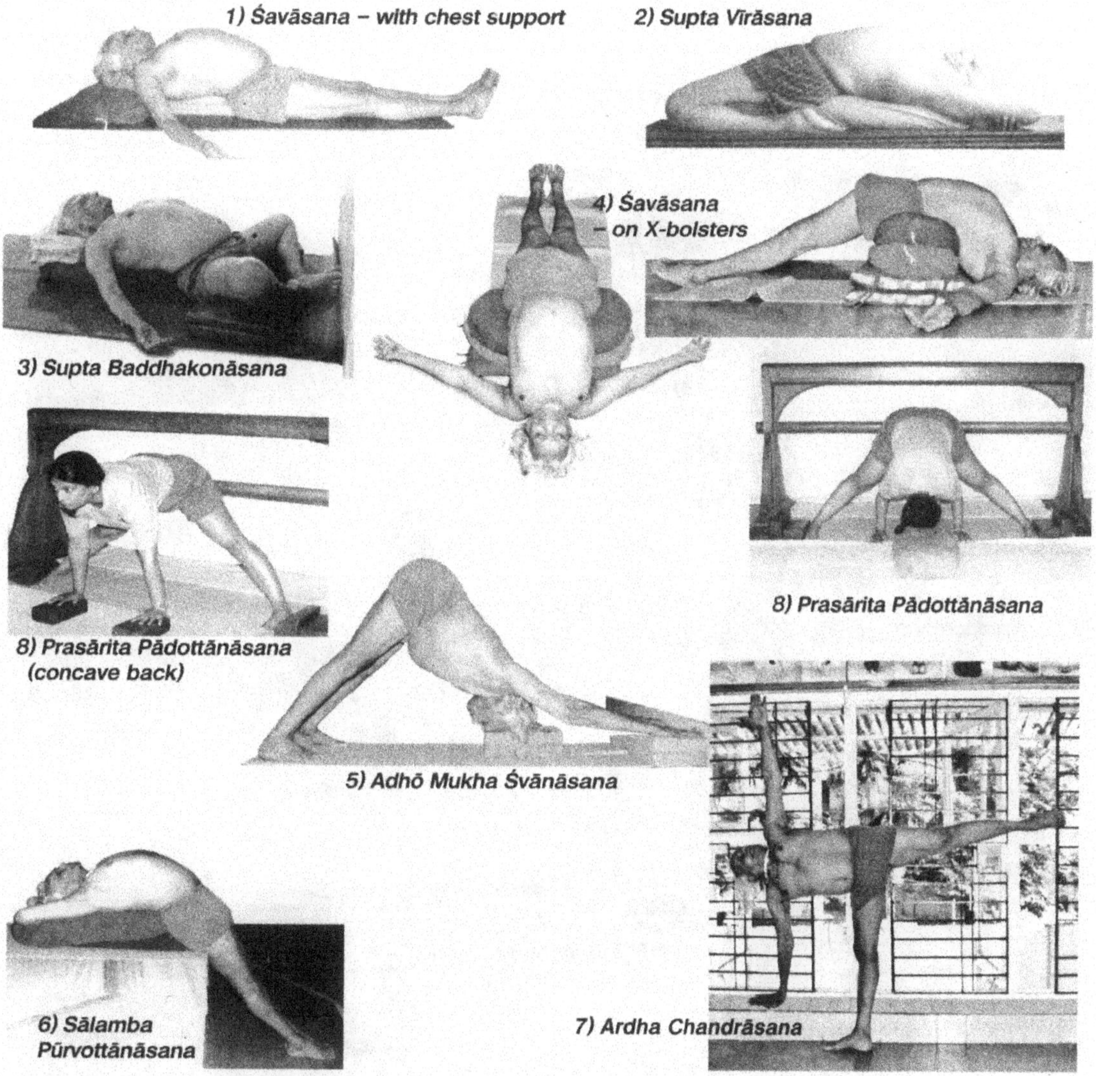

Plate n. 6a – *Āsana* to stimulate the heart without irritation

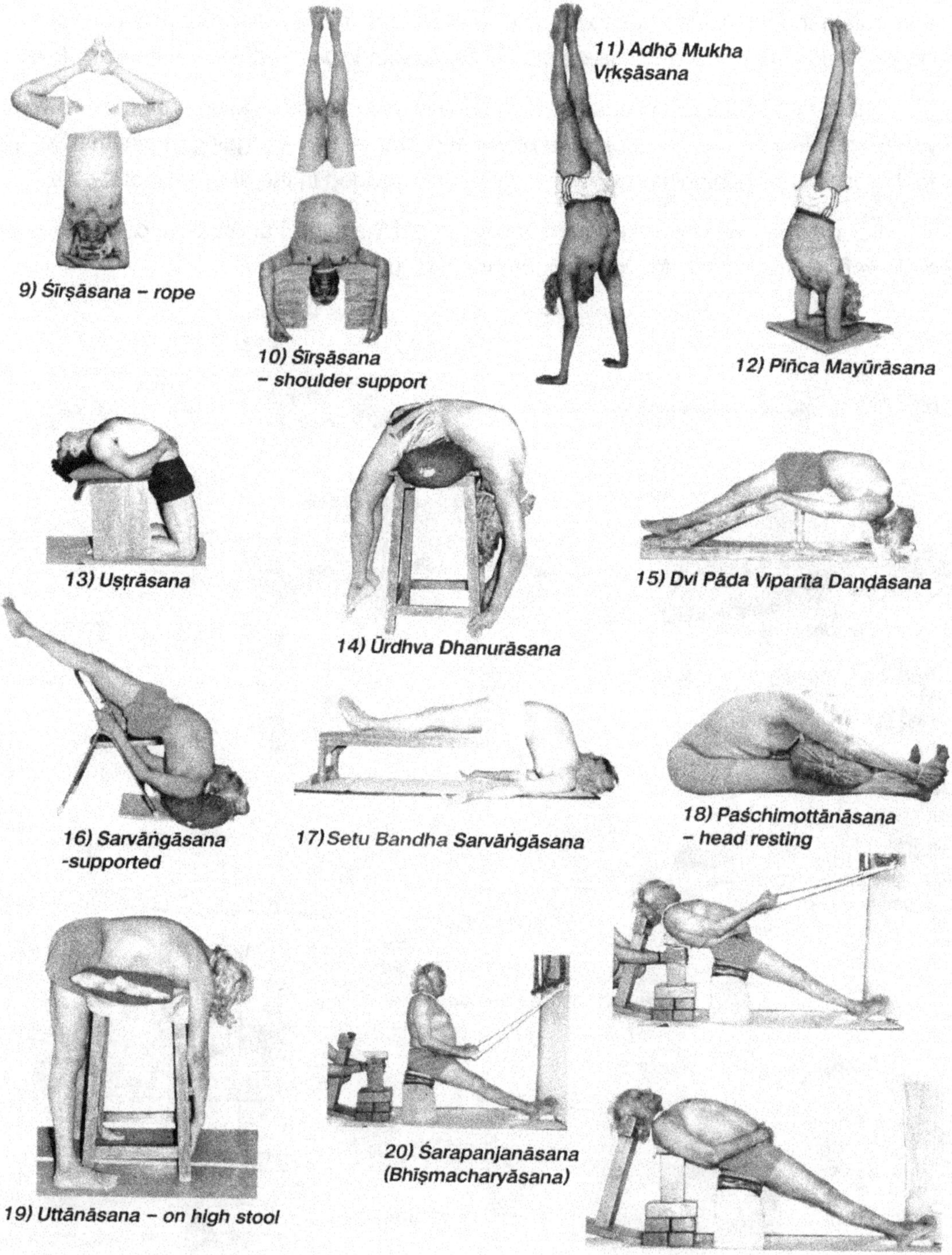

Plate n. 6b – *Āsana* to stimulate the heart without irritation cont . . .

III.4. - *Āsana* - exercise

On account of want of knowledge the majority of people consider *āsana* as just an exercise. The word for exercise in *Sanskṛt* is *vyāyāma*. It means extension and expansion in order to draw the energy with different movements and in different directions. It also means to make efforts to scatter the energy to various parts of the body. *Āsana* helps in gathering and filtering the energy in order to distribute it evenly all over the body.

Yet I cannot deny the fact that when a beginner begins to practise *āsana*, it seems somewhat similar to ordinary exercises. The body which is in a state of inertia needs the energy to vibrate, hence it needs movement. Movements like extension, contraction, adduction, abduction and circumduction in the muscles are considered as exercise. Without the functioning of the joints fully the muscles cannot be flexed, extended or rotated well. Without right and total movement, life force cannot be regenerated. Hence, *āsana* practice at the starting stage appears as physical exercise.

When you attend primary school, the teacher teaches you the alphabet for the sake of learning. In yoga also no teacher introduces the higher aspects at once. The teacher has to begin *āsana* from the rudimentary level where movements assume prominence due to lack of sensitivity. It is a fact that not a single moment passes without a movement. Even a newborn baby moves its body. Obviously a beginner is a baby in the path of *āsana*. Often they do not know how to make right movements in the muscles nor do they know how to create energy and use it to the minimum without wastage.

Beginners show intense interest in yoga but it dies before it sprouts. Yogic practice takes time to bring integration in the body, mind and self. To start with, *āsana* acts as exercise in disciplining and channelling the movements of the body in order to develop sensitivity in the body. This ploughing of the body is *vyāyāma*.

As aspirants are mild, medium, intense or supremely intense, the practice of *āsana* differs on these levels from the rudimentary to the finest points. Generally the *sādhaka* does not apply his mind for changes in the performance that is needed to grasp the depth of each *āsana*.

Though Patañjali's aphorisms seem to be very disciplined, he had a soft spot for some human beings. In *Samādhi Pāda*, he asks the consciousness *(citta)* to have an eagle's swoop to pounce whereas in *Sādhana Pāda* he asks the *sādhaka* to swim like a kingly swan. If *Samādhi Pāda* was meant for the advanced souls, *Sādhana Pāda* was for the average intellectual human beings. Therefore, he asks the *sādhaka* to unveil himself from the physical level to experience the higher levels of growth. In *Sādhana Pāda*, the *sādhaka* has to make all efforts. Practice of *aṣṭāṅga yoga* strengthens the faculty of determination and sows the seed of will power.

According to one's way of thinking and acting, attempts may be slow or fast and quick. Sometimes in the *āsana* the body and mind act willingly together and sometimes the body wants to be in action but not the mind or vice versa. When the body and mind play hide and seek, then the way of practice has to be rearranged.

As a beginner, the consciousness is in a wandering state *(vyutthāna)* and as such he is restless to some extent due to lack of determination.

Hence I make the students do the *āsana* in quick succession so that their minds have no time to calculate. If their minds are lazy, dull, lethargic, I change the sequences to make them dynamic, alert and restful.

Depression alienates the mind. In such cases I make them do *Ūrdhva Dhanurāsana*[1] or *Viparīta Cakrāsana*[2] in quick succession. Similarly *Halāsana* and *Paśchimottānāsana* cycles.[3] This refreshes the body and brings alertness to the mind.

Āsana stabilises and establishes the vital energy *(prāṇa-śakti)* before one proceeds towards *prāṇāyāma*. It is worthy to note that in *āsana* alone, there is vast scope to deal with body, mind and energy.

It is said in the *Haṭhayoga Pradīpikā*, *āsanāni rajo hanti* – the practice of *āsana* destroys *rajoguṇa*, and helps *sattvaguṇa* to expand.[4] In average people mostly the *tamoguṇa* predominates. What they need is to decrease the influence of *tamoguṇa* and increase *rajoguṇa*, and later decrease the predominance of both and increase the dominance of *sattvaguṇa*.

When *tamōguṇa* is dominant, *āsana* practice is like exercise. When one transcends from *tamo guṇa* to *rajoguṇa* and *sattvaguṇa in practice* he penetrates the mind deep within the body to gain a perfect position by re-adjusting and repositioning the *āsana*.

Vyāyāma is an external work but when done with the spread of energy within the body, it is *prāṇa āyāma*.

---

[1] See pl. n. 14, vol. 5, *Aṣṭadaḷa Yogamālā*

[2] See pl. n. 29, vol. 4, *Aṣṭadaḷa Yogamālā*.

[3] See pl. n. 7, vol. 4, *Aṣṭadaḷa Yogamālā*.

[4] See Commentary *Jyotsnā* to the *Haṭhayoga Pradīpikā* I.17 of Brahmānanda.

Water is purified by boiling and filtering and then drunk when it is cooled. Similarly, in *āsana*, the body heats up to refine subtle adjustments to culture the cells. Blood is made to circulate and reach the remotest parts of the body. *Āsana* avoids all unwanted movements wherein the body is made to become cool and quiet.

The first stage of *āsana* practice is like the boiling water. When one gains some control, then one begins to repose body and mind in that position. The *Brahmasūtra* says, *āsināt saṁbhavaḥ* - those who are established well in the *āsana*, for them it is possible to realise *Brahma*.

So long as the mind is petty and contracted, *āsana* is treated as exercise. Once the mind opens and spreads, then the *āsana* is no more a *vyāyāma*. It is *yogāsana*.

III.5. - Yoga or acrobatics

There is a difference between yoga and acrobatics. Acrobatics only flex the body and give it a muscular shape. The involvement of the mind may not be there. Awareness of the breath would not be there. For acrobatics, the body is the main instrument whereas to those who do *āsana* the body, mind, intelligence and consciousness are all important. Without rhythmic breath adjustment there is neither yoga nor *āsana*. Yogic practice is for controlling the body, breath and mind. When we practise a particular *āsana* we have to move the body to achieve the required position. For this, one has to involve one's mind to adjust the position to get the specific effect from specific *āsana*. *Āsana* demands perfect co-ordination of body, mind and intelligence for *samādhāna sthiti* - or equilibrium in body, mind, intelligence and self.

At least I am glad that they do some body movements rather than watching scenes on murders and violence on TV.

My advice to the lovers of acrobatics is to take to yoga which is stimulative and exhilarating.

SECTION IV

ON LEARNING AND TEACHING

SECTION IV – ON LEARNING AND TEACHING

IV.1. – How to be a good yoga student

There are no special qualities required to become a student of yoga but only regularity, determination and discipline are needed. These go with urgency, passion and courage. Besides these, one has to be accepting failures as stepping stones to success and persist in practice with perseverance. A sharp memory is needed for comparing day-to-day practices with watchful attention. One has to connect the mind and intelligence to be in constant touch with each and every fibre and cell of the body. The most important vehicle that is needed is to trace where the mind and intelligence do not touch and how to work to make their attention to flow there. Lastly practice must be done with labour and love. These are the qualities required from a student not only in yoga but in all arts. Remember that yoga begins from the basic art and takes one towards the divine art.

Know that in yoga one has to depend entirely upon self-determination and the ways to tap the inner source of energy and strength through a group of instruments, namely the body, mind, intelligence and will-power to tune oneself fully to the music of life. In other arts like music, dance, paintings, architecture, sculpture and so forth, one has to depend on external resources to express one's hidden light.

IV.2. – One teacher or several teachers

We have several hotels in Pune. If you eat food in different hotels each day, will you really relish it? Maybe you may end up with stomach upset. Right from diarrhoea to food poisoning, anything can occur. Children throw out immediately the undigested or unwanted food that is consumed. Their reaction is very fast. When this can happen to children, you can think what happens to grown ups like you and me whose digestive system functions slowly. The dishes in each hotel will be of different tastes to attract customers. But can we digest such dishes if we consume daily?

It is the same with *yogi* and *guru*. Each teacher feeds you with different *masālā* or spices and a variety of salads to attract the students. Teachers tempt you saying that their teaching is better in quality than others. Some crazy students jump to different teachers as they change hotels according to the whims. Being a child in yoga, such a student who has not even digested the teaching of one *guru* when he switches over to another *guru*, is like a man suspended between heaven and earth. The first principle of a student is to learn, digest and absorb the knowledge from one teacher and assimilate well before he jumps to another *guru* or a teacher. Such students should have some subjective experience to measure the standard of other teachers to decide whether it is worth leaving a teacher or not.

The present day tendency of students shows no difference between the teacher and the pupil. A teacher is a teacher and a pupil is a pupil. This, a student should know. Even Patañjali accepts the need of a *guru* in I.25 and 26, wherein he says that God is the foremost *guru* who passes on knowledge to others. In the very first *sūtra* he says the word *anuśāsanam* – i.e.; discipline. *Śāsanam* means to discipline or to govern. The prefix *anu* indicates "after" or "along". Thus the word *anuśāsanam* means, "already set in or conveyed".

Guru has to be at least two or three steps ahead of the pupil with his *sādhanā* as well as in confidence, clarity, will power, vitality, reflective power and prolific awareness. A pupil should see these qualities in a *guru*. Today's *guru* adjust according to the temperament of the pupils. Many pride themselves saying that they have many *guru* and some like to win many pupils. The reason is that the pupil is keen to acquire knowledge with a number of *guru* instead of actually learning. Pupils demand from the teachers to teach according to their tastes whereas in olden days the *guru* did not impart teaching according to the taste of the pupils. The teachers used to demand and command the pupils. Now, it is the other way round. The pupils demand according to their taste and command over the teacher. My *guru's* demands on me were great. He taught less but demanded non-stop practice from me. This made me learn a lot.

Now pupils decide on their *guru* as well as the type of yoga they want and make the *guru* to fit into their preconceptions. If a pupil knows what type of yoga he needs, then why hunt for a *guru?* If he knows what he wants, then why go in search of a teacher? First of all, one has to determine the path and then search for a *guru* who can help and uplift one. Otherwise, the doubting mind makes him run after many *guru*. Running from one *guru* to another leads the seeker into further confusions and doubts and makes him travel from darkness to darkness only.

When one learns from one teacher, one has a background of that experience. When one enriches oneself with experience, one can weigh the teachings of a new *guru*. Without experience if one goes on hunting from one *guru* to another, God alone knows where one would ends up.

In *sādhanā*, by chance you get a pain, you blame the teacher and begin to dislike him; if you get pleasure you think the pleasure giving teacher is a right *guru*. If I had decided about my *guru* this way, then perhaps I would not have reached my present state and status. Even in that painful state I tried to live with his commands and demands and proceeded. I reflected the play of pain and pleasure on my mind and assimilated through my intelligence.

When you go from one doctor to another for treatment, you need to explain in detail about your health history. A new doctor needs to know your past status of health, constitution, and your reactions to medicines and so forth. If he does not know that you are allergic to some medicines, both of you might end up in trouble. Similarly a teacher keeps an eye on a pupil and watches his nature, constitution, mental set-up, physical ability, intellectual capacity and accordingly he imparts knowledge. In olden days the *guru* used to study the pupils who were asked to stay in the *āśrama* or *gurukula*[1] of a *guru*. They were called *antevāsin*. Now such life in *āśrama* may not be possible but we need a teacher who can judge and decide what is to be taught.

Moreover, when we go to several *gurus* we neither learn nor get clarity. We land up in a confused state of mind. The mixing of methodology and confusion in the mind harms not only the *guru* but also the pupils if ever one thinks of teaching. Take precautions before choosing a *guru*.

In my early days I used to read the name plates of lawyers on some bungalows, Bar-at Law (England returned). Today, yoga teachers in the West are following the East on their advertisements, Yoga Teacher (India returned).

First, work steadfastly with one *guru*, learn, reflect and assimilate. Then you become a *guru* to yourself. Your inner light begins to guide you. The matured intelligence leads you towards the exalted intelligence. That is what Patañjali calls *vivekaja jñānam*.[2]

---

1 The house of *guru* with a residence for pupils. *Gurukula* system: traditional boarding system where the pupil stayed with the *guru* and learnt from him. Such a pupil was called a *vāsin* (abiding in) or an *ante-vāsin* (living near *guru*).

2 *Y.S.*, III.53, 55. Cf. the author's *Light on the Yoga Sūtras of Patañjali*, Harper Collins, London.

After assimilating, if one finds that his first *guru* is stuck without progress, then one can go to another *guru*. Your own consciousness then guides you whether the *guru* that you have chosen is a right one or not.

If your approach is honest and you have faith in yourself, then the guidance comes from within.

IV.3. – Recognising a good yoga teacher[1]

First of all, if yoga is undertaken for generating yoga teachers, it is definitely unfair to yoga. A good teacher will have to be truthful to yoga. He or she has to be a genuine practitioner. This puts a tremendous demand on practice to digest before thinking of teaching. No teacher can be a teacher without proper training and practices. Without knowledge and experience how can one become a teacher? Pupils should demand from their teachers now and then to present what they say and the teacher should be able to see the difficulties in their presentation and correct them at once. Teaching without practice is cheating. Then there is no difference between a teacher and a cheater. Only the order of the letters changes.

The good teacher should be able to bring the required change in his pupils. Mere sweet-talking does not help or uplift pupils. Direct progressive instructions with precepts, enlightening with knowledge and understanding must be the quality of a good teacher.

IV.4. – The *dharma* of a teacher

Yoga is not only an emotional subject but also needs great intellectual intensity to watch over the changes in the student that occur in *sādhanā*.

Teaching yoga from the head is not a *yoga dharma* or a *guru dharma*. Acquired knowledge from the head combined with the experienced understanding of the heart should

[1] See also *Aṣṭadaḷa Yogamālā*, vol. 3, section V, *On teaching*.

be the *dharma* of a teacher. The synchronisation of the analytical intellect of the head with the intelligence of the heart in action is the real quality needed to be a teacher. One cannot become a yoga teacher with gathered knowledge without the background of experiential feelings. Reverential practice under an able teacher and assistance to the students under his guidance are essential to become a teacher.

When one uses the word teacher, *guru* or *ācārya*, one must be sure that one is a good practitioner before one teaches. If I preach and do not practise, then I am only a propagandist and not a teacher in its true sense. Whichever religion a teacher belongs to, he has to follow the ethical *dharma* of teaching on the lines of morality, sincerity, integrity with humane principles of honesty.

Suppose you have a headache and I as a teacher advise you to do *Śīrṣāsana*. My idea in advising you to do this is that there will be good blood circulation to the head and the headache may lessen. No doubt your headache will not be there as long as you are in *Śīrṣāsana*. The moment you come down from *Śīrṣāsana*, the headache may appear again. In some cases, it may not be possible even to keep the head down. This shows that I as a teacher guided you through theoretical knowledge and not with practical experience. It means that I as a teacher am not following the yogic morality needed to qualify myself as a teacher.

In Patañjali's words a *guru* has to be a *tapasvin*, a *svādhyāyin* and an *Īśvara-praṇidhānin* (*Y.S.*, II.1). These are the characteristics needed to be a teacher. As a student, if he has not cultivated zeal and study in depth with devoted action, then I am afraid that he cannot become a teacher.

Have you not seen me admonishing my own teachers? Actually I do not admonish them from my heart of hearts, I correct their behaviour so that they do not repeat such mistakes. Secondly I use force both physically and intellectually on account of the background I have behind the subject. If people say, "Iyengar is very rough on his teachers", have I to follow their dictates or my conscience? Then what would be my *dharma* if I surrendered to hearsay? My *dharma* is to correct my students when they go wrong. I speak to guide, to warn, to reprimand whereas many speak to hear the sound of their own voice. My corrections act as an intellectual prick so that they improve soon for the better. People expect me to speak sweetly because it hurts them in the presence of their students. When a doctor treats the patients with bitter medicine or performs an operation, is it not for the good of the patient? The doctor who do not take a quick action to relieve the patient's disease, do you call such a doctor a dutiful doctor? There is *vaidya dharma* also. In the same way, a yoga teacher has to think of his duty *(dharma)* in his profession. If I do not correct at once the wrong instructions of my students-teachers, know then that I am not an honest teacher but a selfish teacher to earn just their good will. The *dharma* of a teacher is to find ways and means to correct his student's faults immediately.

These days we find teachers who are good in communicating information, but to find those who commune and interact with students is rare indeed.

IV.5. – A real teacher is a pupil within

I do not pat teachers easily though my teachers go out of their way to pat those who come to them. Instead I want them to look to the needs and to remove the obstacles that come in their ways of learning. For this, the teachers need re-learning and re-training in their own *sādhanā* to find ways and means to guide those who come to them as to how they can cross over the obstacles to progress. Expression of gratefulness from pupils is one thing. But to think and find ways for their progress is another. If such students come to me I consider myself a fortunate man, as they act as my eye openers in my practice and I remain grateful inwardly.

Teaching is learning, and re-learning is true teaching. Accept your pupils as a blessing from God for you to re-open your intelligence to re-think and re-act with wide-open eyes. See the generosity of God who sends such students who pay for you to refine your *sādhanā* both in teaching and learning.

Each pupil who comes to you comes with some new problems. No two persons are alike. Therefore teaching cannot be parrot teaching. Each pupil has to be studied. The teacher has to go down to the understanding level of the pupils. The teacher has to get experience by thinking and learning adjustment processes as each different pupil opens new angles of thought.

Do not differentiate between yourself and the pupil. As the mother loves her children, the teacher should show affection in guiding them towards progression. If there is a gap between teacher and student, it creates egoism in the teacher and a communication gap between them. A teacher becomes a teacher because he knows and learns more to impart to his pupils. Teaching does not make one a master of the subject. There may be many unknown things to be known. Compassion, strictness and discipline need to be utilised when necessary. Teaching needs love, compassion, firmness and determination. There is nothing wrong with roaring like a lion on the outside but be a lamb inside. Though he acts as a teacher within himself, he should be a learner.

As a teacher I know one's responsibilities. I may assume a ferocious mantle in order to bring alertness and clarity in students as well as teachers while they are practising or teaching. As teachers when they come to learn from me, I make them forget that they are teachers but pupils because I want them to learn and relearn, reflect and re-reflect on what they practise and teach.

When students come to me to learn I treat them as God, as we are all children of God. From outside I treat them as pupils. As you see yourself in the mirror, I see also myself whether my teaching is correct by watching their faces which reflect their reaction fast. The teachers must be like this in order to develop the quality of right direction.

The teacher has to learn while teaching by blending his head and heart. He has to learn to weigh the intellect of the head and emotional intelligence of the heart in each student which helps him to improve himself in the art of teaching. As a teacher one must be a pupil within. As a teacher some homework has to be done by investigating what was expressed and what was missing in teaching. Observation of errors helps to correct not only the students but also oneself as a teacher. For this to develop, watchfulness and persistent effort are needed.

When pupils commit mistakes, the teacher has to think whether he too commits such mistakes. I did work like this before and I do this even now. This studentship in me has made me to be a good teacher.

So please do not practise yoga with the sole motive to become a teacher. If occasion arises accept to teach. While learning, I never thought that I might have to teach. The circumstances forced me to become a teacher. If pupils did not come to me, I said that it was God's wish that I devote my time for more practice. And when pupils came I was saying to myself that it is God's wish to serve them. In both ways I took it as God's grace.

RECENT INTERVIEWS

FROM DARKNESS TO LIGHT*

Q.– Many people practise yoga but do not seem to be able to take their practice beyond the physical level. When did you realise the deeper meaning of your own practice or were you always aware of the deeper aspects of yoga?

I think I have dealt fully in my Keynote address at Estes Park as well as in *Light on Life* how transformation took place in me and in my practices. I suggest you go through my first book *Light on Yoga* with the latest book *Light on Life* to get a clear picture of my growth in yoga.

When I began yoga I did not know what yoga was and my *Guruji* was not willing to explain it when questioned. He only said: "Good for your health, go ahead." I took this as a *mantra*. As I was ill from birth it took me six years through yoga to experience the sense of health and well-being. As lots of students started coming to me to learn, it opened my eyes to understand that minimum practice and insufficient presentation is not enough to teach. I wanted those who come to me to appreciate the subject. Hence I had to find out means to give the feeling of well being and exhilaration. This made me to reflect on my thoughts as well as practices by watching and studying my mind and body movements where co-operation is and how to associate and bring the union between mind and body in case they do not co-operate. This made me peep into my body and observe its actions, re-actions and non-actions. This made me to develop friendship with the body and mind in my practices. I was cajoling the body when it was not willing to perform but to cajole the mind it took me a long time with all my efforts, I could not get the clue for using the mind while performing the *āsana*.

But the students who were coming to me were highly educated and intelligent than me. They often questioned me on the hidden basic things which helped me to open my eyes and mind to look and feel each and every part of my body in my practice. It took me time to co-ordinate the mind to flow concurrently with the movements of the various parts of the body in different *āsana*. No doubt, in the beginning it was difficult to make the intellectual mind and the

---

* A conversation between Patricia Walden and BKS Iyengar, Boston, Massachusetts, October 9th, 2005.

flow of energy to co-operate and co-ordinate in the body. I succeeded in bringing co-ordination between body, energy and the intellectual mind to be lively while practising. This started igniting me with a sort of exhilaration and jubilation. As I was feeling and seeing my own body with my mind, my intellectual eye began to judge my body movements and mind movements in each *āsana*. When my physical eyes used to fail I took the help of the intellectual eye to perfect the *āsana*. This intellectual involvement gave me the light to discriminate and to discern whether I was practising right or wrong. By this process my intelligence started developing from a dormant state to an evolved state. This involvement of my intelligence stirred my body further to reach the extension and expansion to the fullest possible extent and made me a devotee of *āsana*. Though I was sweating I never practised for contorting the body. On the contrary from this inner observation and attention I was able to eradicate the contorting and distorting movements in the body and illusive thoughts of the mind in all the *āsana*. For this transformation I have to thank my students with their queries, which helped me to learn, re-learn, un-learn and re-learn the *āsana* to acquire a right hold on them and to impart that knowledge to the students.

This acquisition of control over the *āsana* helped me to maintain the anatomical body in the proper and correct position as it is normally structured in a healthy state. For instance when we stand in *Tāḍāsana* our chest remains broad but it collapses in *Śīrṣāsana*, *Sarvāṅgāsana* or *Ardha Matsyendrāsana*.[1] I was questioning myself why should it shrink, or drop or tilt and how to keep the original state of the chest in these *āsana*. These questions began taunting me. With these thoughts of *Tāḍāsana* I worked in all the *āsana* to bring that quality of maintaining the natural anatomical structure without distortion or contortion or refraction. I began synchronising the thinking mind while practising and the working body with the thinking mind. This helped me in balancing the intelligence evenly throughout my body. This is the light of knowledge that I got from this combined effort of combing body and mind.

The river has two banks. Similarly, the body has two banks. If one bank of the body is the skin, the other bank is the intelligence of the self. This river of energy has to flow touching the intelligence of the self and the inner surface of the skin evenly. This process of thinking and observing made me do the *āsana* in such a way that my intelligence began to move closer to the frontier of the body touching the back, the sides and the four corners of the torso including the legs and arms as well as the self. This way I began connecting the intelligence to the four corners of the entire human body in all *āsana* to see whether I could fill the body with the consciousness and the self in the length and width of the body. When I learned this contact of intelligence and the consciousness with the skin of the body I began to realise the consciousness

---

[1] This can be seen in pl. n. 22 of *Aṣṭadaḷa Yogamālā* vol. 7.

expanding and energy spreading all over the body with concord. This contact of intelligence and consciousness running in contact with the bank of the skin of the body ignited to infuse awareness to bring the self *(prajñā)* and *prāṇa* (energy) to unite with the body. This vertical growth of intellect of the head along with the horizontal intelligence of the heart made me trace the middle line throughout my body from the centre of the head to the centre of the trunk, the two feet and arms. This brought me to understand what total awareness means. This study made me realise the state of existence without the knowledge for the presence of the self. That's how I learned from culturing my body, churning my mind and the ways of sharpening my intelligence to feel the intelligence of the self to touch and flow everywhere in my practice. If you all pay attention to the entire cellular system with total attention and awareness while practising, you may experience what I am saying. I have explained how I developed stage by stage to reach this level of union with the trio – body, intelligence and self. So keep the mind away from the impression that *āsana* is just physical. It is pure brainwash from the intellectuals who lack practice. I am trying my best through my progression in *āsana* to remove this branding of *āsana* as physical as utter nonsense. Patañjali has not said it. So I want you to trust Patañjali and not those easy-chair commentators.

The original text says that the dualities, the disparities between body and mind, mind and intelligence, intelligence and self disappear when you have mastered the *āsana*. It makes sense for one to experience the infinite touch of the soul contacting its frontier – the skin of the body. This is the effect of *āsana* that has been explained by Patañjali,[1] where the soul assumes its true form in the *āsana*. No doubt the practitioners have to begin from the physical level but as one goes on in one's practices, one should stir the self through the intelligence and consciousness to go beyond the body level. These neo-yogi, neo-philosophers give this idea that *āsana* is only for physical well-being and a common man takes it for granted without delving into it further.

When Patañjali says that one has to be friendly and compassionate, it is applicable in the learning of the *āsana*. When the body needs friendliness and compassion, be friendly and compassionate. The body has to co-operate with the mind and mind with the body and appreciate this union. When the body tries to overrule the mind, show indifference and proceed with your mind. This embellishes the consciousness and helps in learning the *āsana*.[2] This approach is hidden in *Pātañjala Yoga Sūtra*. I started with this background of the *sūtra* in my practices.

1 *prayatna śaithilya ananta samāpattibhyām* (*Y.S.*, II.47) – perfection in an *āsana* is achieved when the effort to perform it becomes effortless and the infinite being within is reached.

2 *maitrī karuṇā muditā upekṣāṇāṁ sukha duḥkha puṇya apuṇya viṣayāṇāṁ bhāvanātaḥ cittaprasādanam* (I.33) – through cultivation of friendliness, compassion, joy and indifference to pleasure and pain, virtue and vice respectively, the consciousness becomes favourably disposed, serene and benevolent.

Sometimes the mind was rebelling and at other times the body. I used friendliness and compassion when mind and body were not co-operating. When they were co-operating, the practice was conducive and I was experiencing gladness. I was indifferent to both the mind and body when needed. I often overlooked them and used the needle of intelligence in practice which changed my attitude. That's how I learned to integrate the physical body, the mental body, the intellectual body and my conscious body and vice versa throughout the *āsana sādhanā*

Q.– Thank you, *Guruji*. I think you're a mind reader because this leads beautifully into the next question. *Sūtra* I.33.[1] You translate this *sūtra* that "through cultivation of friendliness, compassion, joy, and indifference to pleasure and pain, virtue and vice respectively, the consciousness becomes favourably disposed, serene and benevolent." And the question is: How can the practice of *āsana* and *prāṇāyāma* lead to *upekṣā* indifference, and in *Light on Life* you translate it as neutrality?

This *sūtra* explains how you have to establish contact with yourself as well as the society. It explains how the individual and social health has to be maintained. In society we find good and bad things. There are pious people and there are impious people. Aren't people easily attracted to vices? See how youngsters get attracted towards sexual life, alcoholism, drugs and cigarettes. They know that these are vices but can one abolish drugs, alcohol and tobacco from society? They do not disappear. Virtue and vice dwell side by side. The more one tries to suppress the vice, it rears its hood from another direction. We need to learn indifference, we need to remain neutral, so that these vices do not attract and entangle us. Don't we like to remain healthy and keep the diseases away from us?

In the early phase of my practices people used to call me a madcap. They were laughing at me. Being young and doing *āsana* throughout the day made people call me a madcap but I remained indifferent to their teasing, laughter and criticisms. I never got disturbed or perturbed though it was hurting me inside. I took all comments in my stride and survived. Even now some criticise me but I keep aloof and show indifference to such remarks. Indifference to some extent stands for neutrality.

---

1 See footnote n. 2, on pp. 79

Now, coming to the practice of *āsana* and *prāṇāyāma,* when they are done with accuracy, the mental and intellectual stature transforms to trace the seed that guides towards accuracy. This is the mystical effect of *āsana.*

I have said often that those who were drunkards visiting the houses of prostitutes and wanted to do yoga came to me and I taught them. I never pointed out their vices and weaknesses but remained friendly and taught them compassionately. With the practice of *āsana* and *prāṇāyāma,* they got rid of their problems on their own. As a human being I helped them. They changed and got rid of their weaknesses. I was accepting such men to see whether the practice of *āsana* and *prāṇāyāma* could change them or not. I was happy because rigorous and disciplined practice proved successful.

When you practise *āsana* and *prāṇāyāma* the dualities and conflicts in mind fade out gradually. It is a kind of bio-chemical change and mental clarity that take place in the practitioners. This made me to devote my practices to penetrate intensively to experience what more these two petals of yoga could give. This made me practise with enthusiasm and intellectual application without being caught with emotional upheavals. Even while teaching I have to blend my intelligence of the head with the emotions of the heart without giving chances for emotional weakness to surface. That is why I am considered a strict, tough, taskmaster.

The *Vibhūti Pāda* speaks of *siddhi.* We may come across such achievements. Even simple health is an achievement for us and when we teach others and give them health we feel great. Our ego gets puffed. If we learn to remain indifferent to our achievements and accomplishments, can't we progress further? Let us learn *karma-dharma-saṁyoga.* Do good and virtuous *karma* as a religious and righteous duty and forget about it.

We know that the brain has four lobes and the heart four chambers. As I read and re-read the *Yoga Sūtra,* I thought that Patañjali divides these four lobes of the brain as four parts of intellectual development. These are analytical part *(vitarka),* the part that reasons and synthesises *(vicāra),* the part of bliss *(ānanda),* and the fourth part as the seat of the individual self *(asmitā* or *sāsmitā).* If these parts make man develop his intellect by means of vertical growth to reach the highest level in acquiring knowledge, the four chambers of the heart are meant for horizontal growth of intelligence through friendliness *(maitrī),* compassion *(karuṇā)*, gladness *(muditā)* and indifference to good or bad virtue and vice *(upekṣā).*

Patañjali speaks of the head as an intellectual seat and of the heart as an emotional seat. I used these two faces of the intelligence in practising *āsana.* I worked out ways of how to bring head and heart to co-ordinate in the practice and learnt how they have to co-operate not only with the body but with the consciousness also. This helped me to realise what is harmony, concord and balance. Until then there was turmoil. Often all of us practise with turmoil. The two functions or two hemispheres of the brain which are needed first in *sādhanā* are analysis and synthesis or *vitarka* and *vicāra*. Similarly, we have to make use of friendliness *(maitrī)* and compassion *(karuṇā)* of the intelligence of the heart to function in co-ordination. Normally, intellectual people live only in their heads but their bodies below their brains remain completely in darkness. I've met and taught lots of intellectuals, hence I know what I am saying. Often the yoga practitioners practise with their brain without any background of diffusing the intellect of the head to experience the value of yoga. They have no knowledge of blending the intelligence of the head and the heart.

Patañjali indirectly says, "You have to live not only in the head but also in the heart." So my advice for you all is to read I.17 and I.33 to understand the functions of the head and heart. These two *sūtra*, I.17[1] and I.33,[2] have spiritual bearing for learners like you. He connects analysis and synthesis with friendliness and compassion. The intoxicated intellectual people do not connect to the emotional intelligence of the heart namely; friendliness and compassion. You find in them only pride. They are very proud of their brain. That is why Patañjali uses the word *upekṣā*. When intellectuals get intoxicated with their intellectual prowess ending up with arrogance, he wants them to inculcate indifference *(upekṣā)* to that prowess. He connects the third hemisphere of the brain *(ānanda)* with the third chamber of the heart; gladness *(muditā)*. *Ānanda* of the head and *muditā* of the heart convey the same meaning. Patañjali says that at the time of bliss or gladness the *sādhaka* may be carried away and a downfall may happen as he is caught in the web of that gladness. Then the practitioner may lose the sight of the soul. There he wants one to follow indifference *(upekṣā)*.

Stopping the practice *(sādhanā)* with a wrong notion of satisfaction brings back heedlessness *(pramāda)*, illusion *(bhrānti-darśana)*, missing the point *(alabdhabhūmikatva)*, unsettledness *(anavasthitatva)*. When this happens take guidance from these two *sūtra*.

So even if you have the sight of the soul (it may or it may not come), don't think that you have reached the final level. Take it as a guideline that your *sādhanā* is in the right direction and stick to the *sādhanā*. Don't stop *sādhanā*. I have seen many stopping and become a prey to unhappiness. Remember the *sūtra*, *hānam eṣāṁ kleśavat uktam (Y.S.,* IV.28) – the way the *sādhaka* strives to be free from afflictions, the yogi must handle these latent impressions

---

[1] *vitarka vicāra ānanda asmitārūpa anugamāt samprajñātaḥ* (I.17) – practice and detachment develop four types of *samādhi*: self-analysis, synthesis, bliss and the experience of pure being.

[2] *maitrī karuṇā muditā upekṣāṇāṁ sukha duḥkha puṇya apuṇya viṣayāṇāṁ bhāvanātaḥ cittaprasādanam* (I.33) – through cultivation of friendliness, compassion, joy and indifference to pleasure and pain, virtue and vice respectively, the consciousness becomes favourably disposed, serene and benevolent.

judiciously to extinguish them. Patañjali cautions that even evolved people will have to undergo and suffer afflictions because of their pride in the spiritual light and achievements. The achievement makes one callous. That is the fissure. Hence, I.33 becomes handy as it guides the *sādhaka* to show indifference to such things and continue *sādhanā* so that he develops humility in the heart. I hope you understand when I say *ahaṁkāra-vṛtti nirodha* alone will take one towards *ātmadarśana*.

Q.– Did your wife Ramāmaṇi know about what you were doing and how much you were committed to your yoga practice when she married you?

Absolutely nil! When she got married she asked me about yoga as she had not heard the word 'yoga' at all. She was a musician. She knew about music but she never knew about yoga. She came to know of yoga from me and through my practices. I used to tell her that, "As you sing in rhythm I move the body in *āsana* with a rhythm and that rhythm in performance is called yoga." That's how I made her to understand the practical aspect of yoga as she was a singer. As her husband I had to tell her of my interest in yoga and wanted her to express what interest she had so that we could adjust and accommodate our interests and live amicably throughout our lives. By this exchange of our thoughts we lived together understanding each other well. Seeing my daily practice, she got interested and I was willingly obliging her in teaching this art. This way she became my pupil.

As there was no chance for me to understand whether I was doing right or not, I took advantage of my wife's presence; I wanted her to watch my practice and act as a talking mirror. I explained to her how the *āsana* should be and began guiding her how to see, watch and correct. If she had lived probably she, as a woman would have been the number one teacher in the world in yoga. She was quick to catch the defects and disparities. What I could not see, I gave her clues to see by making her to do the *āsana* and explaining where she had to see the adjustments of the body in the *āsana*. That's how I built in her the art of teaching.

In the 1940s and 50s lots of women wanted to learn but were shy to stand in front of a man. As I trained her she became a yoga teacher teaching women who approached her or me. As they started coming I had to guide my wife what to teach for the problems they were having. As I started yoga from scratch not knowing any theory, I started telling her about it to see from the visible things of the skeletal body, showing how to help those who came to her as well as me, so that she learned the intricacies of each *āsana* to know how they function. Later I made her to become my friend, my guide and my philosopher. Making her to see the right alignment made her to understand the background and philosophy that was behind each *āsana*. Hence, I am grateful to her for her help. She readily kept aside all her work, assignments and wishes whenever I wanted her to help in my *sādhanā*. She used to leave her work halfway whether it was cooking or washing but came to help me. Later she became very much interested in yoga and began learning a great deal. I am talking about her with such elaboration for the simple reason that when I married, I had no maturity of mind or the intelligence to see and feel if I was correct in my practices.

As I settled in Pune I had absolutely no chance of asking or sharing with my colleagues *(gurubandhu)*. I had to depend on my own intellectual level.

If one sees earlier books before I wrote *Light on Yoga*, one will never see the *āsana* presentation matching the techniques. This made me learn alignment of the right with the left body as well as balancing the mind as I went on practising.

My wife also helped me by coming to the studio to help me present the *āsana* for *Light on Yoga* which became a unique presentation. I am hoping for the day when someone surpasses me in presenting the *āsana*. The credit of such a presentation goes to my wife only. Through her observation and adjustment I realised that the exterior and the interior bank of the muscles and skin should be of equall distance without any deviation in all *āsana*. Then I learnt how to create space in the joints and muscles so that the fluid lubricates the joints for the muscles to flex or extend accurately. Without pliability in the joints the muscles could not function and without proper functioning of the muscles, the joints were not functioning. I learnt to intermingle these actions with the senses of perception. By this union of action with the senses of perception I learned to separate motor nerves with sensory nerves creating space without jamming or jarring the spindles of the motor nerves with the spindles of the sensory nerves. This approach immediately made my mind to move to feel how the senses of perception work by re-adjusting the spindles of the sensory nerves to exactly face the spindles of the motor nerves. This union *(saṁyoga)* of the sensory nerves with the motor nerves made my mind conceive the feelings that were taking place in each and every part of the body. This made me bring my intelligence to be attentive all the time. All this training with my wife's help made me directly reflect and re-reflect in each *āsana*. This watching and reflecting and re-reflecting helped me to make good progress in my *prāṇāyāma*, *dhāraṇā* and so forth.

Q.– I have one final question, *Guruji*. In *Light on Life* you say "Failures in life lead to further determination." Would you please elaborate?

When I started teaching yoga my chest was expanding only half an inch. I was an example for anti-yoga though I was a yoga teacher. My chest could not expand nor had I muscles. Only bones were visible and I was skinny. I was not doing the *āsana* as well as they were to be done. I could not do *prāṇāyāma* because of the weak lungs. The presentation of *āsana* was not attractive as the body had no flesh and no shape. How I won over the people of Pune is something which I say is a mystery. Actually I do not know or re-collect how it gained popularity. My students were all elder to me. I was not even eighteen when I became a teacher. The students of mine were adept in sports culture and education. Due to my illnesses in childhood, I had developed tolerance to bear pain. Suffering both physically and mentally developed strong willpower in me. The tolerance to bear pain built endurance in me. I with skin and bone could tolerate the load of work with ease, whereas men of bulky muscles were unable to take the load. The wrestlers and body-builders in Pune used to wonder how I went on practising non-stop in all the classes. My classes were six to eleven in the mornings and four to eight in the evenings. I was conducting several batches each hour. I was practising with each batch and each group without any rest or gap. My students were getting exhausted while I was continuing my practices. This was the only courage shown though I was nervous inside. By the grace of God I faced the disappointment and yet won the battle. I the union of body and mind started settling in me which brought grace and elegance in my presentation of *āsana* as days went by and I proved to disprove those who talked against *āsana* saying that they are contortions. With this determination I proved successful and now see how many millions are doing, when I was a laughing stock in my early days of practising teaching yoga with my skinny body.

One memorable or unforgettable incidence that occurred was in 1984 where the first Iyengar Yoga International Convention was held in San Francisco. The people in the medical field wanted to test my lungs to see my lung capacity. They asked me to do *prāṇāyāma*. I started *Ujjayi prāṇāyāma*. I was inhaling, exhaling, but the machine was not recording; yet the machine was working. So they asked me to use a little force. I said to them, "If I use a slight force I know you can record but that is not *prāṇāyāma*." They said, "We hear the sound but the recording is not happening." So I had to do *prāṇāyāma* with slight force for the machine to record. They took the recording and said that my lungs have the power of a twenty-five year old Olympian." I was sixty-six. Having suffered with so many illnesses, this record of 1984 gave me confirmation for the first time that I have good lungs. The credit of this scientific record proves the fact that I took all disappointments in my stride and stuck to my practices. Do not take stalemates as disappointments. Stalemates are time gaps when we are not making any progress.

In any walk of life whether one is an artist, a musician or a dancer, one suffers facing certain stalemates. If they become negative in these stalemates, then they cannot make progress at all. This stalemate may remain for years. I have also faced this several times without making progress. I was doing everything but feeling empty inside. Nothing was emerging. Nothing was happening. Many artists might have faced such a state. They hate such stale states and are afraid to express these weaknesses. I have taught lots of top class musicians and they admit and took such stalemates as a failure. Failures not only gave me the determination but also showed new light, a new way to progress. I used the tool of disappointment as an appointment for a new assignment.

Actually failures, stalemates and disappointments strengthened my will to pursue the path with determination and God graced me in my path.

FROM *LIGHT ON YOGA* TO *LIGHT ON LIFE*[*]

Q.– After considering *Yoga Sūtra* as a crowning glory what made you come out with this new book *Light on Life?*

It is an interesting question but I have a long story behind all my works.

Never did I ever dream that a day would come for me to venture to write a book on *Light on Life.*

Regarding *Light on Life* it was a sudden demand. Two editors, Doug Abrams and Daniel Rivers Moore (editor of my book *The Tree of Yoga*) along with one of my pupils, John Evans landed at my Institute and proposed that I undertake to write on the evolution and progress of my life through yoga.

The book on *Yoga Sūtra* was a huge amount of work. Many writers have rambled on in an inconclusive commentary that fails to elucidate or illuminate the work in part or in whole. I suffered a lot of fear and frustration in undertaking this. To be honest I went on correcting each *sūtra* dozens of times till it gave me the right sense. No doubt in the end, it turned out very well as a crowning glory in my attempts. With this mature knowledge from the study of *Light on the Yoga Sūtras of Patañjali,* I went on practising and new ideas started cropping up within me.

When these friends told me that Rodale Publishers were interested in my work, I thought I should accept and present my new ideas to yogic students and lovers of its philosophy and so I agreed to undertake this new project. I thought of naming the book *Light on Life.*

I had already written four classic books namely, *Light on Yoga, Light on Prāṇāyāma, Tree of Yoga* and *Light on the Yoga Sūtras of Patañjali.* In this new treatise *Light on Life,* I am presenting the cosmogony of nature *(prakṛti),* with the play of its qualities *(guṇa)* which represents the five sheaths *(kośa)* and five types of energy *(prāṇa* or *vāyu)* in the body. As all these are interwoven and inter-related, I have explained how to recognise and understand these principles

---

[*] This interview was conducted on 7th November 2005, in the Ramāmaṇi Iyengar Memorial Yoga Institute

of nature and their functions so that the practitioners of yoga one day connect all these in order to communicate and commune with the Self or the *ātman*.

I thought of ill-health that began while I was in my mother's womb which caused negative thoughts driving me to the edge of suicide. At the same time I thought how it acted as a boon for me to embrace yoga at an early age in order to gain health which became a religious fervour that intensified my practice with dedication and devotion. With this back-ground I decided to name this new book *Light on Life*. It is the light of yoga that kindled me to face life and illuminated me with its brilliance.

I have been engrossed in yoga since the age of fifteen, explicitly practising *yogāsana* and *prāṇāyāma* although other aspects of yoga remained in latent form for years. In course of time, these aspects surfaced and began revealing the secret and sacred aspects of yoga. Hence this book covers my yogic journey from nescience to wholeness and ultimate freedom.

I began practising with an open mind reflecting on the sparks of light which were interruptedly flashing physically, mentally and intellectually, throughout my *sādhanā*.

It is my *sādhanā* that attracted people towards me for guidance and I unhesitatingly accepted their requests as Godsent and began teaching with what I had learned and experienced through my practices and shared my knowledge with them as per their needs. This sharing of knowledge with my own students opened the horizon of interest in yogic knowledge and experiences.

Slowly but certainly, the word spread from mouth to mouth and the flame of my *sādhanā* took me to various parts of the world. My contacts and communication with the Western intellectual elite helped me in sharing my empirical knowledge, which was flavoured by my life and character.

It was a hard decision for me to make when my friends induced and enthused me to present the essence of my life's experience and self-development that had dawned on me through yoga.

No doubt it was a great challenge but I accepted this task as a springboard and thought it over recollecting on my *sādhanā* from the early days to its present stage. My early life had remained on the bank of total darkness and ignorance but my practice of yoga later made me gradually swim to the other bank of self-knowledge in understanding the purpose of life with its worthiness, loveliness and liveliness.

Q.- If one follows Patañjali's *Yoga Sūtra*, there is a lot there. Then why this new book?

Well many people think that the *Yoga Sūtra* is a highly sophisticated subject because of the name it carries as *sūtra*. *Sūtra* means a thread, a string, a line, axiom or aphorism. So in order to elaborate the depth of the *Yoga Sūtra* for average intellectuals to grasp with comfort I started from the rudimentary state building up gradually towards the subtleties in the subject.

In *Light on Yoga*, naturally I had to deal with the somatic system of the body which is the first element of nature, namely; the *pṛthvī* or earth element or the *annamaya kośa*. Then I wrote *Light on Prāṇāyāma* which is on the vital body, the *āp* element or *prāṇamaya kośa*. Afterwards I brought out the *Tree of Yoga* showing how to confidently face the emotional upheavals of life which arise with the attributes of the world through practice.

No doubt I started first from the body and moved towards the vital organs through the study of the breath. After understanding the breath I presented the emotional aspects through *The Tree of Yoga* which was *tej*, the element of fire and the *manomaya kośa* and from there I thought of presenting the intellectual wisdom, *vāyu* and the *vijñānamaya kośa* through *Light on the Yoga Sūtras of Patañjali*.

Q.- What part of Patañjali's teaching was challenging in your practice and life?

There's no denying that the *Yoga Sūtra* represent a very demanding ethical and spiritual practice, one that challenges even the most highly intellectual wizards. Yet I would like to admit that the *Yoga Sūtra* does not just demand but guides one to begin from the feeble level to the intensive or vehement level. Patañjali instigates, inspires and builds up the faith and courage in the practitioners to proceed from the feeble level to vehement level. Very often the mind, the senses and the body drag the practitioner in different directions and do not help nor co-operate or co-ordinate harmoniously. Hence one thinks that yoga is a highly demanding subject of practice. This thinking is a negative approach in the minds of the practitioners. Another weakness is that very often our mind skips over the parts which are difficult or challenging and we give up our efforts. For instance people see the pictures in *Light on Yoga* and seeing the complicated *āsana* like *Naṭarājāsana* or *Vṛścikāsana* give up. This is no way to go about it. First build the foundation through the simple *āsana* and then proceed towards the complicated ones. In the same way Patañjali advises the *sādhaka* to follow from the basics towards the higher goal of life through yoga. He says that the practice becomes steadfast as one goes on attempting it regularly.[1] Pain in effort stops one from persisting in practice. Pain has to be accepted as a switch towards progress and evolution and for evolution, effort is an essential factor.

The challenge is to practise devotedly with patience in order to unite body, senses and mind as a single unit. Then one does not feel the effort. No doubt my ill-health from birth and want of basic necessities for survival were my real challenges. Even when I started to get better, it took me five to six years to feel the sense of health. But as I practised whatever little I knew it developed in me will-power and determination to practise. I could not tolerate missing practice. I adhered to it. I stuck to the principle of long uninterrupted practice which is said to be the pillar of success. Patañjali says that "Long uninterrupted, alert practice is the firm foundation for restraining the fluctuations."[2] This was relieving the strain of my efforts. There was no condition of time on practice. I knew that effortful, long practice was essential. The triggering of interest arose in me from *Yoga Sūtra* 20 of the *Samādhi Pāda*. It came to me as a guiding hand in persisting in my *sādhanā* with trust and confidence, physical and mental vigour to face failure and dejection. The imprints of memory on my practices whether good or bad, positive or negative made me alter my way of approach in my *sādhanā* and brought me a lot of transformation in my work and thoughts. At the same time I learnt how to remain aloof from the past experiences but watch for what new thoughts would turn out from the practice. This way of watchful re-action built in me strength to write a commentary as per my experiences for pupils of yoga to understand easily the meaning of each *sūtra*.

Q.- It's interesting, *Light on Life* comes when you're eighty-six, right? Do you feel this is a synthesis of your life?

Yes, I think it is so. I brought out my in-depth wisdom that I experienced in practice and the way I lived into *Light on Life*. For example, when *Light on Yoga* received a great response many branded me as a physical yogi. It did not disturb me as I wanted the foundation, the body firm through that treatise.

The body has been divided into five sheaths according to the five elements (earth, water, fire, air and space). These are the *annamaya kośa, prāṇamaya kośa, manomaya kośa, vijñānamaya kośa* and *ānandamaya kośa*. I started *Light on Yoga* enlightening the values of the element of earth, *annamaya kośa*, the foundation of the Self, which has be firm to proceed

1 *tatra sthitau yatnaḥ abhyāsaḥ* (I.13) – practice is the steadfast effort to still these fluctuations.
2 *sa tu dīrghakāla nairantarya satkāra āsevitaḥ dṛḍhabhūmiḥ* (I.14)

towards the Self through the finer aspects of yoga. Naturally I started with this field *(kṣetra)*, the body and presented it through *Light on Yoga* in 1966. But I've gone ahead from there. If people don't read my other books and still brand me as a physical yogi, I have to laugh at their ignorance. I know that it is easy to criticise and attack. But the criticism should be honest, sincere and educative. It appears not. The depth of each *āsana* which I've presented in *Light on Yoga*, I don't think even those who criticise me know about them. Even today to call me a 'physical yogi' is nothing but ignorance in yoga and arrogance in their mentality.

I started for my physical well-being and the first work which came out from me was *Light on Yoga*, based on the anatomical and physiological levels. From then on I proceeded to understand the other sheaths, namely the mental sheath and intellectual sheath. Though I could understand the movement and observation of the mind I was not able to bring the intellectual sheath to dissect and correct the weak points in my practices. I was in doubt and confusion. So I made my intellect see and attend to various parts of my body in order to bring actions for getting the right judgment of each *āsana*.

I was happy that in my *sādhanā* from nowhere the intellectual part began to unveil more and more. Art is from the heart and it is immortal but the practitioners like me are not immortal. Hence I thought I got a chance to share my felt feelings with the readers through *Light on Life*.

Now, let me give you in a nut-shell an overview of this *Light on Life*. It has seven chapters which I have based on the *Yoga Sūtra* of Patañjali, *tasya saptadhā prāntabhumiḥ prajñā* (II.27): These seven states of *prajñā* are: (a) knowledge of the body (*śarīra-prajñā*), (b) knowledge of energy (*prāṇa-prajñā*), (c) study of the mind (*mano-prajñā*), (d) stability and clarity of intelligence (*buddhi-prajñā*), (e) felt experiences (*ānubhavika-prajñā*), (f) re-filtering the experiences into a flavour (*rasātmaka-prajñā*) and (g) the feel of using the Self as a direct instrument in practice as intuitive knowledge (*ātma-prajñā*).

Light on Life expresses the integration in the *sādhaka* from the envelope of the Self to the core of the Self. As these seven states of yogic awareness are inter-related and inter-woven from the envelope of the Self (the skin) to the core of the being, I have acted on it from my heart.

The eight petals of *yoga*, *yama*, *niyama*, *āsana*, *prāṇāyāma*, *pratyāhāra*, *dhāraṇā*, *dhyāna*, and *samādhi* integrate: (a) the body, (b) the organs of perception and action, (c) senses connecting to the vital breath, (d) the vital breath to the mind, (e) mind to the intelligence, (f) intelligence to *ahaṁkāra* (I-form), (g) *ahaṁkāra* to consciousness, and (h) consciousness to the core – the Self.

Circumstances and challenges came to me at the right time and made me reach this state which you all find in this work in my way of living as well as in my *sādhanā*.

No doubt I started yoga with no background of its scientific or philosophical views but my devoted practice poured inside me the yogic knowledge like torrential rain. This made me humble as things which first appeared impossible to reach became possible and led me towards the subtlest of the subtle particles of nature. This helped me to get subdued and the beam of illuminative light began brightening my consciousness.

The first chapter covers a small resume of my early life on how I embraced yoga to come out from the pit of a parasitic, purposeless life leading me towards a purposeful and worthy life. My search and journey began from the physical, material world towards the spiritual world.

The wisdom of Sage Patañjali, being a perfect master has explained both the material as well as the spiritual life, attracted me and gradually made me embrace yoga.

In the second chapter I speak of stability. Stability is of various dimensions. As I explained before with the seven states of awareness (*prajñā*), health also has seven dimensions. These are physical, ethical, emotional, intellectual, conscious, conscientious and divine health.

The five sheaths (*kośa*) of the body are the garments of the Self which create confusion, delusion and a dual state in our body, mind and speech. It is the petals of yoga that lead one from an unsteady body and mind towards a firm and stable body and mind in order to experience equanimity and universality within one and all.

I began to get rid of my ill-health and as I progressed in yoga my understanding of yoga increased. My body became a play ground on life and I dived deep inside the well of the body which to revealed me various aspects of life, namely; health, intellectual clarity, awareness in consciousness and intuitive power, synthesising my thinking powers with the power of actions.

In chapter's three and four, I speak of how energy power and mental power can spread along with stability, vitality, lightness, wisdom and bliss in the *pañcakośa*. They are anatomical (*annamaya*), physiological (*prāṇamaya*), mental (*manomaya*), intellectual (*vijñānamaya*) and bliss bodies (*ānandamaya*). These five *kośa* represent the five elements (earth, water, fire, air and ether) which are supported by five *prāṇa* (*apāna*, *prāṇa*, *samāna*, *udāna*, *vyāna*). *Prāṇa* is energy. It permeates the universe at all levels. It is physical, mental, intellectual, sexual, spiritual and cosmic. Heat, light, gravity, magnetism and electricity are *prāṇa*. *Prāṇa* is the prime mover of all activity.

If *āsana* lead one towards *jñāna mārga*, *prāṇāyāma* takes one towards *bhakti mārga*. We breathe throughout our lives and the breath has the power to create, protect and destroy (what should be destroyed).

The most important and characteristic part of *prāṇāyāma* is that it teaches one to be humble and lessens the un-rhythmic potentialities of the spokes of the emotional wheel, namely, lust, anger, greed, infatuation, pride and envy.

I have emphasised the importance of *āsana* before going into the practice of *prāṇāyāma* as they bring alignment in joints, muscles, breath, mind, intelligence and consciousness. *Āsana* sculpts life from the bone to the brain utilising the intelligence from the skin to the self and from the self towards the skin. *Āsana* taught me and made me to reach the epitome of man by uncovering the physical, ethical, mental, intellectual and spiritual planes.

Then I explain that the body is the child of the seer. Just as the mother protects and helps in educating the children, I showed how *āsana* and *prāṇāyāma* educate one towards evolution in understanding our child (the body) so that it is used as an instrument to earn knowledge and liberation.

As the body is the element of earth (*annamaya kośa*) *āsana* help in building up solidity, shape, firmness, strength to bloom with beauty, charm, grace and intense awareness.

It is my experience that *āsana* do infuse right knowledge with proper understanding (*jñāna*) by synchronising and harmonising motion and action in par with the sensitive intelligence of the self.

These four chapters educate the practitioners to understand the known cognisable elements of nature and take them towards the subtlest of nature (element of touch and sound) to trace the seer to receive itself.

If the readers and practitioners reflect carefully on what I have said, then they realise that the integration *(saṁyama)* of the organs of action, senses of perception and mind takes place between them in their approach to *sādhanā*.

The other three chapters are on wisdom, bliss and the ways of living in emancipation, freedom and beatitude.

Yoga is meant to bring the union of nature *(prakṛti)* with the seer *(puruṣa)* and then the *puruṣa* with the *Viśeṣa Puruṣa* (God). The connecting factors of *prakṛti* and *puruṣa* are breath *(prāṇa)* – the elixir of life, intelligence *(prajñā)* and consciousness *(citta)*.

The intelligence at the core of the Being or the Self sprouts into two branches. One moves towards the heart and the other towards the head. In yoga these two intelligences are made to unite and integrate as a single intelligence which discriminates between the world outside and the world within, transforming *ahaṁkāra* (pride and ego) into *sāttvic* quality as auspicious *asmitā* or *sabīja samādhi*. From here it leads towards *nirbīja samādhi*.

Thus *yoga sādhanā* intermingles the intelligence of the heart with the intellect of the head so that the Inner Supreme Light glows on life with holistic living which is nothing but the "Light on Life".

Life is filled with latent imprints of our previous lives. Yet I have taken *yama* and *niyama* at the end as a part of ethical philosophy to build up right actions and imprints accepting the fruits of past deeds that play their role so that we are guided towards everlasting wisdom (*vedānta*).

If the moral codes of *yama* and *niyama* are one wing, illumination for emancipation is the other wing to evolve in spiritual *sādhanā*. Both wings have to move together. Then freedom and beatitude *(mokṣa* or *mukti)* is felt.

Tapas (burning passion) in the form of *yama* and *niyama* is the hub of yoga for investigation to handle the intelligence *(vijñānamaya kośa)* as this *kośa* is integrated with *(icchā)* will-power but mind depending on memory reacts as per the dictates of memory.

Yoga develops physical prowess *(śakti)*, skilful intelligence *(yukti)* and surrender of oneself to God *(bhakti)* through one's devoted *sādhanā*. Then comes freedom from the aims of life *(puruṣārtha)*, the qualities of nature *(guṇa)* fade out on their own and make the Self to dwell in its exalted state.

This is the light that I have touched in *Light on Life*.

Q.– It's the road map that you have given?

Yes, you are right, it is the road map that I have given for the practitioners to journey from the physical plane towards the spiritual plane.

Challenges do come to the practitioners as many may not know how to proceed and what means to use. I have shown through this book how to face the challenges and gain confidence and faith through their own experiences. I am sure that those who read and re-read develop the capacity to overcome the challenges.

Today nobody wants to work hard and yet each one wants to become a genius. Without inspiration or perspiration nothing can be achieved. No art is impossible to learn if one has will-power. Particularly in learning *āsana*, many misinterpret *āsana* as not requiring any strain *sthira sukham āsanam* (*Y.S.*, II.46). This way of misinterpretation creates doubts and confusions which act as mental pains.

In *Light on Life* I have presented that one has to face and master the subject.

This is, in a way a road map on yoga.

Q.– You grew up in a completely different culture. Now we see a rush to attain a physical, superficial perfection, but is there any possibility to link life towards the spiritual?

If people think that physical perfection is the end in life they are mistaken. Such thoughts are just mental imagination. Their mind is filled with dust *(mala)*.

To be frank with you there is no such thing as spiritual *sādhanā*. We all do various types of *sādhanā* to experience the Self. The Self has no *sādhanā*. This very terminology "Spiritual *Sādhanā*" is itself a misnomer. I'm saying this in order to indicate that Self is pure and it needs no *sādhanā*. The five sheaths which veil the soul or the Self have to be cleansed. As such there is a need for physical purification but that alone is not the end.

Physical fitness or perfection is the first stage to explore the other inner spheres, namely; mind, intelligence and consciousness, to feel the Self. If a temple is ruined no one wants to go there with a divine mind but go as visitors with curiosity. If the bells are ringing and the chanting is on, you are attracted and like to participate listening to the chanting quietly. Similarly when we are doing the *āsana* it is a chanting in action where each and every part and every cell of the body gets purified. Then the joy one gets from such actions turns out as spiritual joy.

Q.– Then how does one deal with the impatience many people suffer from, that it is not happening?

People who complain are not using the five sheaths concurrently in their *sādhanā*. Intellectual inspiration and perspiration is not there in them. Like the measuring scales, the emotional scales sometimes go up and sometimes go down. This is the dust *(mala)* which has to be removed and cleaned as one does not know at what time it gets clouded.

That's why I started with the body, the envelope of the Self. It is a part of the Self as mind and intelligence are parts of the Self. Therefore all the contents of the body put together make up the Self.

I have explained the twenty-four principles of nature, namely; five elements, five atomic qualities of the elements, five organs of action, five senses of perception, cosmic intelligence which form in man as consciousness in which the mind, intelligence and I (the impostor of the Self) cohabit with one facet of *puruṣa* as *jīvātma* or realised individual self, as well as with the immortal, universal *ātman*. Within the body, the *puruṣa* resides and *puruṣa* resides in *Īśvara* or God or Universal Self. All these parts or divisions should merge. This is harmony in action.

Even saints and sages though they are free from ambitions and afflictions go out of their way to help common people like us. They too have physical problems like us. They tolerate and bear their sufferings but we lack that power and I have shown how we can live with them through our yogic practices.

Q.– Now, it has been twelve years. It is estimated that over twenty million people are practising yoga. How do you feel about this?

Yes you are right. I am visiting America after a long time. The practitioners have increased. Though many people do not know me, I gather that they practise my method and when they meet in the meetings, they say that they are practising *Iyengar Yoga*. This makes me laugh though it is embarrassing to hear when I am in their presence.

After a long gap I see their mental attitude has changed which is a good sign in them and for yoga.

– Especially in the Iyengar community, it has grown tremendously... –

Present day people do not know how my way of practice caught the minds of the people then. I used to give public performances thinking that the audiences are my gods. I was presenting for them to witness and join in my classes if it interested them. For me, the audiences are my *ārādhya devatā*. *Ārādhya* means favourable to be worshipped or adored. *Devatā* means God. I stood on the platform as an offering – *ārādhanā* – worship. My presentation was like going to the temple and lighting camphor as worship to God. I was doing the 'camphor work' for these *devatā*. This is what made yoga become popular. I did treat the audiences as gods and in the same way I treated those who came to learn from me as Godsent. Though I was losing my temper with my students yet they all treated me well. *Guru* is considered as Brahma, Vishnu and Maheshvara. As a teacher, *guru* is a trinity of creation, maintenance and destruction. As a teacher these three qualities were required according to the needs of the students. Naturally I had to lose my temper when they were going wrong. I never pampered explicitly if they were good but used to say that they have to work hard to maintain a good standard. I used to generate inspiration as well as showing anger like Maheshvara. If Brahma is the generator, Vishnu is an organiser and Maheshvara is the destroyer of vices. I used to play all these qualities as per the needs of the pupils.

Yoga being the opener of the inner eye (intelligence), these qualities are essentially needed while teaching. Probably my insistence on alignment and balancing the intelligence precisely according to each *āsana* and the effect they obtained enticed the people to practise in such large numbers. I give credit to my pupils who were and are responsible for attracting millions towards yoga.

It has been their appreciation that has encouraged me to present and share my knowledge, from *Light on Yoga* to *Light on Life*.

INTERVIEW WITH THE *TIMES OF INDIA**

Gurujī, thank you very much. Yesterday was very good. Surprisingly I tried what you taught yesterday in my yoga this morning. Since my mother died last year, because of stress I could not move my arm and when I tried your style, surprisingly I could move my arm very easily. Same āsana *I was doing and suddenly my arms started moving.*

Actually I had two things to ask you.

Q.– Everything is perfect. Only one aspect, what is *sthirasukhamāsanam?*

The answer to your question on *sthirasukhamāsanam* is hidden in *Yoga Sūtra,* II.50, wherein Patañjali explains *prāṇāyāma* in detail. There we find out what perfection in *āsana* is; *bāhya abhyantara staṁbha vṛttiḥ deśa kāla saṁkhyābhiḥ paridṛṣṭaḥ dīrgha sūkṣmaḥ.*

What is *staṁbha vṛtti? Staṁbha* means pillars. *Vṛtti* means being, revolving, staying or abiding. Regarding *bāhya abhyantara staṁbha-vṛtti . . .* (II.50), *bāhya* means external *vṛtti, abhyantara (abhyantara* is also called *antara)* means internal *vṛtti.* These three stand for the movement of outbreath, inbreath and restraint on breath. This interpretation fits well on *āsana* also where the external body and the internal body are maintained in the state of stability *(staṁbha vṛtti).* That is *sthira sukham āsanam* (*Y.S.,* II.46).

The inner body covers the organic or the physiological, mental as well as the intellectual bodies. These inner bodies have to be made to remain as stable as the outer body. This is *bāhya-antara-staṁbha-vṛtti* in *āsana. Bāhyendriya* and *antarendriya* should be co-ordinated with equal pressure and stability. This means that they have to co-operate and balance with harmony and concord with each other. This is *sthira sukham āsanam* where stability is maintained between *bahiraṅga, antaraṅga* and *antarātma śarīra. Sthiratā* means stability or *staṁbha-vṛtti* in *āsana.*

---

* This interview with B.K.S. Iyengar was conducted in June 2006, at the Ramāmaṇi Iyengar Memorial Yoga Institute, Pune by a representative of *Times of India,* from Rajasthan.

Q.- But the question is how to attain *sthira āsana?*

It has been explained by Patañjali how the *āsana* should be presented through *prāṇāyāma* techniques. It should be stable without contortion of the anatomical structure without refracting mind, intelligence and consciousness. It means the *āsana* has to be done not just on physical level, but on intellectual level. For this one has to sweat in body as well as sweat intellectually.

Q.- How one can sweat intellectually?

When I say to sweat mentally and intellectually, it means one has to analyse and co-ordinate the thoughts and actions. Patañjali calls this as *pakṣa* and *pratipakṣa bhāvanam*. If *pakṣa* is analysis (*vitarka*) it has to be balanced by reason *(pratipakṣa)*. Analytical thought has to be synthesised exactly in each *āsana*. While performing an *āsana* one has to use the needle of consciousness with its eye, the intelligence for them to synchronise the thinking process with the physical action. While performing an *āsana* if something is in want, the process of thinking may vary between body and mind, mind and intelligence, and intelligence and consciousness. If it is so then is it not *sthira sukham* in *āsana?* In *āsana* one has to use the four pillars of intellect; *vitarka vicāra ānanda asmitārūpa anugamāt samprajnātaḥ* (*Y.S.,* I.17). Unless and until there is no understanding between *vitarka* (analysis) and *vicāra* (synthesis) in *sādhanā, ānanda* (joy) cannot happen. In order to have that joy one has to analyse each *āsana,* then put into action for them to coordinate. When this co-ordinated action takes place then there is joy. This *ānanda* has to arise from the self. Then one experiences stability and joy in the *āsana* as the self is made to get involved in practice.

Q.- Sir, you taught me to experience that, yet when I tried to do this morning, I felt pressure, I mean I was aware of the pressure, so those pressures ...

The answer for you is in your question. Pressure means physical force. Please dp not see pressure on the physical level. See it from the intellectual level. No doubt practitioner has to use his *karmendriya* (organs of action) and *jñānendriya* (senses of perception), which in the modem science are known as motor nerves and sensory nerves. Sensory nerves *(jñānendriya)* are afferent nerves which carry messages to the brain and nerves of action *(karmendriya)* known as efferent nerves, receive messages for right action. While performing the *āsana,* there should be no rubbing or jamming of the motor nerves with the sensory nerves or the sensory nerves with the motor nerves. This is *sthira sukham āsanam* (*Y.S.,* II.46). If the motor nerves are overextended, sensory nerves become dull and numb and if sensory nerves overact, it pressurises the motor nerves. Then the co-ordination between them is lost and as such *sthiratā* and *sukhatā* is lost in *āsana.*

Q.– So when you told me yesterday I felt the energy flowing and when I did *Vīrabhadrāsana* today, I felt pressure especially on one hand, and do you think it was energy flowing?

It is true that you felt the pressure because that hand was bent in the presentation of the *āsana.* Yours was an insensitive practice. If you charged you feel the evenly measured sensation not only in the hands and legs but the entire body. In *Vīrabhadrāsana* I you never looked at your arms where one elbow is straight while the other remains bent. It means that your intelligence on one hand makes it to stretch straight while on the other hand, the same intelligence moves zig-zag or remains insensitive. That insensitivity makes the energy to deviate in its flow in that arm. Attend to the motor nerves on the bent hand. It stretches up straight and connects to the sensory nerves which in turn make the energy to flow vibrating evenly in both the arms. This perfect union between the spindles of action and spindles of the skin spurts the mind to attend there. This sense of feel and action has to be felt evenly in whatever *āsana* you do.

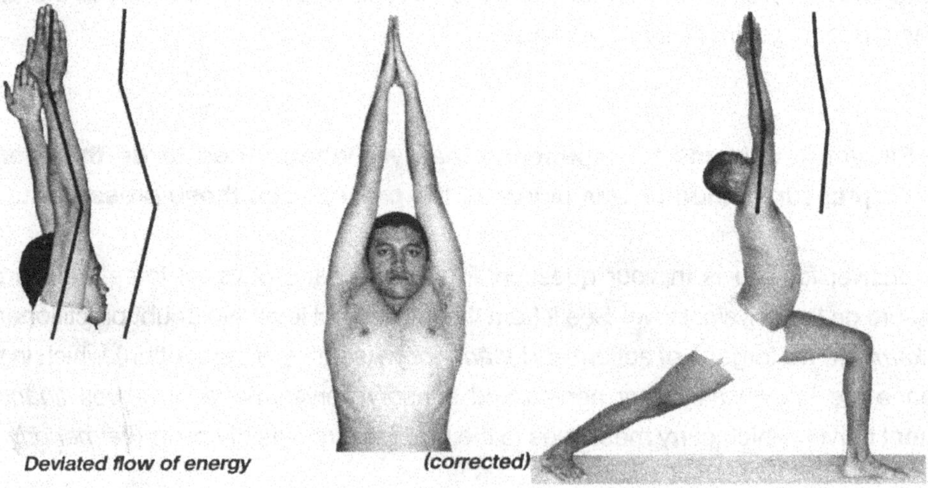

Plate n. 7 – Way of correcting the deviated energy flow in *Vīrabhadrāsana* I

If you do not adjust space between the motor nerves and sensory nerves then reflection of action gets lost. Then it is not at all to be called an *āsana*. *Āsana* has to stimulate the mind and intelligence and to trigger the consciousness. Each *āsana* has its own characteristics and these characteristics have to be brought out by the intellectual analysis and practices for the consciousness to establish itself as absolute.

Q.– When I did *Naukāsana (Paripūṇa Nāvāsana)* I had freedom on one side and on one side I had some kind of hardness like a stone. Do you think that this is blocking of energy?

Hardness means blocking of energy. If you feel hardness then where is *sukhatā* in your *āsana* practice? While doing this *āsana* see which hand is stretched forward and which hand remains dull and inactive. Bring that dull hand to stretch forward from the back of the torso and see what happens. Stretch both sides of the arms identically in the *āsana*. Then see how the hard part becomes soft. This means intellectual discretion is essential while practising the *āsana*.

Q.– This means that when the alignment is complete you don't feel the deviation in body or mind.....

Correct. Alignment is enlightenment. It enlightens the practitioner. This is *ānanda*. When one practises one does not see or use one's intellectual judgement but just does it. Hence many brand *āsana* on a physical level. No one likes to give a thought of even balance on the right and the left sides of the body measuring from the centre to balance evenly. This requires alertness in the intelligence and active functioning from the inner body. Otherwise the *āsana* becomes a stagnated *āsana*. Hence energy and intelligence remain in a stagnated state. For example re-do *Nāvāsana*. See one buttock is firm and short while the other is in the air. Rest both the buttocks on the floor. Now feel whether the one which was in the air is alert and active or is it in a state of stagnation.

See the moment I re-adjusted the *āsana*, your hand and the buttock that were retarding came up and removed the stagnation and retardation of the buttocks and in the arms. Not only did you feel the change in the *āsana* but your energy and intelligence became alert. If you practise this way then you understand the feel of *sthirāsana* and *sukhāsana*.

Q.- It is fantastic. I was never, never guided by experts when I approached them. I have never come across this energy theory and muscle theory together; this is only in Iyengar Yoga. When I read your book initially I could not understand the theory of muscles. But when I talked to you I read your book again .....

Each *āsana* has its own identity which you have to attend and bring to surface. Actually my teaching is on *śakti, yukti and bhakti.* I have *bhakti* (devotion) for the *āsana* and I do it with *yukti* (intellectual skill) using the power of the body as *śakti.* It is to bring three into one in each *āsana.*

Q.- How is *bhakti* related to the *āsana?*

God exists anywhere and everywhere as ether or space. Therefore I feel that God exists for me in the *āsana.* I see *āsana* as my *Iṣṭadevatā,* I treat the *āsana* with respect. My intellectual skill *(yukti)* guides me how I have to develop my physical power *(śakti)* in my *sādhanā.*

Q.- When you started in the 30s, with what *āsana* did you start?

I started only with one or two standing *āsana* and *Sarvāṅgāsana* as I was ill by birth. I was taught to do non-straining *āsana.* I was taught *Trikoṇāsana, Parśvakoṇāsana, Prasārita Padottānāsana, Sarvāṅgāsana* and *Paśchimottānāsana.*

I remember the first lesson where my middle finger tips could not reach my knees. This is because I was lying supine on the bed for years together. So the back had lost its elastic power.

Q.- And when you started *āsana* was your breathing normal?

How can you expect a tubercular man to breathe with ease? It took me years to start *prāṇāyāma* and if you read my book *Light on Prāṇāyāma* you get an idea of how I struggled to learn. My lungs were very tender.

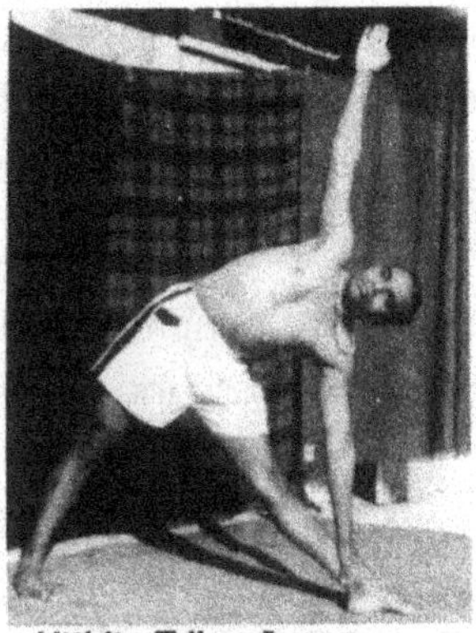

Utthita Trikoṇāsana

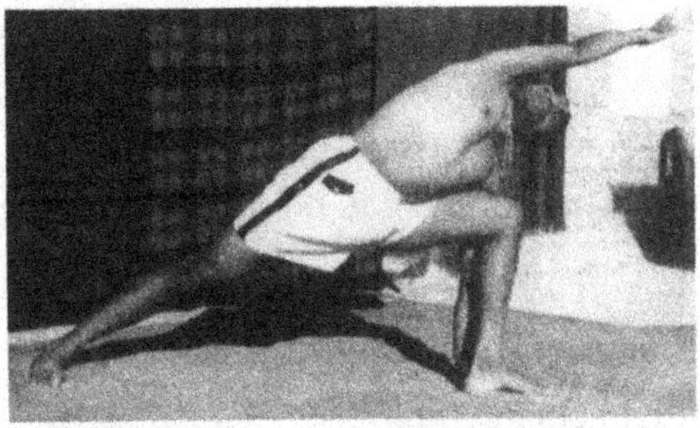

Utthita Parśvakoṇāsana

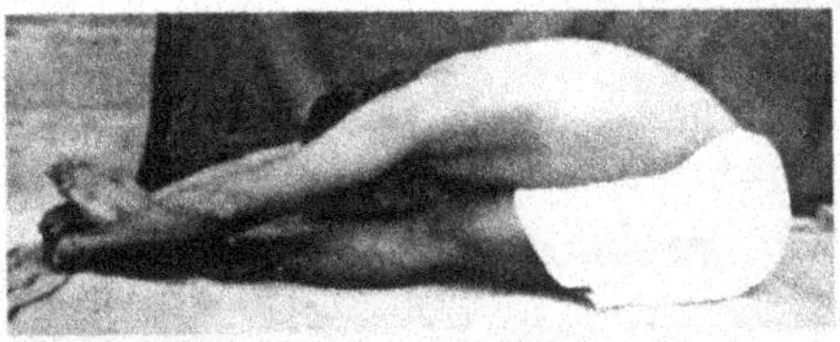

Paśchimottānāsana

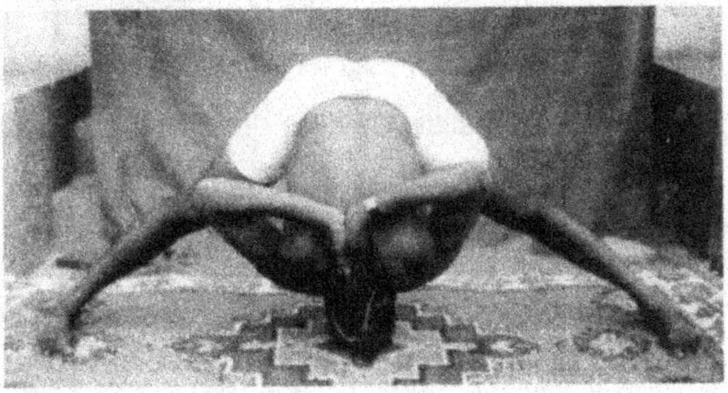

Prasārita Padottānāsana

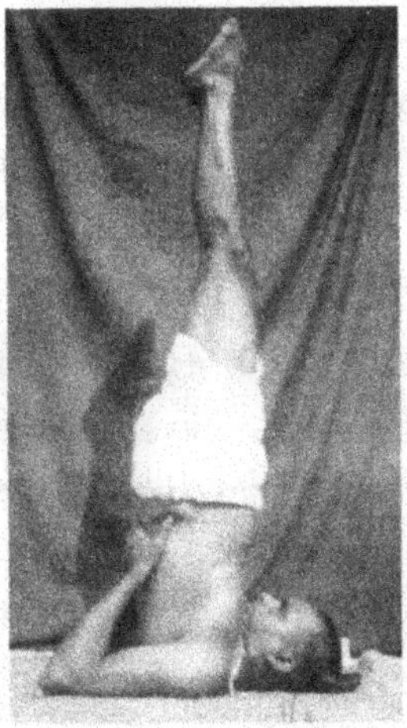

Sālamba Sarvāṅgāsana

Plate n. 8 – *Āsana* for beginners

Q.– Should *śakti, yukti* and *bhakti* be a part of some *āsana* or all?

First, one has to know the anatomical structural position of each *āsana* and one has to balance this anatomical functional action as per the anatomical structure of the body. Both have to co-operate and co-ordinate with equal attention while practising the *āsana*.

Take any book on *āsana* from my library. I will explain to you whether the presentation of *āsana* is adjusted or measured according to the anatomical structure. Presentation of each *āsana* needs correct calculation. *Āsana* is like mathematics where addition, subtraction, multiplication and division have to be worked out accurately.

See my *guru's* book *Yoga Makaranda* and my book *Light on Yoga*. Compare his presentation of *Utthita Trikoṇāsana, Utthita Pārśvakoṇāsana, Śīrṣāsana, Sarvāṅgāsana, Halāsana* to my presentation. See the difference. I have maintained the *āsana* without distortion of the anatomical structure and function.

You said that you are fond of *Naukāsana (Paripūṇa Nāvāsana),* compare my *Gurujī's Naukāsana* to the *Naukāsana* in *Light on Yoga*.[1] Know that I learnt from him. But the progress in presentation is evolution. I evolved from where he left off though he initiated me. I am showing how knowledge progresses as there is no end to knowledge.

I was lucky to work under Dr. V. B. Gokhale, a retired civil surgeon from whom I learnt the functioning of the anatomical body. I utilised his knowledge in my *sādhanā* to do the *āsana* without contorting the structural skeletal body.

Q.- Now I understand that one should feel the flow and energy flowing evenly without interruption or wrong presentation of an *āsana*.

You are correct and it should be observed to spread evenly everywhere. It should not be uneven. Look at the *āsana* again from both the books. Though the *Paripūrṇa Nāvāsana* is the same, it has differed in presentation. Using my guru's thoughts I worked to remove contradiction to a great extent between external presentation and inner action.

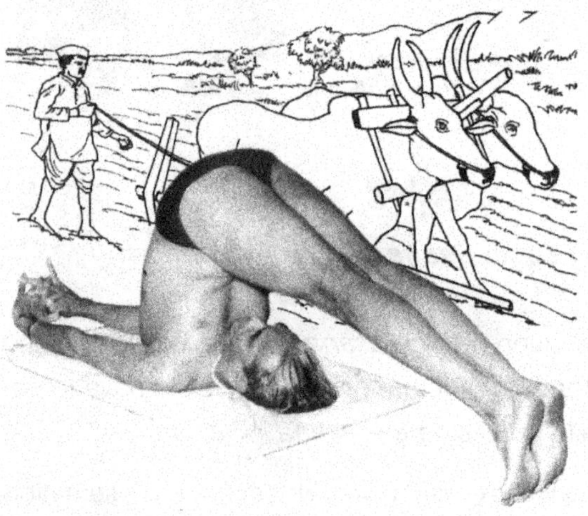

Plate n. 9 – *Halāsana*

Take *Halāsana*. One has to view the *hala* which means a plough. The plough is used to till the land. You must have seen how farmers use it on the field, tilling with bullocks to dig the earth through the plough making the soil soft in order to sort out weeds that grow deep under the earth. Hence in *Halāsana* the two bullocks represent our legs, the arms behind our back represent the farmer gripping the plough and the neck, the actual plough. This way of thinking and doing *Halāsana* makes one to circulate the blood and energy to seep deep in the body for good health and contentment.

Q.- Sir you said just now the flow of energy in the *āsana* should be there and it should be even. When you say there is flow of energy, where is it?

[1] See this comparison in pl. n. 22 & 23, *Aṣṭadaḷa Yogamālā*, vol. 6.

It is hidden. The cosmic flow of energy exists both outside and inside. But many of us do not know that it remains dormant and it has to be tapped through *āsana* and *prāṇāyāma.* Patañjali says that *avidyā* is dormant, attenuated, active-passive, fully active. On this same scale one has to know that energy remains dormant, attenuated or may be active-passive or fully active. Even diseases also roll the same way. They may be dormant; they may be fully active. One says, "Oh! He is suffering from the third stage of cancer". But how is that one cannot trace cancer in the first stage? Only when it is advanced, is it traced. This is what Patañjali means when he uses such words. Due to inactivity in certain parts of the body, the energy remains dormant. He wants it to be tapped from the dormant state so that it flows evenly from the source of the inner body towards the extremities of the body. Core is the being – the life force. So the life has to touch everywhere like the rays of the sun which reach the earth when the sky is clear.

Q.– When I understood your explanation, when I felt the blockage in *Naukāsana,* I should have known by myself that my buttock is slanting to one side. The moment I lifted it in par with the other one, the catch is gone. It means I allowed the energy to move where it was not moving.

Yes! The way you were doing was that one buttock was at a red light and the other moving with green light. While your other parts of the body were moving with green light, only one buttock remained at the red light without any motion or action.

– This is wonderful. Suppose a beginner starts; does he have to put all the pressure or...... –

It is not a question of pressure; it is the question of adjustment and alignment of muscles, joints, mind, energy and intelligence in each *āsana* and in each breath.

Q.– How to see adjustment and alignment?

Learn to see the right side and left side of the body from the centre. Find out which part is dull, whether the dullness is even or casually active at some places or whether one is intelligently active everywhere in the body.

Q.– This is a very difficult differentiation to understand.

It is not difficult to trace the differentiation. It needs attention and a pliable intelligence. You did *Naukāsana*. In that, one buttock was dull and the other active and lively. You did the *āsana* with disparity between one buttock with the other expressing healthy feel on one side and an unhealthy feel on the other side. That's why a teacher is advised who can show these disparities and correct towards parity. The teacher makes his students to adjust and align to feel the vibration that takes place in practice. This feel of vibration is nothing but the flow of energy. This flow of energy triggers the intelligence to be awake and aware.

In your own *Naukāsana* did you find out life in the toes? Were they alive or senseless?

- I feel about fifty percent senseless. -

Then why don't you think of that fifty percent, the senseless part and work it out to get the same sensation? Now spread the skin at the bottom of the feet. Stretching the skin I see the feet raising and feel the energy moving. This is attention in action. Look at the kneecap which is turning out. Turn it in and feel the flow of energy changing its avenue.

- I feel the energy, it is moving in. -

This is a guide for you to know what is storing or sapping of energy. Turning the knee out made the energy to let go. Moving in made one to feel the storing of energy.

- So these are the intricacies in āsana sādhanā. -

Keep in mind Lord Krishna's words *Samatvam yogamuchyate. Samatvam* means equanimity. It means equanimity between the right and left side of the body to bring in par with the centre. So be dynamic in thoughts and action and not mechanical.

Q.- Sir, mechanically and dynamically - that is a very wonderful terminology... what is mechanical?

Mechanical means just a cultivated habit and live in that habit. Practising year in and year out in the same way is mechanical. Whatever the body dictates, the mind follows. But one does not give a thought to it. Doing unintelligently is mechanical. Thinking intellectually and synthesising the action is dynamic action.

See in *Śīrṣāsana*, many keep their legs loose. In that case does the energy move in an ascending or in a descending order? See my book whether you see two legs seperately or two legs as one? Are the legs straight or bent? Is energy sinking or extending in the legs? This is study. This is direct perception.

Q.– Sir, I had a chance to learn Iyengar Yoga from some lady from London and she could not explain these intricacies of your yoga. This is the first time. I was under the impression that Iyengar yoga is because 'you' are teaching it but now I think that this is really a yoga propounded because it has got these characteristics, it is not just the name.

If you pay attention to the median line from the fibre to fibre, muscle to muscle, joint to joint, then a new light may flash in your mind and intelligence to do better and better.

Q.– When you are doing it, how do you see yourself, how do you know....

I just used the word vibration. You have to learn the *āsana* in two ways according to Patañjali. One is through the sight of the eyes and the other through the vibration listening from the ears.

What can be perceived by the eyes has to be corrected by looking and adjusting from the median line. What can be heard and felt but cannot be seen has to be adjusted by intelligence. It took time for me to understand how to use the sight and how to use the ears to feel. For example, *āsana* has to be done by using the eyes and the ears. It is the same with *prāṇāyāma*. Though you close the eyes, you have to learn to see the inner body.

– Sir, would you call it inner awareness? –

Intellectual eye is the inner eye which brings inner awareness. You may call it as attentive awareness, not just awareness. Because attention may remain but awareness may fade out.

Q.– Sir, when I see yoga philosophically and when you say attentive awareness, does it imply that you are the observer.....

You have to be an observer, a spectator and at the same time an actor and a witnesser.

– This is the highest thought of Veda... *–*

That is what it says, *dṛṣṭa ānuśravika viṣaya vitṛṣṇasya vaśīkārasaṁjñā vairāgyam* (Y.S., I.15) and one has to live like this.

– When you do Iyengar Yoga you have to evolve yourself.... –

Yoga is an evolving progressive subject. Whether you do my method of yoga or any other. You have to look, observe, eflect on the re-actions on actions which helps you to develop your intelligence and understanding to re-do the *sādhanā*. This teaches alignment so that you know the wrong and stop repeating it. This way of study leads towards enlightenment.

– But to reflect... –

You have to do the *āsana* and wait for some time to feel at what and where you are engrossed and where and why you are not engrossed. Exchange the attention and awareness on places where you are not attending without losing attention where already it is focused and awareness on the engrossed place of the body. This is reflection and re-reflection *(biṁba – pratibiṁba saṁvāda).*

– You start observing yourself with attention and you become aware –

First I have to observe the *āsana* to become aware of it. We have been gifted with two visions. One is through seeing with physical eyes and the other through intellectual vision. Use both these visions together, both observation and rectification become easy. I made you do *Vīrabhadrāsana* I and asked you to look at your hands. One hand was straight and the other was bent. When you do on your own, do you see like this?

– No –

It means you just did it mechanically without reflecting on it. If you learn to look and do the way I just showed, then you see the deviation in presentation vanishing, electrifying the intelligence. Use your vision this way to look, reflect and re-adjust. This is the way of cultivating knowledge, attention and awareness.

Q.– So when I did *Naukāsana*, you mean to say the foot pointing in *Naukāsana* is not right?

Foot pointing was correct but was there any life force moving? Do it again and see your big toe nail. One is broad and powerful and the other appears non-existing. Observe the length of the big toe nail of the left and of the right, which is long and which is short? Also see one toe is above whereas the other is not. They do not run parallel to each other.

– No. –

Now look at the toes separately and bring them to be active. Is your movement there different or the same?

- Different -

This is observation, and observation induces reflection. This is how you have to see each *āsana* in your practices.

- But these small details are very difficult to....... -

Samatvaṁ yogamucyate (*B.G.*, II.48). Then what is the use of quoting that evenness in yoga?

Q.- I can see with my eyes what you taught me but what about what you cannot see.....

I told you of vibration. Now do your *Vīrabhadrāsana*. You have sensation in one hand and not so much in the other. Stretch and lift the bone up and see whether you made your hands straight and even.

- But I felt the sensation but not the flow of energy...... -

First sensation has to come. Then you have to bring life in the motor nerves. Then energy moves spirally circularising the entire arm. Learning to study the spiral movement of energy by moving each muscle circularly straightens the intellect in the arms.

- Now not only do I feel the energy moving but also the touch of intellect -

Yes. You are right. Feeling of sensation is from the senses of perception and movement of energy from mind and intelligence.

This is how you have to see and know. Study the skin, muscles, joints and bones. Bring them to function in unison. Observe and feel carefully like this again in *Vīrabhadrāsana*.

- This is a miracle, unbelievable. -

Yes. Seeing is believing, this is attentive awareness in the *āsana*. You have to reflect on what you feel. Transfer the soma (body) as psyche (mind).

Q.- I have never seen anywhere this way of p[resenting... this is what people should basically be aware of. You know there are so many yoga centres but I have not heard these words of hidden wisdom.

Yoga is a highly evolved subject, but people don't read or observe or practice.

– I had a chance to visit Bihār school of Yoga which is.... –

Satyānanda is my very good friend. He has seen my practices. We have mutual respect towards each other.

Q.– Earlier when I met that lady in London, I thought it was only a kind of Power Yoga and I was convinced that Iyengar Yoga is only in the name but today since I talked with you for two days I am convinced....

My friend, in my early visits to West in the 1950s and 1960s my system was treated as physical yoga. Even today my method of practice is considered as physical but those who criticise me do not know the hidden secret of each *āsana* which by the grace of God I acquired.

Q.– That's why I want to bring it out because of the feeling I have felt myself when I discussed with you. Sir, your system is wonderful! I am not saying this because of you; it is a wonderful system and every yoga practitioner should be aware of this system...

We talk of knowing the known in order to know the unknown. Actually we don't know the known fully. When we do not know the known things well, how can you think of knowing the unknown? The known dissolves or submerges in the unknown and the unknown alone shines forth. This is the eternal Self. This is what I learnt from my practice of *āsana* which helps me to trace the hidden unknown things.

– And when you start feeling the sensation you take it louder and louder....

That is light. When that light comes you work for the better to reach the best. This is refinement of body, senses, mind and intelligence to move closer to the Self.

– Today I see the secret and my realisation is different. It is a new revelation for me. –

Body has to align with the intelligence and intelligence has to align with the body and that is actually *sthira sukham āsanam (Y.S.,* II.46).

When I use the word *sukha* – it connects to the intelligence, not to the body. *Sukha* is connected to the intelligence and *sthira* to the body. This is *staṁbha-vṛtti* in body, mind and intelligence. This stability is the sign of a perfect *āsana.*

Q.– Now I have felt more *sthira* in myself when you corrected me whereas I was shaking before. So the earlier meaning of *sthira sukham* was...

Patañjali has defined the characteristic of an *āsana* that whatever *āsana* has to be done, it has to be done with stability and comfort.

– Yes wonderful... –

When people talk of performing the *āsana* according to one's comfort, one has to achieve to reach that comfort. Real comfort can only be experienced when the *āsana* has been fully achieved.

Patañjali says, *prayatnaśaithilya,* which means that the effort has to reach that *sthira sukham,* when that *sthira sukham* is reached, that effort becomes effortless. It means that *āsana* is mastered.

Q.– Now sir, when you say you have talked about muscles – this muscle intelligence, bone intelligence, now when I come to think of the internal body, say my nervous system, say my heart.....

I have already told you to start from what you perceive. After right perspective action, you conceive. After conceiving all points, deliver them in each *āsana* and in each breath in *prāṇāyāma.* Move the intelligence of the head towards the intelligence of the heart and from the intelligence of the heart, perform the *āsana.* Deliver the *āsana* from the intelligence of the heart which is nothing but the Self.

Q.– Sir, I have understood you but the question is, suppose I have to exercise my liver or if I have to exercise my stomach, then how do I.....Do you treat them as muscles or differently...?

No, no, they are organs. They belong to *prāṇamaya kośa.* Muscles are skeletal body. Muscles are just like the construction materials of a house. Body is a house. It has to be constructed and plastered to get a fine finish.

Do your *Naukāsana.* Now roll the skin of the body inwards attend to the spine to remain straight as needed in the *āsana* and see what happens to the liver or stomach. They act as the skeletal body adjusts.

- Now I can see a very big difference. -

This is learning. If you do not experience the purpose of *Naukāsana*, is it your fault or the fault of yoga?

Q.- So, in this *Naukāsana* as you say if I raise my legs to 60 degrees my intestines work, when I raise the legs to 30 degrees the liver and pancreas work, so do I have to know all these?

Without knowing the functions of the skeletal body, you cannot make use of the organic body. I have just shown you in *Naukāsana* that as the legs turn in the energy also turns in which you do not observe or attend to.

Now when the legs are at thirty degrees the liver stretches outwards. Roll the skin, flesh and bone inwards keeping the body at thirty degrees. Now observe whether the liver is working or not?

- Yes. -

Therefore you have to use your intelligence as to how to make use of the structural body for the organic body to function well.

Q.- Time is constraint now. How to adjust yoga?

Well, a minimum of thirty minutes a day has to be spent. Don't say that people have no time. They can gossip on the road. You mean to say you can waste time with your friend. You can sit around order toast which takes fifteen minutes to come. You waste that thirty minutes and you say you don't have fifteen or thirty minutes to spare for yoga?

Q.- In those thirty minutes what can you do?

I have given the sequence of *āsana* in lots of books according to the timings.

Q.- Sir, now there is a lot of talk about *sūkṣma* and *sthūla*....

My friend, yesterday I explained to you *sūkṣma prāṇāyāma – dīrgha prāṇāyāma*. If you act from the soul, it is *sūkṣma*. If you act from the peripheral mind and body, it is *sthūla*. It is so simple.

– It is very simple, I agree, but how do I act? –

Do *Naukāsana* again. Just one *āsana* I am guiding you. Where is the mind or the soul? Move the mind or the soul close to the legs. What do you experience? You forgot the body and brought the self closer to the legs. This is the wholeness of the *āsana*.

Q.– If you chant a *mantra* during the *āsana*, does it have positive or negative effect?

My friend, when you speak of concentration and meditation, how can you do two things at the same time? Can you smoke and meditate together? Such things are going on. I like to tell you that Duryodhana and Dharmarāja were there at the same time. Duryodhana was a very powerful and a dexterous man and his cousin Yudhiṣṭhira (Dharmarāja) who was honest to the core had to suffer a great deal. Duryodhana followed the wrong and his wrong was superseding the right. It took thirteen years for Yudhiṣṭhira to relinquish Duryodhana to become the King. For an honest man like Yudhiṣṭhira it took so much time. So it is the same with right method of practice of yoga. Even in the yogic field you may find Duryodhana and Dharmarāja.

Q.– I am coming to a very, very important point. People are getting diplomas and becoming yoga teachers. So my first question is can yoga be harmful if not done properly?

Yoga needs a matured head and emotional heart to teach. It takes years of practice to get maturity. Today yoga is treated like ready-made food. Hence I am not happy where diplomas are given in short courses which may in the long run affect those who learn from such diploma holders. Though ill effects of wrong *āsana* may be felt after a long time, the ill effects of wrong *prāṇāyāma* will be felt soon.

Q.– How do I know if I am doing *prāṇāyāma* correctly?

Your practice of *prāṇāyāma* is wrong if you get irritated every now and then. First sign of wrong *prāṇāyāma* is irritability, and restlessness leading towards intolerance. If somebody does wrong instead of guiding, if one flares up at once, then it is an indication that the nerves are disturbed and mind does not tolerate. First disturbance comes in the nerves. *Āsana* may take a longer time to affect the body and the mind. Right practice of *prāṇāyāma* soothes the nerves and quietens the mind

Q.– When you taught me *prāṇāyāma* I felt quiet instantly, it's wonderful. When you do *Kapālabhāti*...

Bhastrikā, Kapālabhāti have nothing to do except for clearing the nostrils.

– So it can be done... –

Just for a few minutes. They are not basic *prāṇāyāma*.

In order to learn some of the complicated *āsana* such as *Śīrṣāsana, Sarvāṅgāsana, Matsyendrāsana,* one has to start with simple *āsana* as all cannot do the above *āsana* at once. Similarly subtle *prāṇāyāma* like *Nāḍī Śodhana* cannot be done at once. One has to learn *Ujjāyī, Viloma prāṇāyāma* before *Nāḍī Śodhana prāṇāyāma*.

Q.– Sir, when is it told breathing by the mouth and exhaling through your nose...

In traditional yogic books *prāṇāyāma* is done by mouth only in *Śitali* and *Śitkārī*. It is suggested to do this in the summer months because it keeps one's breath cool.

Q.– And what about when you make use of *mudrā*...

Mudrā are meant to connect the mind with the single thought. Don't tell me that *jñāna mudrā* affects concentration. If so the world would have only intelligent people. *Mudrā* is a seal-support in order to see that my mind does not get disturbed. It comes in the *āsana* also.

Q.– What is *dhyāna?*

Patañjali says, *ekatānatā dhyānam. Dhyāna* is uninterrupted attentive awareness or one single flow of thought. As oil is poured from one vessel to the other it runs without any disturbance, so *dhyāna* is an uninterrupted attentive awareness. We learn this in *āsana* also. When the *āsana* and you become one, it is meditation in *āsana.* To experience this union, you have to become a *bhaktan* or a devotee.

Thank you.

- Hopefully people of Rajasthan and Delhi will be highly benefited. -

Definitely.

YOUTH'S INQUISITIVE INTEREST IN YOGA*

First of all I have to thank you all for your adorations on me though I don't think I am worthy to receive this.

For seventy years I have spoken on yoga. My brain has reached a state of blankness and I find it hard to speak on the subject, which is dry and difficult to understand and follow.

I am open today for youngsters. Consider me as a senior sādhaka *and not as a master of yoga. The only difference between you and me is that if you are raw or medium students, I am a senior-most student. Being a senior most-student, I may be able to guide the youths like you who can keep your body and mind in a balance and concordant state through yoga. Our minds have constructive aspects as well as destructive aspects. You have to study the destructive thoughts first in order to change these into constructive thoughts to build up confidence in yourselves to move towards the finer points in the field of yoga as well as nature to experience the absolute state of consciousness without any deviation.*

Though I am nearing ninety, I am numerically nine years old. I don't think I can explain this thought to you in a mature way as God has made me young. Considering myself young, I am with you to know how a youth's mind thinks on yoga.

Youths are not only inquisitive but courageous enough to question me. Grown ups have complexes of being superior or inferior. Secondly, as the grown ups don't want to expose themselves I ask you as youngsters on how you feel about practising yoga. Your minds are not tainted and you may ask questions which may surprise all of us. Therefore I have taken the responsibility to answer your queries instead of exposing myself as an orator or a master! I thought that I should deal with you as your minds are fresh and at the same time it may help me to educate myself through your questions. I stand to answer your questions and I hope my replies will create interest in you all.

---

* These questions were asked of B.K.S. Iyengar on the occasion of the celebration the Ramāmaṇi Iyengar Memorial Yoga Institute, Annual Day celebrations, January 2008.

Q.- While practising *āsana*, we deal with the muscles, joints and skin. The practice is then followed by breath. How and where does one feel the touch of the breath in *āsana* since we breathe through the nose? Can you also tell us about the feel of the mind, intelligence and the consciousness and how to experience those in the *āsana*?

It is true that we just do or stay in *āsana* and give up when they are painful. Yoga is a spiritual or *ādhyātmic* subject. If we give up or practise it with interruptions, how can we understand the subject or go closer to it? The question is that many of you are unstable to practise any subject seriously.

Each one has to begin the subject from the foundation to understand the principles of nature (body) and the *ātman* (soul) and how they work in co-ordination within himself. The subject appears difficult as we have to journey from the external body (the envelope) towards the contents of the internal body.

First of all we should know the principles of nature or *prakṛti*. Our bodies are made of five *bhūta* or elements, namely, earth, fire, water, air and space.[1] The atomic qualities of these five elements are odour, taste, form, touch and space or sound. The first principle of nature is *mahat* (cosmic consciousness). This becomes individual consciousness, as *citta* (mind) in each one of us. We have five organs of action, five senses of perception, mind, intelligence and ego *(ahaṁkāra)*. Besides these, nature has been provided with the characteristics of *triguṇa (tamas, rajas, sattva)* which represent inertia, vibrancy and goodness as well as virtue.

We have *pañcakośa* (sheaths) corresponding to the five elements, anatomical, physiological or vital organs, mental, intellectual and spiritual. In the same way we have *pañcavāyu; apāna, prāṇa, samāna, udāna, vyāna* concurrent to the five elements. The five organs of action are hands, legs, mouth and generative and excretory organs, and the five senses of perception are eyes, ears, nose, tongue and skin.

While practising the *āsana* you have to activate all these principles of nature hidden in the body (microcosm) to function according to their connections with the elements to bring harmony and balance in all the principles of nature (macrocosm), co-mingling the power of the Self to get the right impression in each *āsana*. The principles of nature have to feel the presence of the *ātman* everywhere in the body in each *āsana*. This is *sthira sukham āsanam* (*Y. S.*, II.46).

---

[1] See *Aṣṭadala Yogamālā*, vol.2, pp. 274-287.

After understanding the connection between nature and soul, there are two ways of practising the *āsana*. One is to go compartmentally step by step. complementing and supplementing the skeletal sheath *(annamaya kośa)*, the physiological sheath *(prāṇamaya kośa)*, the mental sheath *(manomaya kośa)*, the intellectual sheath *(vijñānamaya kośa)* and the abode of the Self or the core of the being *(ānandamaya kośa)*.

You cannot jump to the final point of yoga without undertaking to practise what is perceptible to the senses of perception. You have to learn first what you can perceive from the five senses of perception and five organs of action. These act as external senses *(bahiraṅga)* for acquiring knowledge. The initial stage of learning for you is to understand the muscles, joints and skin *(āraṁbhāvasthā)*. Then you have to bring your mind to conceive or learn how they should function while doing the *āsana*. To start anything, you have to begin with the perceptible things as they are easy to understand through the muscles, joints and skin because they are closer to your minds.

Yoga has eight aspects, namely, *yama, niyama, āsana, prāṇāyāma, pratyāhāra, dhāraṇā, dhyāna* and *samādhi*. Some are exhibitive and explicit while others are inhibitive and implicit.

The explicit part of yoga is *āsana* and *prāṇāyāma*. The other parts of yoga are implicit while *yama* and *niyama* are the ways which show what to do and what not to do ethically and morally. *Āsana* and *prāṇāyāma* are the only two parts or petals which can be practised by bringing the attention on the senses of perception and action on each and every part compartmentally or wholly. Just as a mason keeps the bricks one above the other in line without deviation, you have to learn to place hundreds of joints and hundreds of muscles in concord with each other in each *āsana*. Therefore my suggestion is to begin your practice through your senses of perception. You have to study and balance each and every joint, bone, muscle as if each of them is a single brick standing on its own. Create action in each *āsana* without deviating the positions of the joints or the muscles.

The first thing to learn is, "Can I maintain the *āsana* without disturbing the anatomical structure?" The length of the inner and the outer muscles, the space between the ankle and the knee, knee and hip, side ribs, front ribs and skin have to be adjusted by balancing them evenly. While doing the *āsana* there should be a thorough communication between the organs of action and the senses of perception. Performance of the *āsana* is like the mother understanding you and you understanding the mother, which helps one in maintaining lovely and lively feeling between you and the mother. I am making you to understand to maintain such connections while performing the *āsana*. The skin which is the sense of knowledge must be studied and understood while doing the *āsana*. You have to see how the sensory nerves react with the actions of the motor nerves without jamming and jarring each other.

There are vibrations felt in each and every *āsana* at certain places of the body whereas at certain places they are not felt. As such, the intention in presenting the *āsana* is to watch and balance the vibrations to be felt evenly on both sides and then to extend these vibrations to reach further depth through further action in extension and expansion. When the thought of extending and expanding the vibrations strikes the mind, you begin to act surprisingly with an attentive mind. Till then, the mind does not really start to function and therefore the senses of perception try to adjust on themselves without the involvement of the mind. When there is a harmonious communication between the sensory nerves and motor nerves, then the mind gets the message but fails to grasp the message. At this time it calls its trusted friend, the intelligence to guide to act as a bridge between the fibres of the muscles and the fibres of the skin to conceive the action and reaction from each other. The intelligence tries to balance these two. Once you work from the intelligence; the mind, the organs of action and senses of perception listen and surrender to the dictates of the intelligence and follow. At this point, the compartmental practice begins to fade out and wholeness in practice sets in.

Now let me tell you something about the breath. Today, *prāṇāyāma* courses are taught anywhere and everywhere. If you carefully observe the contact of the breath in different *āsana*, you observe that the breath touches different parts in different *āsana*. Even if you take a deep in-breath or a deep out-breath, the touch of each breath in the torso differs each time and will not be the same. Each breath touches sometimes the inner parts and at other times the outer parts or the middle parts. When a deep inhalation or a deep exhalation is taken, you like to be in touch only with that part where the breath touches and neglect the other parts allowing these areas to remain dry and senseless. If the land is dry, it cracks. The same thing happens here: wherever the breath touches, that part gets nourished and the non-attended parts remain undernourished. It means there is progression on one side and regression on the other. While doing the *āsana* learn to observe that the breath taken in or out touches the torso evenly.

For example, in *Trikoṇāsana*, the breath touches the body at certain places, while in *Utthita Pārśvakoṇāsana* it touches at some other places. It is the same in *Vīrabhadrāsana* I. When you do *Trikoṇāsana* on the right side, the inner part of the right side of the lung absorbs the breath as it braces that part. The left side of the lung feels the breath as it touches the peripheral top part, though that side shows greater expansion and expression. Therefore while doing the *āsana* on the right, try to fill the breath on the inner part of the left side of the chest with attention and also attend to fill the breath on the peripheral part of the right side. This is balancing of the breath evenly between the right and the left sides of the trunk. This way follow the process of breath in all the *āsana*. If you think and act in this manner, then I am sure you learn to sustain deep breath in each *āsana* without strain. I don't want you to draw the breath by force deeply. Learn to grasp the touch of breath in each *āsana* and amalgamate and try your best so that the breath braces evenly each and every part of the torso.

Though *Śīrṣāsana* and *Sarvāṅgāsana* are inverted *āsana*, the touch of breath is different in *Śīrṣāsana* to that of *Sarvāṅgāsana*. Though *Ūrdhva Dhanurāsana* and *Viparīta Daṇḍāsana* are both back bends the movements of breath vary. In *Jānu Śīrṣāsana* the touch of breath is felt only on the side where the leg is kept straight. Therefore each of you have to study the feel of touch of breath in standing *āsana*, sitting *āsana*, balancing *āsana*, twisting *āsana* or back-bending *āsana*. Each *āsana* opens certain areas of the torso for the breath to occupy. By this you learn various areas of the torso through the touch of breath. You may gauge now the reason, why all yoga texts including Patañjali, insist that *prāṇāyāma* has to be practised only after gaining some perfection in *āsana*.

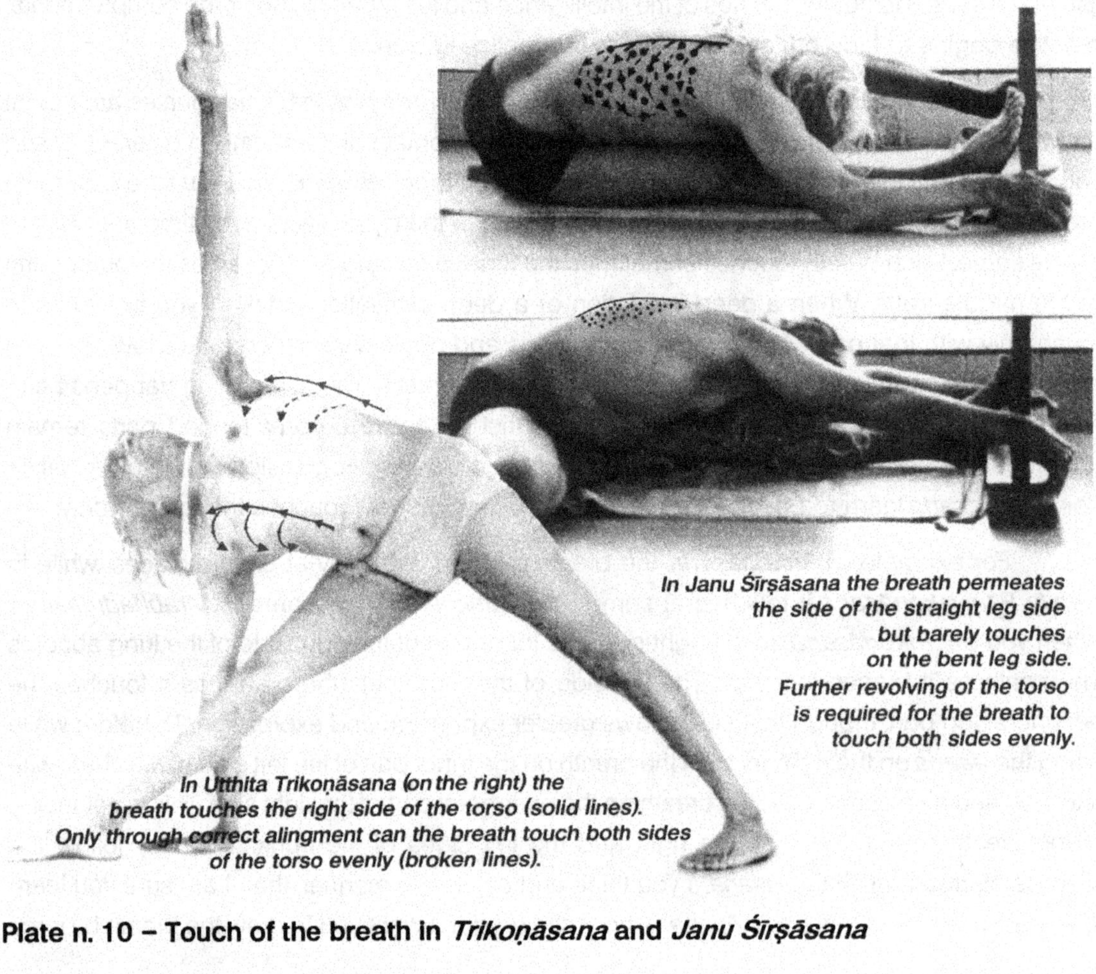

In Janu Śīrṣāsana the breath permeates the side of the straight leg side but barely touches on the bent leg side. Further revolving of the torso is required for the breath to touch both sides evenly.
In Utthita Trikoṇāsana (on the right) the breath touches the right side of the torso (solid lines). Only through correct alingment can the breath touch both sides of the torso evenly (broken lines).

Plate n. 10 – Touch of the breath in *Trikoṇāsana* and *Janu Śīrṣāsana*

When you know that breath touches different areas in different *āsana* then you like to work out to feel the touch of breath evenly and wholly in the entire torso before you begin *prāṇāyāma*.

Don't mistake deep breath with *prāṇāyāma*. Deep breath is different from *prāṇāyāmic* breath. Deep breath is known as *śvāsāyāma*. In the in-breath, you keep the throat half open so that you may not gulp the air. You create a dyke at the throat to take the in-breath in a sustained way wherein the mind gets completely involved in drawing the senses of perception inwards. This is the beauty of studying how the breath has to be followed in the *āsana* before you adopt the deep breathing in them. Each and every teacher insists on deep inhalation and deep exhalation in the *āsana*. Many oscillate the trunk forward in inhalation and backwards in exhalation. But I am suggesting to do deep inhalation or deep exhalation after maintaining the body in an undisturbed position in the *āsana*. Then the deep breaths in each *āsana* have a tremendous effect in learning *prāṇāyāma*.

Q.- Can you tell us now about the feel of the mind, the consciousness and the intellect?

Consciousness usually remains in a state of dormancy. It's the mind that dominates. As the mind dominates, intelligence and consciousness get compressed and take back-seats and remain in latent and dormant states. In order to awaken the sheaths of the body you have to start from the seat of the spiritual heart, *hṛdaye cittasaṁvit* (*Y.S.*, III.35). The seat of the consciousness is *hṛdaya* (the seat of the Soul). Measure or learn to feel the expansiveness of the body and mind in *Trikoṇāsana*, *Parśvakoṇāsana* or any other *āsana* from the centre of the heart and not from the brain as yoga is a stabilising subject of head and heart.

While doing the *āsana* do not feed the intellect of the brain but make it descend to the seat of the consciousness at the heart so that the consciousness with its intelligence guides the brain to use its brilliance for even balance and firmness from end to end in the body.

Unfortunately, we do the opposite. We use the brain in the *sādhanā* and keep the intelligence of the consciousness empty whereas the *āsana sādhanā* has to be done with the fullness of the consciousness by making the brain quiet as a receiving instrument to act when things go wrong in the body.

No doubt, you have to start to work with the brain, studying compartmentally whether the foot is straight or not, the toe is in line with the metatarsal or not, the foot is in line with the heel or not, and so on. These are all essential parts needing to be observed with the help of the brain. The moment you reach the final state of the *āsana*, then you have to forget the brain and begin to study from the intelligence of the consciousness. This controls the mind as well as aggressive stretches in the body.

As one starts with the skeletal body *(annamaya kośa),* which is *bahiraṅga,* the *āsana* is called *bahiraṅga sādhanā.* But *āsana* is not really an external quest as the term conveys. It is meant to bring the *bahiraṅga* (external body) closer to the *antaraṅga* (inner body), the *prāṇamaya kośa, manomaya kośa* and *vijñānamaya kośa.* Even after years of practice many of you continue *āsana* or *prāṇāyāma* with the *annamaya kośa* but do not move inwards to come in contact with the interior *kośa.* When we sprinkle water on a hot oven, the moment it is sprinkled on it the oven absorbs the water. Similarly, the *bāhya śarīra* should be absorbed towards the inner body through *tejas tattva,* the mind. Through the mind you have to reach the other two finer and subtler elements; *vāyu* and *ākāśa. Pṛthvi* and *āp* are the gross elements. They are the *annamaya* and *prāṇamaya kośa.* Elements of *vāyu* and *ākāśa* are *vijñānamaya* and *ānandamaya kośa.* In between is the *tejas tattva* which is the mind and the mind has to balance the external body *(bahiraṅga śarīra)* as well as the inner body *(antaraṅga śarīra)* so that without one overstretching or understretching, the five *kośa* and the five *bhūta* reach the *antarātman* or *antaryāmin.* That's how one has to learn to perform the *āsana* for the mind to balance evenly *pṛthvī* and *āp* on one side and *vāyu* and *ākāśa* on the other. If one practises *āsana* this way, then the flow of *prāṇa* not only do not disturb the nervous system but taps the *prajñā* to move with its flow.

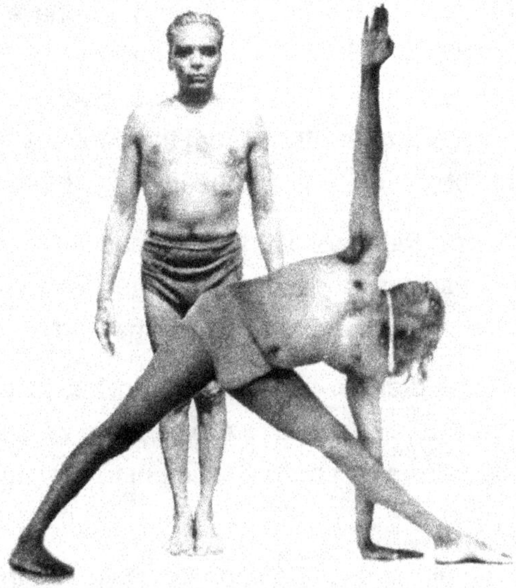

Plate n. 11 – Torso in *Tāḍāsana* and *Trikoṇāsana*

For example, take the simple *āsana* – *Tāḍāsana.* How many of you know that the metatarsal of one foot moves out and the other moves in? The one which moves in, *prāṇa* flows inwards and where the foot moves out, the *prāṇa* moves out.

Similarly, take *Trikoṇāsana.* Whichever side you work with, the outer ankle goes out like an abscess but you don't bring that in line towards the inner ankle. Question yourself, "How come in this *āsana* it goes outside?" This way when you start studying and adjusting the *āsana,* then you bring the mind to that part to act and adjust as it should be. In order to adjust you need intelligence. In order to make the intelligence work, the *prāṇa* (energy) has to present itself to act. In this *āsana*, as the ankle on the right side drops out, the energy spills out. Therefore it is for you to look and adjust the outer ankle to reverse the energy to move inwards. For this, the intelligence alone has to be brought to attention to guide and reverse the process of energy by re-working on the ankle. This is how the *āsana* have to be done and mastered.

Q.– Regarding *guṇa*, how can one increase the *sattva guṇa*?

The body is *tāmasic*, mind is *rājasic* and self is *sāttvic*. If you do the *āsana* from the seat of the consciousness you control the *rajoguṇa* and *tamoguṇa*. Brain is *rajas*. The consciousness at the heart is pure, and hence *sattva guṇa* is there but dormant. Brain calculates and becomes the seat of pride and pride is *rājasic*. Hence, you as yoga practitioners have to use your intelligence as the centre for measuring the accuracy of the *āsana* and the brain for motion and action. The brain may create confusion and doubt while the intelligence of the consciousness removes confusion and replaces it with the light of knowledge. As the seat of consciousness is the heart *(hṛdaye cittasaṁvit)*, awaken the consciousness and make it flow through the entire body so that the hidden light of wisdom surfaces.

As a beginner you have to perceive through your senses and mind to adjust the *āsana*. If the senses of perception reach the ultimate level of adjustment, then start observing from the intelligence of the consciousness to conceive the right position of the *āsana* and move the muscles or joints accordingly. This way, reach the final stage in the *āsana* without oscillation but with stability and confidence.

As I said earlier the last two elements namely, *vāyu* and *ākāśa* belong to *vijñānamaya kośa* or the brain and *ānandamaya kośa*, the consciousness. The quality of intellect of the brain is to be attentive and the quality of the intelligence of the consciousness is to be aware from the core to its frontier *(tatra pratyaya ekatānatā dhyānam Y.S.,* III.2). This indicates that *dhāraṇā* and *dhyāna* have to be followed in the presentation of an *āsana*. *Dhāraṇā* is to look at each and every part to focalise. After looking at each and every part of the body with its contents in the *āsana*, bring the intellect of the head to extend vertically and the intelligence of the consciousness to expand horizontally. In this equi-state of extension and expansion there is zero gravity. As you draw a circle from its central point the centre of the consciousness, the seat of the heart acts as the central point from where you have to move measuring attention and awareness without any difference. This makes you understand *ākāśa* or the space between the self to the skin. Ether has a power to expand and contract. Naturally you have to bring the intelligence of the head or the brain and the intelligence of the consciousness to see each and every *āsana* where you have to extend, expand and where you like to contract to get firmness and elegance in *āsana*.

For example when you present *Trikoṇāsana* on the right side observe the left foot, which appears shorter than the right. The bottom skin on the left foot shrinks which makes the foot to float in the air. This means consciousness has shrunk in that foot. Know that it is not the body that has shrunk but the consciousness has narrowed which makes the limb appear narrow. While on the right side, the intelligence is alert and as such you try to stretch the bottom skin of the foot which makes that foot appear longer. But you don't look at the other foot because you do not use your experimental intelligence *(vijñāna)* on the other foot. Therefore the consciousness goes to dormancy in that foot because the experimental intelligence is made dormant. See to what length the right foot extends and touches the floor in *Trikoṇāsana* and with what length the left foot touches the floor. You feel and realise that expansion is in the front foot, while the rear foot is in contraction. This means the element of ether is contracted. Hence spread the left leg away from the right until it feels the firmness of the earth element. This way if you learn to observe, correct and maintain, you have not only learnt *Trikoṇāsana* but live in the *āsana* with experiential wisdom. When you begin to see, feel and adjust then *sattva guṇa* sets in on its own in the legs. The moment you spread the constricted left foot by extending the leg, your mind at once becomes attentive on the left side.

You can easily perceive your right foot and correct it from the senses of perception but you do not perceive the left foot from the senses. As such you have to bring the mind to observe for corrections and adjustments. You have to open and broaden the arch of the left foot through mental conception. When you do this, it means that *sattva guṇa* has entered that foot for it to become long. This is how you have to learn to bring the *sattva guṇa* in the *āsana*. Wherever the consciousness is narrow remember that your practice is of *tamoguṇa* on that side. It may appear to be illuminative outside but that is a partial stretch because of partial attention. The moment you open the constricted side, *rajoguṇa* surfaces and you begin to feel the space on the right side becoming narrow to give room for the left foot to spread out to create space. This is the art of balancing the *guṇa* to reach the *sattva* state, or the principle of being in the *āsana*.

Q.– How does one deal with the esoteric anatomy and physiology?

I think I have already covered this. Esoteric anatomy conveys that it is intended only for a small number of people who show interest in it. In short it means going inwards to know the body fully from the skin to the Self. Though both anatomy and physiology are biological, anatomy happens on its own while physiology is to know and understand the functions of the living organisms. *Āsana* works not only on the structural body but also works on balancing the living organisms to function accurately.

As you begin to learn to balance the skeletal body to remain in their positions while doing the *āsana*, you also have to learn to adjust the physiological body without creating any difference between anatomy and physiology as if they are one though they appear as different subjects outwardly. For example in *Tāḍāsana* you turn your foot slightly out, the liver dips down. Bring your foot inwards; you feel the adjustment at the bottom of the liver and diaphragm. This is how they are co-related. Suppose you have skeletally adjusted your limbs in *Trikoṇāsana*, you have to keep the front sternum in line with the navel as well as the corners of your legs in line with the chest and the navel. If any part of *Trikoṇāsana* slightly bulges in or out, you feel the imbalance taking place in the poistion of the organs.

Again, how many of you observe the pelvic girdle while doing *Trikoṇāsana* on the right side? Here the right side of the pelvis remains in line with the right side while it bulges like a boil on the left side, whereas it should be in line with the trunk. This understanding guides you how the skeletal body must be placed in the *āsana*. If you refine adjustments in the anatomical body (the skeleto-muscular body) the physiological body co-operates while performing the *āsana*. In turn, they work effectively on nervous and glandular systems. The process of penetrating inwards makes us to go from the grossest sheath towards the subtlest sheath of the body. Hence, the energy is made to reach the subtlest as well as the remote areas of the body.

That is why yoga is an esoteric subject. In *Trikoṇāsana* on if the pelvic girdle of the left bulges up and out , this means you have place the the skeletal body wrongly. Distance is wrong as the knees and ankles do not run parallel to each other. If the legs are closer the lower leg of the left will be longer and the thigh appears short. You have to know the space required on the left side of the pelvic girdle when you are doing this *āsana* on the right side. Learn to lengthen the space between the legs, you maintain even weight on both legs. While doing *Trikoṇāsana* nature works on its own on the right leg, while you have to bring the intelligence of the *puruṣa* to work on the left leg for adjustments and corrections as nature does not work on the left side. Similarly, the same things happen when you change the *āsana* on the left side. This is how you have to learn when and where to use the intelligence of *prakṛti* and when and where to use the intelligence of *puruṣa*. If these two powers act in co-ordination there is unity between *prakṛti* and *puruṣa*. *Prakṛti* remains stable *(sthira)* and *puruṣa* in bliss *(sukha)*. As you start observing these then you adjust the anatomy and physiology to balance evenly together. The human body is touched or felt by an unknown entity within. The body as an outer instrument is perceived easily by the new sophisticated instruments but we have our own inner sophisticated instrument (the Self) which opens up through practice and you begin to look at the body from inside.

Q.- Can they happen on their own?

If they can happen on their own then there would be no room for diseases. As they cannot happen on their own yoga comes handy in reconstructing the ingredients of the needs of the body and mind through *āsana* and *prāṇāyāma*. Then work with ethical discipline to gain further benefit from practice for the cultivation of psycho-spiritual life.

Q.- Can one understand the *pañcabhūta,* the *pañcavāyu* and *cakra?*

Modern science says the hormones control the body. The yogi say the body is controlled by the *cakra*. *Cakra* are mystical words which you may find difficult to understand. As there are seven plexi in the body there are seven *cakra*. *Cakra* collect and store *prāṇa* that is distributed in the nervous system. Though medical science has advanced beyond what one would have imagined, I'm not sure whether they have full knowledge of the nervous system.

Nervous system is an electrifying flow of energy in the system. Though anatomy and physiology have been explained clearly I don't think the nervous system has been explained so clearly for people like us to understand and consolidate it. The yogis have said that they are like tubes wherein air, blood and energy *(prāṇa)* flow. They call them *nāḍī, dhamani* and *sirā*. At least they have divided and say that. The *nāḍī* act like avenues wherein the wind, blood and energy flows. If *nāḍī* is the pumping station of air, circulation of blood flows in *dhamani* which vibrates. The energy or *prāṇa* flows in *śirā* which is within *dhamani*.

The blood has many components like haemoglobin and so forth which carry chemical elements. These chemicals that flow in the blood produce a new energy as *prāṇa* commonly known as bio-energy. These energies are stored in the *cakra*. As it is hard to explain the ductless glands for those unfamiliar with medical science, it is difficult to explain *cakra* as they are invisible to our eyes. If the glands and plexi are outside the spinal column, *cakra* are in the spinal canal.

Yogi use the words like *iḍā nāḍī* or *candra nāḍī, piṅgalā nāḍī* or *sūrya nāḍī,* and *agni nāḍī* or *suṣumṇā nāḍī,* and they crisscross each other at the seat of each *cakra* pouring out the energy which is stored there to stir *prakṛti* and *puruṣa* in the seventh *cakra* to unite.

Q.– What are *pañcamahābhūta?*

Pṛthvī, āp, tej, vāyu and *ākāśa* are the *pañcamahābhūta*. With this background of *pañcamahābhūta* the yogi divided the body into five layers *(kośa), annamaya, prāṇamaya, manomaya, vijñānamaya* and *ānandamaya*. By this it is possible to understand the close connection between the skeletal body which is known as *annamaya kośa* or *pṛthvī tattva* (earth element), physiological body as *prāṇamaya* or *āp tattva* (water element), mind as *manomaya* or *tejas tattva* (fire element), intelligence as *vijñānamaya* or *vāyu tattva* (air element) and absolute consciousness as *ānandamaya* or *ākāśa tattva* (ether element).

The *mahābhūta* are basic, visible and tangible matter. *Mūla prakṛti* is the root matter with three *guṇa*. These *guṇa* are invisible whereas the five elements are cognisable in the process of evolution.

Though each cell of the body is made of five elements, we need to use them properly while doing *āsana* and *prāṇāyāma* in order to maintain balance of these five *tattva* in the cells. For instance while doing *Trikoṇāsana* on the right side, the right foot is in the *annamaya kośa* as it acts as a foundation to perform the *āsana*. Besides the smell, the quality of the earth is heaviness. Quality of water is lightness and taste. Actually in *Trikoṇāsana* the right foot which has to be in earth element remains in a fluid state or *āp tattva*, whereas the left foot which should be in *vāyu tattva* acts as if in *pṛthvī tattva*. This makes the legs unsteady in the *āsana*. Your minds are caught in between the feet. If you give a thought and make the right foot to be in *pṛthvī tattva* and left foot in *vāyu tattva*, then it is possible to move the left foot to bring equal weight on both the legs balancing the *āp tattva* to flow evenly in both the legs. Otherwise right leg stretches more than the left making the left leg appear dull. To bring this understanding for right balance, *tejas tattva* (mind) is needed. You have to bring the mind like the scales of justice. The mind being exactly in the middle of the five *tattva* has to measure the *āsana* with the gross elements of earth and water on one side and *vāyu* and *ākāśa* on the other side. While doing *Trikoṇāsana* on the right side, your right hand remains heavy, firm whereas the top left hand oscillates forwards and backwards. As it oscillates you have to bring *pṛthvī tattva* in the left hand so that it gains firmness to remain, straight and heavy. Then the *pañcabhūta* are balanced on that left hand. As you make the arm that rests on the floor heavy, learn to lessen this heaviness in order to make the left arm heavy. Unless you lighten the heaviness of the lower arm the firmness in the left arm does not come. This way you have to learn to interchange the *mahābhūta* in the *āsana*.

Suppose you are doing *Śīrṣāsana*, you feel *pṛthvī tattva* in the lower arms which remain steady, but the legs wobble. The moment you feel wobbling or oscillating forwards or backwards you have to charge the legs with *pṛthvī tattva* by making the upper arms to move into *āp tattva.* Without *āp tattva* in the upper arms, the legs remain loose. The moment you charge *āp tattva* judiciously in the upper arms the legs receive *pṛthvī tattva* and gain firmness. This way the interchanges have to be learnt while doing any *āsana.* Each *āsana* has a certain way of balancing the *pañcabhūta.* If you know the usage of *pañcabhūta* I need not speak about *pañcavāyu* as they follow the *bhūta.* Study the close relationship of *pañcabhūta* with *pañcavāyu.*

As I have explained this interchange in *Trikoṇāsana* and *Śīrṣāsana* you should follow them in the other *āsana* by studying the principles of *bhūta* with the principle of *vāyu.*[1]

The *vāyu* work like a fuel, heat, magnetism, light, gravity and electricity as far as the functions of the body are concerned. The *vāyu* help the *bhūta* not only with the functioning of the physical body but also with the *cakra.* In yogic terminology it is converted to power, vigour, strength and vitality as *prakṛti śakti.*

Patañjali indicates *siddhi* or accomplishment which we feel or experience in our practices. He says, *udānajayāt jala paṅka kaṇṭakādiṣu asaṅgaḥ utkrāntiḥ ca* (*Y.S.,* III.40) – by control on *udāna vāyu* you can walk on water, swamps and thorns. Tongue does not become dry. The seat of *udāna vāyu* is the throat. When you are doing the *āsana* keep the tongue and throat passive and quiet as if it is in a sleepy state. Unknowingly you block the throat passage and make *udāna vāyu* to be over-active in your practice and therefore you neglect to attend to the other *vāyu.*

Observe *Śīrṣāsana.* The tongue goes up immediately and closes the upper palate blocking the *prāṇa vāyu* to flow with ease. Keep the root and tip of the tongue on the lower palate in its natural position. Then the *udāna vāyu* allows *prāṇavāyu* to flow with ease and experience the lightness in the brain. Similarly, observe the tongue in *Trikoṇāsana.* If you are doing on the right side you turn the head to look up at the extended arm of the left. At that time you will be surprised to notice that the tongue moves up faster than the head to look up at the left arm. Though *Sarvāṅgāsana* is meant to quieten the *udāna vāyu* it happens the same in *Sarvāṅgāsana.* It happens in all the *āsana* non-deliberately. Learn to create space between the throat and the tongue and maintain it in its natural position in the presentation of all *āsana.*

Kaṇṭhakūpa (see *Y.S.,* III.31) is the well at the root of the throat. *Kaṇṭha* is throat; *kūpa* is the well. Keep space in the well of the throat where the tongue has its root. Then the *samāna vāyu* moves with ease. Otherwise one feels the burning sensation in the chest. Even it may burn out the energy which makes one to feel exhaustion and tiredness. The moment you feel the

[1] See the interview *A Subject of the Heart,* in *Aṣṭadaḷa Yogamāla* vol 6, plate n. 11(a &b), pp 69, 70.

sense of tiredness you have blocked the *udāna vāyu* in practice. Then *samāna vāyu* functions instead of *udāna*.

In order to keep *samāna vāyu* under control keep the seat of *udāna* quiet. *Udāna* belongs to the air element or *vijñānamaya kośa*. *Samāna* belongs to *tejas tattva* which represents form *(rūpa)* and warmth. If you adjust these two *vāyu*, the other three act with freedom. The function of the *vyāna* is to create space for expansion or contraction.

When you do *Śīrṣāsana* have you ever thought of the *vyāna* which is on the extremities, the skin which makes the muscles to extend, expand or contract? In *Śīrṣāsana* many of you spread the elbows instead of taking them in. If the elbows spread out one feels the pain in the neck. It means *pṛthvī tattva* is collapsing. Move them in the pain goes and you create space in the neck. *Prāṇa* at once moves in the neck. The throat is free from tension. By this you learn how *vyāna* helps *prāṇa* to function better.

If all the windows and doors of a house are closed while you are in, can you breathe freely? You suffocate. You at once open the windows and doors to breathe fresh air. That is the character of the *vyāna vāyu*. While doing the *āsana*, understand whether the *vyāna vāyu* opens the pores of the skin and allows *prāṇa* to move freely in the system. As *prāṇa* is the generating force, *vyāna* complements it in creating exhilaration and not exhaustion.

In *Śīrṣāsana* the legs have to move inwards. The moment the legs move inwards, the interlocked arms, biceps and forearms get longer because they are supplied with *prāṇic* energy. This removes dryness felt in the legs and arms. This way one has to learn to balance the *pañcavāyu* in an *āsana* keeping the throat and the diaphragm soft and well adjusted so that there are no ill-effects from practice.

It is not a simple thing to balance the *pañcavāyu* in each *āsana*. You have to reach a state of maturity to create that state of poise and maturity. *Samāpatti* is a transforming state in bringing equanimity from the physical, physiological, mental, logical and intellectual levels into *ākāśa tattva* as that *tattva* is *ātmā*. *Ākāśa* means clearness and space. While doing the *āsana* the skin acts as *mahat ākāśa* and the self acts as *citta ākāśa* or *cidākāśa*. *Prayatnaśaithilya* in *āsana* means that you are doing the *āsana* not only to remove the difference between the *mahat tattva* (macrocosm) and the *citta ākāśa* or the *cidākāśa* (microcosm), but to close the distance in between them. *Mahat tattva* is *brahmāṇḍa* (macrocosm) and *citta ākāśa* or *cidākāśa* is *piṇḍāṇḍa* (microcosm). The Self that covers the entire body like the sun in each *āsana* from any point to any point without deviation is *prayatnaśaithilya ananta samāpattibhyām* (*Y.S.*, II.47). Here the core starts guiding directly and you forget your *bahiraṅga* and *antaraṅga* bodies. This is *tataḥ dvandvāḥ anabhighātaḥ* (*Y.S.*, II.48).

Patañjali explains the *guṇa parva,* namely; *viśeṣa, aviśeṣa, liṅgamātra* and *aliṅga* (*Y.S.,* II.19). This *sūtra* explains the *prakṛti* of our existence from outside in. The *prakṛti* as *viśeṣa* gets connected to the body, which are the five *karmendriya,* the five *jñānendriya,* the mind and the five *pañcabhūta.* The *aviśeṣa* are the five *tanmātra* and *ahaṁkāra.* Then *liṅgamātra* is *mahat* and *aliṅga* is *mūla prakṛti.* When *viśeṣa, aviśeṣa liṅgamātra* get submerged in *mūla prakṛti,* then there is hope of having *ātmadarśana.* Often you are caught in *āsana* as a posture and you end the *āsana* on that level.

The nineteenth and twentieth *sūtra* of the second chapter are the foundation or the base for the entire yogic system. As such *tataḥ dvandvāḥ anabhighātaḥ* (*Y.S.,* II.48), *prayatnaśaithilya ananta samāpattibhyām* (*Y.S.,* II.47), convey that you are using the vehicles of nature *karmendriya, jñānendriya, manas, ahaṁkāra* and *buddhi,* which are part and parcel of the *prāṇa* as it exists in all these and vibrates in them. The *pañcavāyu* are not only connected with body but also with *manas, ahaṁkāra, buddhi, citta* and *viveka* as well. In *dvandvāḥ anabhighātaḥ,* the *pañcabhūta* and *pañcavāyu* help each other and support one another in such a way that the dualities do not affect *prakṛti* or *puruṣa.* The effect of *āsana* is the breaking of the conjunction of *pṛakrti* and *puruṣa* or the meaning of *prakṛti* or *puruṣa* so that they do not interfere with each other. The practitioner is not affected any more by dualities such as heat and cold, honour and dishonour, or pain and pleasure as the body submerges in the soul in precise presentation of all *āsana. Prāṇa,* which is in the form of *pañcavāyu* has its reach from the cell to the soul.

In the practice of *āsana* the *pañcamahābhūta* are activated and vitalised through *pañcaprāṇa.* The balance between these two connects the body and self as practice of *āsana* sublimates *prakṛti.* As *citta* associates or disassociates the body and the soul, *pañcaprāṇa* too associate or disassociate the *pañcabhūta* and *puruṣa.*

Q.– You have talked about *dharma kṣetra* and *kuru kṣetra* as the seats of the heart and the head. You have said if the heart is uncultured ego sets in. How to practise *āsana* and *prāṇāyāma* to culture the heart?

I have already answered advising not to do *āsana, prāṇāyāma* or *dhyāna* from the head but from the heart. Keep the throat passive the brain becomes light and observant. Keep the eyes open without tension so that the brain remains quiet. Move the ears inwards the mind becomes quiet. Do not perform *āsana* with closed eyes because you may lose control. But reverse the vision of intelligence inwards *(antar-lakṣya).* Perform *prāṇāyāma* with closed eyes, so that your vision of the eyes and intelligence moves inwards. Do *Adho Mukha Śvānāsana* and observe how the eyes go inwards and observe the back body. Feel the eyes in *Ūrdhva Mukha Śvānāsana*, they bulge out. Study the differences as well as the physical and chemical changes that happen in each *āsana* and learn to act against the current sometimes as well as to move with the current as needed. Observe in *Chaturaṅga Daṇḍāsana* the middle of the eyes are active. In *Ūrdhva Mukha Śvānāsana* the cornea is active. In *Adho Mukha Śvānāsana* the extremities and the middle of the eyes move in. This way of studying in each *āsana*, teaches the behavioural pattern of the eyes and ears. By observing the movements of the eyes in these three *āsana* you study and understand which part of the eye is passive and which part is active. Interchange and feel the effect. It is the same with the ears. You have to learn to hear the vibrations that happen in each *āsana* and not with the eyes. If you hear from the eyes, study what happens. Similarly inter-act and inter-change the sheaths as they are inter-woven and inter-related. Bring this relationship to surface through *āsana*, *prāṇāyāma* and *dhyāna*.

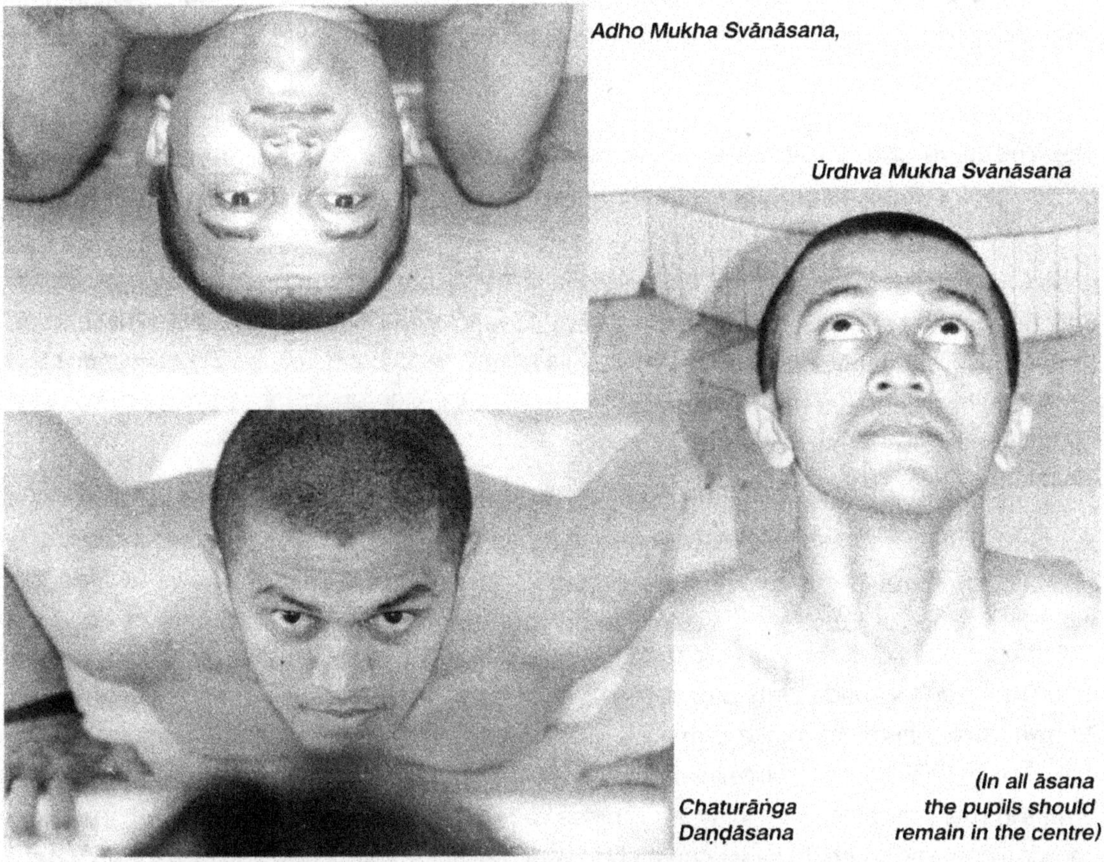

Adho Mukha Svānāsana,

Ūrdhva Mukha Svānāsana

Chaturāṅga Daṇḍāsana

(In all āsana the pupils should remain in the centre)

Plate n. 12 – Change of eyes in *Adho Mukha Śvānāsana*, *Ūrdhva Mukha Śvānāsana* and *Chaturāṅga Daṇḍāsana*

This way of study makes you to become a true pupil directing your *sādhanā* as a teacher. This is *svādhyāya* or *jñāna mārga* of yoga.

See how many times the brain jumps from one thing to the other in your *sādhanā*. This flickering in the brain creates thought waves in the heart. If the thinking seed is the head, the seed of thought waves is the heart. Thought takes the mind to the past and thinking process takes one towards the future and you lose the present. If *citta-vṛtti nirodha* is from the head, *praśānta citta* is from the heart. The stress to be or not to be is played in the head which is nothing but a war of words. Hence this seat, the brain is *kurukṣetra*. Serenity has to come from the conscientiousness of the heart, hence it is *dharmakṣetra*. For example a characterless man never says that he is characterless but in his heart it will be pricking. That is why it is called *dharmakṣetra*.

Do all the *āsana* from the *hṛdaya-sthāna*. Then the brain becomes quiet. As the brain becomes quiet, it is nothing but a state of meditation as you are acting from *dharmakṣtra*.

Q.- You have spoken about how *āsana* and *prāṇāyāma* develop *jñāna*. What is the *jñāna* that one should be looking for?

Nobody can look for *jñāna*. When you switch on the plug the light comes and when you switch it off the light disappears. I have already shown you the method that all the *āsana* have to be done primarily from the subtler two elements, *vāyu* and *ākāśa*, and secondarily from *pṛthvī* and *āp*. No doubt a beginner has to start from *pṛthvī* and *āp*. After toning these two elements start from the other end. Then *jñāna* starts sprouting.

In doing *Trikoṇāsana* on the right side that foot falls out. If the foot that has fallen out is brought in line as it should be in *Tāḍāsana*, it is *jñāna*. If you don't observe this, then there is only *ajñāna* in *sādhanā*. The moment you see bulged out ankle and adjust to move in, then this attentive practice is *jñāna sādhanā*. You bring your *jñāna* on the ankle. This way extend the *jñāna* to see the knee, thigh and so forth. Start practising like this in making the ankles, patella, side torso, side legs, side arms and so forth, to run in line with each other, then *jñāna* sets in on its own. Look where you make a mistake and correct at once. This way every now and then strike the matchstick of the intelligence to illuminate so that light of knowledge and wisdom dawns in your practices. Then this *jñāna* guides you later into *prajñāna* or knowledge of wisdom showing how and where to look accurately in your practices. This is how you move from *ajñāna yoga* practice into *prajñāna yoga* practice.

We have been given five senses of perception. We have also been given the intelligence, memory, consciousness and awareness to conceive knowledge. All these instruments are to see the outer objects of the world to gain worldly knowledge *(laukika jñāna)*. If we have to learn to look within ourselves, then the same attention has to be turned inwards from the body towards the self. Then we gain spiritual knowledge that is eternal *(vaidika* or *ādhyātmika) jñāna*.

Study of inner sensitivity comes through the practice of *āsana* and *prāṇāyāma*. Then the awareness begins to set in to see, feel, perceive and conceive the body, mind, intelligence, consciousness, conscience and self. This is the real *jñāna* we all are looking for. When these inner knowables are known, then the knower is left alone. There is no instrument to know the knower, as knower is the root of all knowables. Knower is *jñātā*. To know the knower is *jñāna*. When this *jñāna* reaches the *jñātā*, nothing remains to be known.

As we sharpen the knife as an instrument to use, we have to strengthen the instruments from body to conscience through the intelligence of the head and heart to reach the self that can never be cut by weapons, nor burnt, neither wet with water nor dried by wind (see *Bhagavad Gītā*, II.22 and 23).

Q.- How can one learn to move from merely inhaling and exhaling to practising *prāṇāyāma*?

After the mastery of the *āsana* Patañjali suggests *prāṇāyāma*. After explaining *āsana* as a state of *prayatna śaithilya ananta samāpattibhyām* (*Y.S.*, II.47) and *tataḥ dvandvāḥ anabhighātaḥ* (*Y.S.*, II.48), Patañjali says that one should start *prāṇāyāma* and defines *prāṇāyāma* as *tasmin sati śvāsa praśvāsayoḥ gativicchedaḥ prāṇāyāmaḥ* (*Y.S.*, II.49). Patañjali explains the characteristic of the *āsana* and not the names which is an enigma to all. Unfortunately many misread and say to do the *āsana* with comfort.

Whether you do *Gaṇḍa Bheruṇḍāsana*, or *Vṛschikāsana*, or *Tāḍāsana*, there should be *sthiratā* and *sukhatā* in every *āsana*. He explains *prayatna*, which means effort and discipline to bring all the five sheaths of the self in harmony and concord where the effort ceases on its own. When this happens you don't pay attention to the body but move towards the self and make the self to reach and touch each and every part in each *āsana*. This is the characteristic of each *āsana*.

As *sthira sukham āsana* is an enigma, it is the same with *prāṇāyāma*. Patañjali has not named *prāṇāyāma* as *Ujjāyī, Śitali, Nāḍī Śodhana, Sūrya Bhedana, Candra Bhedana* and so forth. Probably these various types of *prāṇāyāma* came later. He begins with a simple definition as, *śvāsapraśvāsayoḥ gativicchedaḥ prāṇāyāmaḥ:* it means that you have to observe the flow of breath which is zigzag and to make it flow smoothly and softly both in inhalation and exhalation. Some may get that smooth and soft flow in inhalation and some in exhalation. Studying the difference between the flow of inhalation and that of exhalation and then making the in-breath and out-breath move uninterruptedly and softly makes you become a *guru* in your *prāṇāyāma* practice.

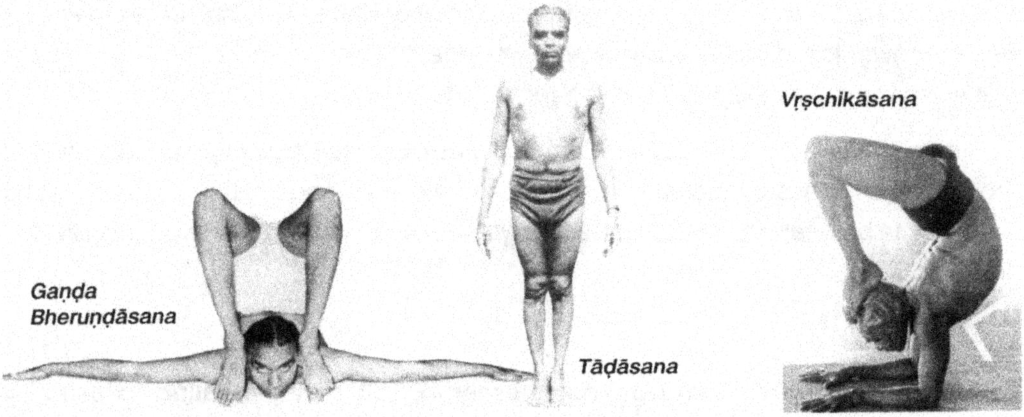

Plate n. 13 – *Gaṇḍa Bheruṇḍāsana, Vṛṣchikāsana* and *Tāḍāsana*

This question has surprised me. Patañjali defines *prāṇāyāma* as *tasmin sati śvāsa praśvāsayoḥ gativicchedaḥ prāṇāyāmaḥ* (Y.S., II.49), and then proceeds with *bāhya ābhyantara stambha vṛttiḥ deśa kāla saṁkhyābhiḥ paridṛṣṭaḥ dīrgha sūkṣmaḥ* (*Y.S.*, II.50).

He explains *abhyantara* or *antara-vṛtti* as *pūraka* or inhalation, *stambha-vṛtti* as *kuṁbhaka* or retention and *bāhya-vṛtti* as *recaka* or exhalation. Then he explains the qualitative practice of *prāṇāyāma* through *deśa, kāla* and *saṁkhyā*. Many people say *deśa* stands for the country they live in, *kāla* to the weather condition and *saṁkhyā* for the length of practice.

For me *deśa* means the torso, *kāla* means the longevity of the flow of inhalation and exhalation and *saṁkhyā* means precise movement. These three, *deśa, kāla* and *saṁkhyā* represent *guṇa; tamas, rajas* and *sattva* respectively. *Deśa* is the entire body of five elements which is the field *(kṣetra)*. If the field is unattended it becomes barren and dull. *Kāla* is *lakṣaṇa*. It means the moment the cultivator attends to the land by digging, watering, ploughing and sowing the seeds for harvesting, he transforms the *tāmasic* quality of the land to *rājasic* quality. *Saṁkhyā* is *avasthā* or the harvest which is the *sāttvic guṇa* of the field. Read *Vibhūti Pāda, sūtra* 13, which says, *etena bhūtendriyeṣu dharma lakṣaṇa avasthā pariṇāmāḥ vyākhyātāḥ*

(*Y.S.*, III.13).[1] This *sūtra* indicates that your body, mind and senses undergo transformation in the process of upliftment as it happens during deterioration. These transformations are known as *dharma pariṇāma, lakṣaṇa pariṇāma* and *avasthā pariṇāma*.

The *prāṇāyāma* vitalises and purifies the *prāṇa*. *Dharma pariṇāma* or virtuous transformation of body *(deśa)* is brought as the various areas are touched, felt and sensitised by *prāṇa*. This sensitisation is the transformation of *deśa* which otherwise remains in the *tāmasic* state. We know the inner body exists but we do not feel it. As the longevity of inhalation and exhalation progresses there comes the marked and significant change. This transformation is *lakṣaṇa pariṇāma*. We animate the inner body to feel its vibrations. It means that we are transforming the *tāmasic* body towards *rajo-sāttvic* body. This change brings purification. Thus *kāla* in *prāṇāyāma* brings *lakṣaṇa pariṇāma*. Then comes *avasthā pariṇāma* which happens due to the improved state with qualitative changes in the elements of the body and cells towards the *sattva guṇa*. This transformation has to be permanently maintained and retained through uninterrupted practice of *āsana* and *prāṇāyāma*. We have to be persistent in our *sādhanā* to live throughout in *sattvaguṇa*.

The word *gativicchedaḥ* indicates the cessation of breath. In *gativicchedaḥ* one has to study whether the in-breath, out-breath or retention are *sāttvic, rājasic* or *tāmasic*. If the inhalation or exhalation is fast and rough, it is *tāmasic*, if it is strong and long but not rough *(dīrgha)*, it is *rājasic*. If the movements of breath are soft, smooth, subtle and long *(sūkṣma)*, it is *sāttvic*. It is the same with retention. If the chest in *kuṁbhaka* is puffed with stress on brain, it is *tāmasic*. If the *kuṁbhaka* is done by taking or lifting the muscles and skin of the chest every now and then, it is *rājasic*. If the self holds and remains steady bracing its frontier – the skin – firmly with softness in head and eyes, it is *sāttvic*.

I am speaking of the *guṇa* here, because in the next *sūtra* he says, *bāhya ābhyantara viṣaya ākṣepī caturthaḥ* (Y.S., II.51). What is *viṣaya ākṣepī*? When one reaches the state of luminosity in *antara-vṛtti, staṁbha-vṛtti* and *bāhya-vṛtti* with fineness, at that time there are no movements of thought waves *(viṣaya)*. Then the disc of the consciousness is without any rays of thoughts and therefore the breath becomes effortless and non-deliberate. Here the breath transcends as if *viṣaya* and *prāṇa* are no more felt or existing.

Later yoga savants studied various methodologies on *prāṇāyāma* emphasising *dīrghatā* and *sūkṣmatā* to get the best effects and coined names for different types of *prāṇāyāma*. For

[1] Through these three phases, cultured consciousness is transformed from its potential state *(dharma)*, towards further refinement *(lakṣaṇa)* and the zenith of refinement *(avasthā)*. This way, the transformation of elements, senses and mind also takes place.

example *Nāḍī Śodhana* helps to gain some control over subtle flow *(sūkṣmatā)*, while in *Ujjāyī* deep flow *(dīrghatā)* takes place.

In *Ujjāyī* the atmospheric air is drawn without filtering whereas in *Nāḍī Śodhana* the placement of the fingers traces the passage *(prāṇa nāḍī)* of the breath in the nostrils, narrows the space at the passage for the carpet of the membranes in the nostrils to hold the dust of the atmospheric air and allows the filtered pure air to pass through the *prāṇa nāḍī* into the lungs. This way one can trace differences in various *prāṇāyāma*. Unfortunately those who practise *Nāḍī Śodhana*, *Sūrya Bhedana* or *Candra Bhedana* place their thumb and fingers in such a way that is as if one is doing only *Ujjāyī prāṇāyāma*.

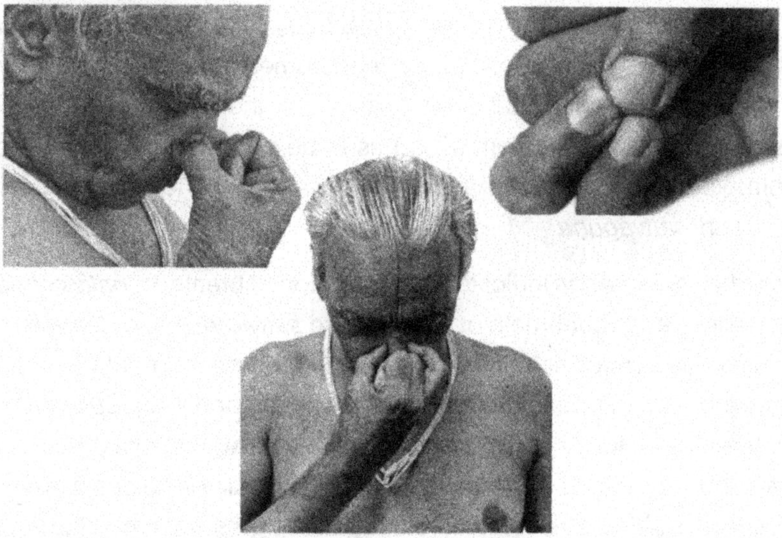

Plate n. 14 – Placement of fingers for digital *prāṇāyāma*

The yoga texts explain not to use the index and middle fingers on the nostrils but do not explain how the thumb, ring and little fingers are to be used. This is another enigma. But it is for us to find out how to use the digits – the fingers, to filter the gross atmospheric air.

For the scientific mind the *prāṇāyāma* is a science. The practitioners have to study with a scientific mind to trace how the digits have to be placed on the nostrils for the in-breath and the out-breath to get cleansed, refined and purified before it enters the lungs or while leaving the lungs. The thumb is wide. If one joins the ring and little finger tips folding the index and the middle finger towards the middle of the palm, then they get the equal width to that of the thumb and ring and little fingers run parallel to each other. Here one feels a better co-ordination between the fingers and the thumb as well as in measuring the flow of breath. In fact, the non-interference of the index and middle fingers co-ordinates the digits with *prāṇa nāḍī*. The way some practitioners place their fingers on the nostrils makes the breath move with hardness and roughness. Without tracing first the *prāṇa nāḍī* in the nostrils, *Nāḍī Śodhana* (purification of the *nāḍī*) cannot take place.

The study of the *guṇa* in *prāṇāyāma* has also to be traced. The digital *prāṇāyāma* enhances the quietude, placidity, serenity which belong to *sattvaguṇa* whereas holding the breath *(kuṁbhaka)* for a minute or so is sheer ego. It is *rājasic* practice. It is not holding the breath long that is important. In retention, the core that is lifted has to be held steadily without allowing it to sink is *staṁbha-vṛtti*. As long as the core is in contact with the skin, it is *sattvaguṇa kuṁbhaka*. The moment the self loses this contact with the skin, it is no more *kuṁbhaka*. Most of the *sādhaka* are not *śodhaka* (inquirer, scrutiniser) and therefore fail to reach the *sāttvic* state in *prāṇāyāma* that is explained in *Yoga Sūtra* II.51.

Therefore the right way of practice of *prāṇāyāma* certainly helps one to remove the veil that covers the intelligence to build up that illuminative wisdom. See *tataḥ kṣīyate prakāśa āvaraṇam* (Y.S., II.52). Hard and deep breathing cannot do this. Hence one has to find ways and means to derive the effect of *prāṇāyāma* that has been explained by Patañjali. The veil is *ajñāna* and the moment the veil is removed it brings *prajñā* (attention and awareness) in the intelligence and makes it a fit instrument for *dhāraṇā*, *dhāraṇāsu ca yogyatā manasaḥ (Y.S.,* II.53). This word *yogyatā* has not been used anywhere except in this *sūtra*. *Yogyatā* means eligibility. *Prāṇāyāma* is not merely the inhalations and exhalations but an instrumental cause to remove the veil that covers the intelligence of the self for it by comfort to move towards concentration *(dhāraṇā)*.

As the body is a huge mass, *āsana* break the awareness of this mass into a subtle awareness. It is the same in *prāṇāyāma* where one starts with *sthūla* (gross) *prāṇāyāma* and then moves on towards *sūkṣma* (subtle and finer) *prāṇāyāma*. When the *sthūla prāṇāyāma* transforms into *sūkṣma prāṇāyāma*, then one experiences a state without the rays of thought in the consciousness. That is why *prāṇāyāma* is called the hub of yoga.

Q.– Does quietness and silence in the mind mean silence in the *citta*?

The mind, ego and intelligence are encased in the consciousness. As it is encased in the consciousness whether you quieten the mind or soften the ego or keep the intelligence pensive, it means that you have quietened the *citta*. The subtlest part of the consciousness is the ego *(ahaṁkāra)* and it may take a long time for a *sādhaka* to subdue it. Many of you have experienced the quietness of the mind in *Śavāsana*. But to move from the quietness of the mind towards the quietness of the consciousness needs deep attention.

Q.- What is the difference between mind and *citta*?

I have already said that *citta* is the container of mind, intelligence and *ahaṁkāra*. Therefore, mind is the gross part, intelligence, the subtle part, while *ahaṁkāra* or ego is the subtlest part of the consciousness.

Like the stars of the galaxies that are impossible to count, the rays of thought waves from the disk of consciousness are difficult to count. So, instead of moving the mind in the rays of thought waves the *sādhaka* has to tap the source of these rays. Then it is possible for him to reach the mother of the mind - the consciousness, and the father - the Soul.

The only difference between mind and consciousness is that as the mind is gross *(sthūla)*, intelligence and *ahaṁkāra* are respectively subtle and subtler *(sūkṣma)* and the consciousness is the subtlest.

Q.- How to differentiate between them?

One cannot differentiate them as they are interwoven together and are close to each other, remaining in gross, fine, finer and finest states. If the mind is gross, intelligence is fine, *ahaṁkāra* the finer and consciousness - the finest. The aim of yoga is not only *citta-vṛtti nirodha* but to reach the auspiciousness and purity of the consciousness.

Q.- What is the role of mind in *prāṇāyāma*?

Cale vāte calaṁ cittaṁ niścale niścalaṁ bhavet (H.Y.P., II.2). It is said that mind moves as the breath moves and where the breath is there the mind is and if the breath remains steady, the mind remains steady. Again in chapter IV, verse 23 of *Haṭhayoga Pradīpikā* it is said, "When the mind becomes stilled, breath is stilled and when *prāṇa* is restrained the mind becomes stilled."

mano yatra vilīyeta pavanastatra līyate I
pavano līyate yatra manastatra vilīyate II

Hence, *prāṇāyāma* plays a major role in quietening the mind. We have to understand that *prāṇa* and *manas* go hand in hand. In *prāṇāyāma* the mind gets focused on the length, breadth and subtleness in the flow of the breath and gets merged in it. As the mind gets merged equanimity or the *sattvic nature* is felt in the mind.

This is how the *sādhaka* has to do the *sādhanā*. *Sādhanā* is a research ground for the *sādhaka* to study yoga. According to the grades of *sādhaka (mṛdu, madhya, adhimātra* and *tīvra)* the quality in understanding the *sādhanā* differs. Yet yoga is the only channel to understand the functions of *prakṛti* and rectify them so that they move closer towards the Soul or the Self.

Prāṇāyāma first removes the difference between the mind and consciousness and takes one's individual consciousness to merge into the cosmic consciousness or universal consciousness.

Q.– Can *Ujjāyī prāṇāyāma* take one towards for example *tataḥ kṣīyate prakāśa āvaraṇam* (*Y.S.*, II.52)? What is the road map of *prāṇāyāma*?

I have explained the road map already. Whatever *prāṇāyāma* you do it has its effect. One cannot deny that. We have got two hemispheres of the brain. We have *nāḍī* like *iḍā*, *piṅgalā* and *suṣumṇā*. As they are all inter-connected, the problem in *Ujjāyī* is that many who practise this *prāṇāyāma* unknowingly or nondeliberately inflate and harden the brain. Hence one has to check and keep the brain quiet and start taking the breath from the seat of the consciousness. If *Ujjāyī* is done with a right intellectual judgement, it certainly gives the same effect. Yet I like to explain the difference between *Ujjāyī* and *Nāḍī Śodhana prāṇāyāma*.

In *Nāḍī Śodhana* you take the breath from the right nostril which moves towards the left side of the brain and when done from the left nostril the energy touches the right side of the brain. As such this *prāṇāyāma* balances the two hemispheres of the brain with its four chambers. The main effect of *Nāḍī Śodhana* is that it cleanses both the hemispheres of the brain and keeps the brain energetic as the filtered and pure air enters which seeps into the cells of the brain and this in turn quietens the brain and keeps the consciousness alert, aware and active. No doubt *Nāḍī Śodhana* is the best of all *prāṇāyāma* because it brings equanimity *(samatvam)* due to the interchanging action that takes place in the hemispheres of the brain. *Ujjāyī* cannot make the two hemispheres to receive the energy or to act evenly though you experience quietude in mind.

I am happy to have interacted with you all and I hope you explore further from this educative talk and grasp everything from *annamaya* to *ānandamaya kośa* in your *sādhanā*.

RECENT THOUGHTS

ON YOGA

BLOOD – A GEM

The river of energy that flows in the human body is unlike natural rivers. Rivers flow through inorganic rocks and sands; the crimson river flows within us through living tissues. But substances like minerals and salts flow in our blood as well as in the rivers.

Vedic traditions speak of a rich heritage of gems that form in the human embodiment. In order to understand the qualitative gems that constitute the human body, our *sādhanā* should be deep to reveal each facet or gem that exists within the blood stream.

From One Precious Life Come the Gems

The life story of Prahlāda is well-known in Indian epics. Prahlāda by his *bhakti* not only purified himself but wanted his progeny to imbibe these noble qualities.[1] Prahlāda's grandson, Bali, became a very powerful demon king with good motivations.

According to the Vedic lore a famous king Ambarīṣa, enquired from his ministers about the creation of the gems *(ratna)* in the human body by the Lord. At that very moment the famous sage Parāśara (Vyāsa's father) happened to arrive there. The king thought it prudent to put to him the same question. The sage answered the king that even Pārvatī had the same curiosity on gems and asked her lord about them. Lord Shiva began revealing the various gems, some belonging to heaven *(svarga-loka)*, some to earth *(mṛtyu-loka)* and some to hell *(pātāḷa-loka)*.

He said that *svarga-loka* contains four gems named as *Chintāmaṇi, Kaustubhamaṇi, Rudramaṇi* and *Syamantakamaṇi*. *Pātāḷa-loka* has nine different-coloured serpents yielding gems in various colours like black, blue, yellow, green, white, red, rose, cream and khaki, whereas *Mṛtyu-loka* (earth) has twenty one gems.

---

[1] In the 10th chapter (stanza 30) of the *Bhagavad Gita*, Lord Krishna says that "of all the daityas, I am Prahlāda." *Prahlādaśchāsmi daityanām.*

Then he began narrating the story of Bali (Prahlāda's grandson) who had many redeeming qualities. He was virtuous *(śīlatā)*, righteous *(dhārmic)* and well-known for his philanthropy and nobility. He would go to any length to keep his word but had one ambition to be the Lord of the world.

Rājā Bali being a religious-minded king used to perform many *yajña* (sacrificial fires). By these, he imbibed not only internal strength but expanded his empire usurping kingdom after kingdom. Rājā Bali's subjects were in a dilemma and often prayed to Lord Vishnu to help them.

Knowing his power and strength, Rājā Bali decided to perform a *mahā-yajña* (a great sacrificial fire) to propitiate the gods and to become the monarch of the heavens. At that time Lord Vishnu decided to manifest himself on earth[1] in the form of a dwarf (Vāmana).

As a dwarf he turned up in the form of a priest at the *yajña* and demanded a gift *(dakṣiṇā)* from the King. True to his innate calling and propriety, the king assured the dwarf-priest that his demands would be fulfilled. The Lord asked just three strides of land. Despite opposition from his *guru* Śukrācārya, Rājā Bali said that he had given his word and he would fulfil it at any cost. He invited the dwarf to take the three steps.

As the story goes the dwarf grew until he spanned the sky. His first step covered the entire planet (earth) and the next the heavens. (This transfiguration of dwarf is the *avatāra* - incarnation of Trivikrama.) Lord Trivikrama asked the king what would he offer for the third step. Bali humbly offered his own head. The moment the lord kept his third step on Rājā Bali's head, his body became *ratnamaya* (laden with gems) by the touch of the Lord's feet. Then Lord Vishnu

---

1 "Whenever the righteousness is on the decline and the un-righteousness is in ascendance I appear in the form of embodiment. I am born from age to age as an *avatāra*, for the extirpation of evil doers, and for establishing righteousness *(dharma)* on a pious footing", so says Lord Krishna promising us his presence and reappearance in *Bhagvad Gītā* -

yadā yadā hi dharmasya glānir bhavati bhārata
abhyutthānām adharmasya tadātmānam sṛjāmyaham
paritrāṇāya sādhūnām vināśāya ca duṣkṛtām
dharma saṁsthāpanārthāya saṁbhavāmi yuge yuge

IV.7,8.

Accordingly his ten *avatāra* are 1) Matsya - fish, 2) Kūrma - tortoise, 3) Varāha - boar, 4) Narasiṁha - man-lion, 5) Vāmana - a dwarf, 6) Rāma - the hero of Rāmāyaṇa, 7) Paraśurāma - a man with *paraśu* (a sickle or curved knife) to fight whenever necessary for the self-protection from warriors, 8) Krishna - Lord Krishna, 9) Balarāma - the incarnation of Adiśeṣa or Buddha - Gautam Buddha who wanted to stop the violence that was occurring on the Earth. Both the *avatāra* are accepted, 10) Kalki - the last appearance which has yet to come until the human race drowns completely in the ocean of sea. The *avatāra* of Vāmana happened during Baḷi's time.

upheld the king's body on the points of four *triśula* (or tridents) thus ensuing the creation of the twelve zodiac systems *(rāśī)* and nine planets *(navagraha)*.[1]

Early mention of the use of gemstones can be traced in the *Ṛgveda, Agnipurāṇa, Devi Bhāgavatam,* and *Mahābhārata.* The poetry of Kalidāsa also mentions the use of gemstones. Today however I do not need to tell you the use of these precious stones but to rediscover the gems within us and make them sparkle through *āsana* and *prāṇāyāma.* We all know how the blood enriched with oxygen reaches the remote areas of our body. *Varāha Upaniṣad* mentions blood as *ratna-pūrita dhātu.*

Yoga has the power to change and transform the *ratna-pūrita dhātu* of the body through *aṣṭāṅga yoga sādhanā.* The gems emitted from Bali's body are related to the human body suggesting that they are to be worn when human beings suffer from problems and they correspond to different areas of the body.

Let us give a thought to these various gems in the body, particularly to this part of blood that is termed as *ratna-pūrita dhātu.*

As the above story shows, the gems were created corresponding to various parts of the human embodiment. The human body according to *āyurveda* is made up of *tridoṣa* (the three humours), *sapta-dhātu* (the seven ingredients) and *trimala* (the three waste matters). The *tridoṣa* are *vāta* (wind), *pitta* (bile or gastric fire) and *śleṣma* (phlegm). The three humours *(tridoṣa)* of wind *(vāta),* bile *(pitta)* and phlegm *(śleṣma),* are to be evenly balanced to gain perfect health as imbalances in them cause diseases. The *saptadhātu* are *rasa* (chyle), *rakta* (blood), *māṁsa* (flesh), *meda* (fat), *asthi* (bones), *majjā* (marrow) and *śukra* (semen). The *trimala* – waste matter – are: faeces, urine and sweat. These three aspects *(doṣa, dhātu, mala)* are primarily elemental. Our *karmendriya, jñanedriya, manas, buddhi, ahaṁkāra* and *citta* – subtle part – have their own *mala.* Our aim is to convert and transform these various ingredients of the body into gems through *yoga sādhanā.* Patañjali indicates how the body and mind are transformed from their potential state to the esteemed state of refinement which are termed as *dharma pariṇāma, lakṣaṇa pariṇāma* and *avasthā pariṇāma.* Keeping these three transformations *(pariṇāma)* as aims or goals, let us see how we experience through health the activation of these gems.

---

[1] The twelve zodiac signs *(rāśī)* are: 1) Aries *(meṣa),* 2) Taurus *(vṛṣabha),* 3) Gemini *(mithuna),* 4) Cancer *(karka),* 5) Leo *(siṁha),* 6) Virgo *(kanyā),* 7) Libra *(tulā),* 8) Scorpio *(vṛśchika),* 9) Sagittarius *(dhanura),* 10) Capricorn *(makara),* 11) Aquarius *(kuṁbha)* and 12) Pisces *(mīna).*

The *navagraha* are: 1) *Ravi* (Sun), 2) *Candra* (Moon), 3) *Maṅgala* (Mars), 4) *Budha* (Mercury), 5) *Guru* (Jupiter), 6) *Śukra* (Venus), 7) *Śani* (Saturn), 8) *Rāhu* and 9) *Ketu* (the comets).

Balancing the Elements Within

Balance is the key word while practising *āsana* and *prāṇāyāma. The sādhaka* has to review the various constituents that function within the body. Then he has to study and learn to balance the various systems of the body covering the five sheaths, three humours, seven *dhātu* and various *mala* for overall health. Within a healthy body there is a proportionate mix of the elements of earth, water, fire, air and ether. It is not water alone which is excreted through urine and faeces. These waste matters have salts, minerals, chemicals, fats, urea, certain enzyme secretions, gases and bacteria. This is why urine and stool tests often reveal the state of the health and disease in a person.

My stress is more on the elemental adjustment and management in the performance of *āsana* and *prāṇāyāma.* If the elements are well balanced, the other gems in the body follow them. You recall the story of *amṛta manthana*[1] the angels and demons churning the ocean to draw out the nectar of immortality. Before churning, they dumped raw materials like trees, herbs and grass to blend them together and churned till the nectar came out of it. In the same way *āsana* and *prāṇāyāma* churn the five elements, their counterparts, the seven *dhātu,* mind, intelligence, consciousness and conscience to get properly mixed and then blend into an elixir of life.

Interestingly the five elements of nature - *pṛthvī* (earth), *āp* (water), *tejas* (fire), *vāyu* (air) and *ākāśa* (space) are to be found in all the important terrestrial and celestial creations.[2]

The *navagraha* or the nine constellations, the twelve zodiac signs and all the creatures that inhabit our world are made up of these five elements. From this perspective the elemental harmony follows in living and non-living things. The body contains *agni* (we often refer to the gastric 'fire' in the belly) which has to be conserved and efficiently used. The gems contain *ratna-agni* and *śarīra-agni* (or *vaiśvānara-agni),* another name for *viśva caitanya śakti.* When *ratna-agni* and *vaiśvānara-agni* are synchronised and properly coordinated, then that person gets invigorated.

There is a science behind the widespread use of gems in different forms like rings, ornaments, bracelets, lockets, charms and other artefacts. For example, *firoza* created from Rājā Bali's blood, is said to be a good grounding stone to balance the physical and the spiritual sides, as the sky connects the heavens to the earth. It is believed that the usage of gems helps

[1] See *The Tree of Yoga,* p. 115.

[2] These elements are of a superior quality in the celestial regions and inferior in the nether regions. The seven celestial regions are: *bhūloka, bhuvarloka, suvarloka, mahāloka, janōloka, tapōloka* and *satyaloka.*

The seven nether regions are: *atala, vitala, sutala, rasātala, talātala, mahātala* and *pātāla* (see *Light on the Yoga Sūtras of Patañjali, sūtra* III.27).

in reducing premature ageing by strengthening the immune system. It helps in preventing nightmares and panic attacks. It is said to be a powerful force in healing arthritis, gout, rheumatism, respiratory and immune weaknesses and blood disorders.

The Blood-Enriched Jewelled Body

In *Light on Prāṇāyāma* I have mentioned that the *Varāhopaniṣad* calls the blood a 'jewel' *(ratna-pūrita dhātu)*.[1] In *prāṇāyāma* the essential ingredient *(dhātu)* called blood is enriched and refined like a jewel as it absorbs the various energies. We have seven ingredients. Out of these seven, *Varāhopaniṣad* singles out blood as *ratna-pūrita-dhātu*. Only when the humours of the body function properly and maintain their respective balance, then the seven ingredients imbibe their purity. The food that we eat is transformed into *rasa* (chyle) and its next immediate transformation is into *rakta* which absorbs maximum essence *(sāra)* of the food that is taken. Through *rakta* the other ingredients get formed. It roughly takes four days for an ingredient to get converted into the next one. This way it takes twenty-eight days to form semen/ovum from the base *dhātu*. Blood is the base or the mother ingredient for the other *dhātu*.[2]

Even *Suśruta*, the famed philosopher-surgeon of ancient India has categorised blood as the fourth *doṣa* (*doṣa* refers to the humours of the body). In addition to the three *doṣa* namely *vāta*, *pitta* and *kapha*, *Suśruta* added *rakta* or blood as the fourth to take into consideration. The introduction to the *Suśruta Saṁhitā* states that "blood which forms as one of the fundamental principles *(dhātu)* of the organism may be designated a *doṣa*. When the blood gets congested in any part of the body, it brings disturbance.

The *doṣa* vitiate the seven ingredients as well as the three waste matters namely, urine, sweat and stools. The blood has a major impact on all the other ingredients or *dhātu*.

I have often emphasised the need to have fully potent respiratory and circulatory systems in order to maintain the health. All *āsana* as well as *prāṇāyāma* (directly and indirectly) work towards improving the quality and flow of this mighty stream of blood within us. Our blood contains various components like plasma, immunoglobulins, fibrinogen, erythrocytes, haemoglobin, leucocytes, platelets and other hormones and proteins. Every sixty seconds,

---

[1] See also *Aṣṭadaḷa Yogamālā* vol 1, *Yoga and Peace*, pp. 141.

[2] This indicates how the menstrual cycle occurs every 28 days. The ovum breaks and the bleeding occurs as the waste matter (known as *ārtava*) is thrown out. Similarly the sperm is the *ārtava* of male reproductive energy. These *ārtava* should not be held in and their disposal from the body should be facilitated. However, the semen has to be held in which *ojas* and *tejas* shines in the intensity of *sādhanā*. Thus Patañjali says, *brahmacaryapratiṣṭhāyāṁ vīryalābhaḥ* (*Y.S.* II.38) – when the *sādhaka* is firmly established in chastity, knowledge, vigour, valour and energy flow to him.

1,440 times a day, our blood travels through the 60,000-mile or 96,000k.m. system of the human body. These tidal waves of blood smash against the aorta, the body's largest artery, seventy times a minute, delivering their blows 2.5 billion times during the average life span. Rigid metal pipes could not withstand this battering for long.

Yet, due to constant abuses they take their toll. Yogic practice does undo the damage that happens and puts the system back on track. Right from the standing *āsana* to the inverted and back bending *āsana,* the practitioner mobilises the muscles, joints, bones, tendons, tissues and fibres to squeeze, rinse, dilate, pulsate and filter the blood through the immense network within the body. Sometimes wearing a ruby is said to help proper blood circulation for those who are anaemic. *Āsana* help first to have a healthy blood circulation in every nook and corner of the body and to revitalise the different *dhātu* to reach their essential form.

The practice of *āsana* and *prāṇāyāma* not only maintains the fine balance between nerves and muscles but also between head and heart.

How *Āsana* Help in the Production of Gems

a) Take the effects of *Prasārita Padottānāsana* II. In this āsana the hamstring and abductor muscles get fully extended and this makes the blood to flow to the trunk and the head, stimulating the adrenals and islets of Langerhans. It also increases digestive power.

b) In *Padmāsana* the blood is made to circulate in the lumbar region and the abdomen, toning the spine and the abdominal organs.

c) Forward bending *āsana* stimulate the spine by improving blood circulation and relieve backaches. In these *āsana* the blood is made to flow around the navel and genital organs so that they get saturated with blood. These *āsana* also massage the heart, the spinal column and the abdominal organs and rest and refresh the mind. As the pelvic region gets oxygenated blood, they keep this area healthy and helps the gonad glands to absorb the required nutrition from the blood.

d) *Śīrṣāsana* and its variations transform and purify the blood and allow the flow of enriched blood to the brain cells. This acts as a tonic for people whose brains tire out quickly. Its regular practice will show marked improvement in the haemoglobin content of the blood.

e) *Sarvāṅgāsana* and its variations amazingly have a direct effect on the thyroid, parathyroid and adrenal glands; the glands and help them to function properly. As the body gets inverted in *Śīrṣāsana* and *Sarvāṅgāsana* the venous blood flows to the heart without strain due to the force of gravity. Besides these effects they exercise the liver, pancreas and spleen ensuring a generous blood supply to these areas to remain healthy

f) *Supta Pādāṅguṣṭhāsana* I, II & III help in circulating the blood rejuvenating the nerves in the legs, abdomen and hips.

g) *Ekapāda Śīrṣāsana* cycle helps not only in strengthening the spine but in eliminating toxins in the body .

h) Back-bends make blood to circulate round the pubic region keeping it in a healthy condition. The thyroids, parathyroids, adrenals and gonads receive a rich supply of blood and this increases one's vitality. As the blood supply to the spine is increased, the nerves do not degenerate.

i) The various types of *prāṇāyāma* help in enriching the blood circulation, as well as strengthening the nervous system. It makes the glandular systems to function to function in a balanced state, and at the same time keeps the mind clear and clean. The pure air channelled through *prāṇāyāma* enriches the blood.

Yogāsana – Their Scope & Impact on Blood

Different groups of *āsana* help us in understanding the scope and depth of the body. They not only improve circulation but nourish and tone the body by eliminating toxins.

These different groups of *āsana* work in different ways to provide a mechanism for blood circulation to reach the arterial network of heart, lungs and brain for them to work efficiently which the modern day limited exercises cannot do. *Āsana* like *Śīrṣāsana, Sarvāṅgāsana, Setu Bandha Sarvāṅgāsana* and *Uttāna Padma Mayurāsana, Viparīta Daṇḍāsana, Pincha Mayurāsana* and *Adho Mukha Vṛkṣāsana* help in increasing the T-cells and B-cells (the T-cells are produced by the thymus gland and are involved in the immune response and the B-cells are the antibodies within the bloodstream.) These *āsana* affect and access different centres in the brain and body helping the immune system through increase or decrease of the circulation in the vascular system. The blood contains cells, plasma, water, salts, proteins and other debris and *āsana* as well as *prāṇāyāma* improve their quantity and the quality which is vitally important for sound health of the body and mind.

Take *Vīrāsana*. It effectively drains the blood from the legs and tones the quality of the blood vessels (arteries and veins) and then reorients the circulation in the legs and the hip region.

The thymus gland, known as the master gland of the immune system produces certain hormones said to stimulate T and B-cells and increases immunity against microbes and tumours. *Uttāna Padma Mayurāsana* has a direct impact on AIDS patients. T and B cells break the cholesterol in the blood flow. Even the spread of cancerous cells can be curtailed by strengthening the defence system through the improved quality of the blood.

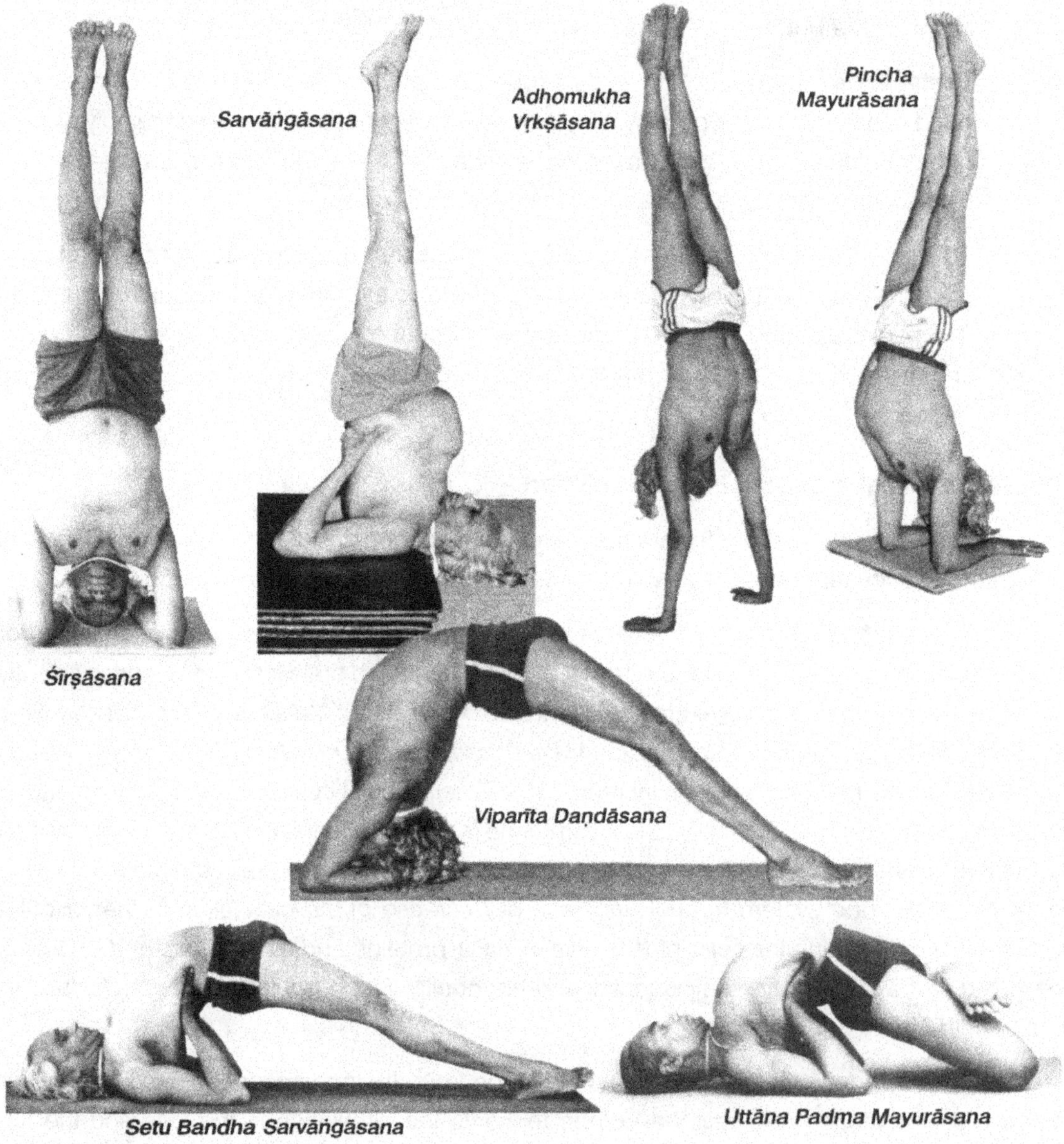
Sarvāṅgāsana
Adhomukha Vṛkṣāsana
Pincha Mayurāsana
Śīrṣāsana
Viparīta Daṇḍāsana
Setu Bandha Sarvāṅgāsana
Uttāna Padma Mayurāsana

Plate n. 15 – *Āsana* that help increase T-cells and B-cells

Glands	Effective *Āsana*
Pineal	Inversions
Pituitary	*Viparīta Daṇḍāsana,* other back bends & inversions
Thyroid / Parathyroid	*Sarvāṅgāsana, Halāsana* & variations
Thymus	Back bends & *Setu Bandha Sarvāṅgāsana*
Adrenals	*Uṣṭrāsana, Rājakapotāsana, Kapotāsana, Śīrṣāsana* (variations)
Pancreatic glands (Islets of Langerhans)	*Nāvāsana, Ubhaya Pādāṅguṣṭhāsana,* all forward bends, *Krounchāsana*
Generative glands	Inversions, back bends and seated, *Baddha Koṇāsana, Upaviṣṭha Koṇāsana*

Table n. 1 – *Āsana* effective for glands

You Become What You Eat and Think

The saying 'you are what you eat' is incomplete. Sometimes 'how you eat' becomes equally important. Actually even the mind behind the food that is prepared and consumed has some good consequence. Food made by the person who is pure in mind and served with love, affection and compassion, becomes *sāttvic.* Even *sāttvic* food may become non-nutritious and/ or poisonous when prepared with a vicious, wicked and crooked mind. Similarly one has to eat with a contented *(santoṣa)* mind. Therefore, one who cooks and serves as well as one who eats both need to have *śauca* – cleanliness in body and mind, contentment, with the feel of offering or sacrifice.[1]

Traditionally and ideally, the food prepared was made as an offering to the gods and eaten as *prasādam.* This ensured that the *yama* were naturally followed: one ate only the food which was congenial to yoga practice, and what the body could absorb easily *(ahiṁsā)* was eaten with a grateful heart *(satya-brahmacarya),* and the food was rightly earned through one's efforts *(asteya-aparigraha).*

In conclusion, everything from *āhāra-vihāra* and *ācāra-vicāra* should influence the blood within and ultimately for life-imprints. If the imprints have to be created by dint of yoga practice, you have to think and act to circulate the blood stream to bathe in pure blood throughout the body. See, this *ratna-pūrita-dhātu* is constantly enriched with right yogic practices so that it ultimately churns out the real jewel – the life force.

1 *śauca santoṣa tapaḥ svādhyāya Īśvarapraṇidhānāni niyamāḥ* (*Y.S.,* II.32) – cleanliness, contentment, religious zeal, self-study and surrender of the self to the supreme Self or God are the *niyama.*

WHAT IS *STHIRA SUKHAM ĀSANAM?**

Patañjali explains in *Yoga Sūtra* that the quality of an *āsana* in a very simple language as *sthirasukhamāsanam.* On the surface it means that *āsana* should be stable *(sthira)* and comfortable *(sukha)* in its presentation from the start to the end. When the *sādhaka* gets acclimatised to staying longer in any *āsana,* Patañjali says that he can proceed towards *prāṇāyāma* and from *prāṇāyāma* and *pratyāhāra* to *dhāraṇā, dhyāna* and *samādhi.*

As practitioners of *āsana* many of you may be facing difficulties that come in the way of learning. Not only do you feel stiffness of the body or pain in the back, knees, shoulders or spine but there are a number of obstacles that prevent you making any progress in practice.

I said that reading of the *sūtra* about *āsana* appears simple but its meaning has great depth. To learn and assimilate an *āsana* is undoubtedly a complex matter and to get the right feel of each *āsana* is not that easy at all.

First of all you should know that Patañjali has explained the characteristic *(dharmi)* of an *āsana* and not its character *(dharma).* You need to understand the difference between *dharmi* and *dharma. Dharmi* is like base gold. *Dharma* stands for various ornaments that are made from the base gold. Similarly while practising various *āsana* one has to come to its fundamental principles of the five elements, their counterparts, mind, intelligence and consciousness which have to be co-related and balanced evenly in all the five sheaths of the body, namely, skeletal, physiological, mental, intellectual and the self. When all these are properly balanced in an *āsana,* that *āsana* becomes *sthirasukham.*

In order to understand *sthira sukham* in *āsana,* you have to refer to so many other *sūtra* apart from the two *sūtra* concerning *āsana.* First is, *prayatnaśaithilya ananta samāpattibhyām* (*Y.S.,* II.47), the second is *tataḥ dvandvāḥ anabhighātaḥ* (*Y.S.,* II.48). It is for you as *sādhaka* to trace what are the things implicit and hidden in understanding to feel the meaning implicit in the *sūtra.*

---

* Talk given on Hanumān Jayanti day, 2007, Pune, India.

All the eight aspects of *aṣṭāṅga* yoga are interlinked and interdependent and as such you have to inter-relate to bring out the effect of each aspect of yoga. If one part of yoga loses its inter-relationship the other aspects go wrong.

Āsana has to be perfect if *prāṇāyāma* is to be performed well. If *dhāraṇā* is to happen *prāṇāyāma* has to be perfectly mastered. This is how the interlink goes on but often as *sādhaka* you do not link them. Hence I like to draw your attention to study think and re-think properly on each of the *sūtra* several times and put them into your *sādhanā* and see what experiences you derive.

Now new terms have surfaced. Hence re-thinking is essential to understand each *sūtra*. Also you have to think in order to understand the particular *sūtra* that you choose by connecting the ideas of other *sūtra* which communicate the meaning.

Sthirasukhamāsanam indicates not only the focus on our body and mind in each *āsana* but on the very being. Being comfortable in any *āsana* is a mis-representation of its meaning which may mislead you as practitioners.

While explaining nescience Patañjali speaks of *sukha anuśayśī rāgaḥ*. The *sukha* that is explained here is not the same *sukha* that he has dealt with while explaining *āsana*. Here, he says that this *sukha* leads towards attachment. When you are attached to things that you like then you like to derive happiness more and more and if that happiness does not come, then that leads towards *duhkhānuśayī dveśaḥ* which means unhappiness and envy.

I think many have taken the meaning of the *sukhatā* of the *āsana* to the *sukha* that leads towards attachments. Many of you are attached to the body and therefore you do not like the body to suffer from pain, hence you dislike the *āsana* and jump to something else. If *āsana* is pleasurable *(sukha)* you enjoy it but *sukha* is not the same as steadiness.

Patañjali uses three terms, *duḥkha*, *sukha* and *ānanda*. In the first chapter, *sūtra* 17, you come across the word *ananda*. You should know that there is a vast difference between the word *sukha* and *ānanda*. *Sukha* means comfort and pleasing while *ānanda* means delight, joy and bliss. Normally we mix up these words and treat *sukha* and *ānanda* as happiness. *Sukha* is felt at the level of the senses while *ānanda* is a spiritual quality. While performing *āsana* the *sukha* conveys the feel of pleasing sensation as *rāga* or attachment. *Ānanda* is an unbiased happiness or delight in the self. In *āsana*, *sthira* and *sukha* both stand for *ānanda* on the spiritual level.

No doubt many of you take to yoga as you have attachment to the body. You dislike pain in *sādhanā*. Many of you are satisfied with your practices as long as you feel comfortable. This is considered as fulfilment of desires. You continue the practice as long as this comfort remains, but the moment the comfort fades out you give up.

Some come to yoga to get rid of their diseases. When they get alright, they give up. In both cases the involvement is in seeking pleasure. Obviously such *sādhaka* cannot experience the real meaning of *sthiratā* or *sukhatā* which should sprout from the self as *ānanda*. Sometimes you may achieve *ānanda* in the *āsana* and suddenly if some unpleasant sensations arise, you get frightened. It is all in your frame of mind. Practising *āsana* within the sphere of the mind is *sukha* and practising beyond the sphere of the mind is *ānanda* or unbiased bliss – joy. Therefore *sukhatā* in *āsana* is not merely a sense of comfort or a non-painful state. You have to seek *ānanda* or the blissfulness in the self and not in the senses.

The word *sthiratā* means stability, firmness, steadfastness, permanency, lasting, calmness, quiescent and composed. To stay in the *āsana* without oscillating the contents that are within the body is stability. For me *sukhatā* and *sthiratā* are realised when you bring the self to establish and cover the entire body in performing the *āsana*. Then it is *sthirasukhamāsanam* as it leads you to experience *tadā draṣṭuḥ svarūpe avasthānam* (*Y.S.*, I.3). This should happen in each *āsana*. When I am in *āsana* I establish my self in each and every part of my body. I make the self to ring its bell expressing that it is present everywhere. This is *svarūpa-pratiṣṭhā* as far as my understanding of the *sūtra* conveys. This is *sthairya* for me in my practice of *āsana*. When my self is benevolently established in its entire frontier without any deviation or contortion in the *āsana*, I consider it as *sthirasukhamāsanam*.

The succeeding *sūtra* after the definition of *āsana* is *prayatnaśaithilya ananta samāpattibhyām*. *Prayatna* means effort and *śaithilya* means laxity. This is another word which creates an idea of stretching and relaxing. If stretching and relaxing is understood like that, then does it convey stability or oscillation? For me it conveys effortless effort. When the effortful effort fades out, effortless effort sets in. This is *prayatnaśaithilya*. If *prayatnaśaithilya* means stretching and relaxing in each *āsana*, then it should apply to *prāṇāyāma*, *pratyāhāra*, *dhāraṇā*, *dhyāna* and *samādhi*. But does it happen?

Regarding *prayatnaśaithilya*, Vyāsa says, *prayatna uparānt siddyati iti āsanam yena na aṅgamejaya bhavati*.[1] *Aṅgamejayatva* is shakiness of the body to which Patañjali refers in the first chapter under the topic impediments causing the distractions (*Y.S.*, I.31). When there are impediments or sickness, the body shakes, the nerves throb, the breath goes fast and fear sets

1 By relaxation of effort, the *āsana* is perfected by which there is no trembling of the body.

in. *Asthira* and *asukha* end only when effortful effort transforms into effortless effort. Just laxity in effort does not convey *sthira sukham.* But *prayatnaśaithilya* has to terminate in *anantasamāpatti. Ananta* is the soul. *Samāpatti* is the transformation in which *citta* gets transformed to its original pure form. This *sūtra* is proof enough to know that *āsana* is not limited to the physical level and it should not be looked at on the physical level only. See the difference between present day commentators and the commentators like Vyāsa.

We have got five *vṛtti* and five *kleśa.* The *kleśa* entangled not only you and me but the wise men also. Among the *kleśa* namely, *avidyā, asmitā, rāga, dveṣa* and *abhiniveśa,* the last one is to be underlined since it does not leave even the wisest of the wise. *Svarasavahī viduṣaḥ api tatha ārūḍhaḥ abhiniveśaḥ* (*Y.S.,* II.9). Here he uses the word *viduṣaḥ api,* which means – "even the scholars (*viduṣaḥ* is a learned, wise and scholarly man) are affected easily", by this *kleśa* but the next *sūtra* suggests that even the *vivekin* (who has attained discriminating wisdom) is also affected.

Again Patañjali repeats that *pariṇāma tāpa saṁskāra duḥkhaiḥ guṇavṛtti virodhāt ca duḥkham eva sarvaṁ vivekinaḥ* (*Y.S.,* II.15) – The wise man knows that owing to the fluctuations, the qualities of nature, subliminal impressions and pleasant experiences are tinged with sorrow. So he keeps aloof from them. Hence a *vivekin* trains to keep himself aloof from pains and pleasures practising the eight aspects of yoga continuously without interruption.

In referance to *avidyā* as *kleśa* and *nidrā* as *vṛtti,* the states of *avidyā* and *nidrā* lack any feel or sensitivity. As *avidyā* or nescience keeps one in the dark, the feel of non-beingness in sleep keeps one in the dark. People are almost numb and dumb in *avidyā* and *nidrā.* Similarly *pariṇāma-duḥkha, tāpa-duḥkha* and *saṁskāra-duḥkha* keep people in the dark. When you are soaked in *duḥkha* you remain in an insensitive state.

Identifying the instrument of the power of seeing as the real Seer is pride, says Patañjali (*Y.S.,* II.6). It is also a sign of insensitivity. How many of us express the *ahaṁkāra* when we are practising *āsana?* Is this not a perverse *(viparyaya)* and illusory knowledge on *āsana?* Have you ever seen the *āsana* with *pratyakṣa pramāṇa* i.e., direct perception with conception and experience? As such *pratyakṣa pramāṇa* has to be the highest goal in the presentation of *āsana* so that each and every part factually intimates the self exist and feel in each and every part of its territory – the body, both within and without. When one does the *āsana* some parts are in the *nidrā* state, some parts remain in the state of memory *(smṛti).* Many of you like to practise and continue to live with past experience not caring to see and live in the present state. One projects the knowledge of *viparyaya* in *āsana* at certain parts while on some parts one oscillates with the illusory knowledge of *vikalpa.* Some do not want to go beyond their frame of reference due to fear complexes while others like to go beyond the frame of mind and experiences.

For example when I ask people to stand on the edge of the stage or a stool for *Uttānāsana*, they fear that they may topple before knowing whether they topple or not. First one has to try before coming to any conclusion. Therefore, while practising the *āsana*, one has to be free from *vṛtti* and *kleśa* except *pratyakṣa-vṛtti* to understand the *sthiratā* and *sukhatā* of the *āsana*.

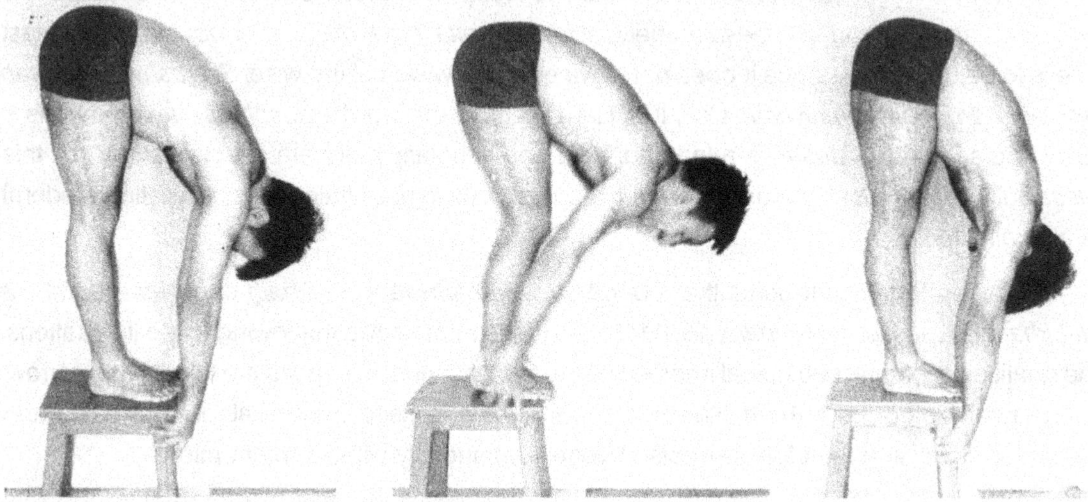

Plate n. 16 - Fear of toppling in *Uttānāsana*

Why I am saying this is because attachment *(rāga)*, hatred *(dveṣa)*, sorrow *(duḥkha)*, fear *(bhaya)* may lead one towards psychosomatic diseases which need to be avoided. Practice of *āsana* must be in such a way that one does not feel the separate existence of the body or the mind.[1] Then the result of doing like this brings an end to the division between body and mind, mind and intelligence, and intelligence and Self.

As I have said earlier that the base for *yoga sādhanā* is covered in *Sādhana Pāda* (*sūtra* 19 and 20), practice of *āsana* and *prāṇāyāma* melt the principles of nature for the soul to establish itself on its own. It means that you as practitioners move from *prakṛti jñāna* towards *puruṣa jñāna*.

As the tree grows from a seed into a tree, so does the tree of *prakṛti* . *Puruṣa* only witnesses. Though *puruṣa* is pure it sees without questioning whatever has been done by *prakṛti*. That is why the whole and sole responsibility falls on *prakṛti*. We have to deal with *prakṛti* as Patañjali refers to it in the third chapter (*sūtra* 45 to 50), where he speaks of *bhūtajaya*,

---

1 *tato dvandvānabhighātaḥ* (*Y.S.*, II.48). - from then on, the practitioner is undisturbed by dualities and is fit to begin *prāṇāyāma*

tanmātrajaya, śarīrajaya, indriyajaya and *manojaya* for the seer to attain supreme knowledge of all that exists and all that manifests.

Sthūla svarūpa sūkṣma anvaya arthavatva saṁyamāt bhūtajayaḥ (*Y.S.* III.45);[1] *tataḥ aṇimādi prādurbhāvaḥ kāyasaṁpat taddharma anabhighātaḥ ca* (*Y.S.,* III.46).[2] Here, he has control over *tanmātra.* Then perfect control on body: *rūpa lāvaṇya bala vajra saṁhananatvāni kāyasaṁpat* (*Y.S.,* III.47),[3] and *grahaṇa svarūpa asmitā anvaya arthavattva saṁyamāt indriyajayaḥ* (*Y.S.* III.48).[4] First he speaks of *bhūtajaya* which belongs to *viśeṣa parva. Parva* means a joint in the body or a section. Then he comes to the atomic qualities of nature and *ahaṁkāra (aviśeṣa parva)* and speaks about the body *(kāyasaṁpat)* which is again a section of nature *(viśeṣa parva).* Later he climbs down to hold the senses of perception *(indriya)* under control and then the *manas.* He says the moment the mind *(manas)* comes under control the *mahat* is under control, and when the *mahat* comes under control, then the *ātmā* shines on its own. *Tato manōjavitvaṁ vikaraṇabhāvaḥ pradhānajayaḥ ca* (*Y.S.,* III.49).[5] But we find it hard to capture the words of Patañjali where he guides us to understand *prakṛti* and *puruṣa.* In *Sādhana Pāda* he guides with what to look at in order to undergo *sādhanā* and in *Vibhūti Pāda* he speaks of where the *sādhanā* leads the *sādhaka.*

The question is not about conquest and accomplishments. The question is about what one acquires in the *āsana.* He acquires the four-fold evolutory process of *prakṛti (viśeṣa, aviśeṣa, liṅgamātra* and *aliṅga).* See how important the *āsana* and *prāṇāyāma* are to bring the parts of *prakṛti* under control. Today the *sādhaka* has totally forgotten the advice given by Patañjali on *tapas, svādhyāya* and *Īśvara praṇidhāna.* No one has the zeal or the burning desire or ambition to penetrate the depth of the subject in order to trace what is hidden in *sādhanā.* One's mind should be blazing when one is practising.

How many of us know and practice the *āsana* as they should be done? Each *āsana* has to be arithmetically calculated like addition, subtraction, multiplication and division. Each *āsana* has a form and shape. Each part of the muscle fibre, bone or tissue of the body has to take the formation that is needed according to the architectural demand of the *āsana,* but never

---

[1] By *saṁyama* on the elements – their mass, forms, subtlety, conjunction and purposes, the *yogi* becomes Lord over them all.

[2] The *paramāṇu* of *bhūta* and *ahaṁkāra* comes under control.

[3] Perfection of body consisting of beauty, grace, strength and compactness sets in.

[4] Through *saṁyama* upon the purpose of the conjunction of the process of knowing, the ego and nature, there is mastery over the senses.

[5] By mastery over the senses of perception, the *yogi's* speed of body, senses and mind matches that of the soul independent of the primary causes of nature. Unaided by consciousness, he subdues the first principle of nature *(mahat).*

adjust the *āsana* to the convenient flexibility of the body. Many of us practise *āsana* according to the behavioural pattern of the body making the mind accept as it presents but never give time for the mind to question whether the body is sending a right or a wrong message according to the name of the *āsana*. One does not allow the intelligence to think and discriminate whether the five sheaths of the practitioner *(annamaya, prāṇamaya, manomaya, vijñānamaya, ānandamaya)* are rightly connected and measured by the intelligence to balance these sheaths in concordance with each other.

Take *Śirṣāsana*. *Śirṣāsana* is nothing but a reverse *Tāḍāsana*. How many apply their minds and intelligence to perform *Śīrṣāsana* like *Tāḍāsana* maintaining all the qualities of *Tāḍāsana*, I am also not sure how many perform *Śīrṣāsana* in plumb line to the floor?

Take *Utthita Trikoṇāsana*. It literally means a triangular *āsana*. According to the dictionary a triangle means a figure with three straight sides and three angles or a thing shaped like a triangle. It also stands for right-angled triangle. The very *āsana* name signifies three-sided base giving the clue that the three sides of the body represent the unequivocal exactitude directing the three forces to function and act equally.

Look at *Utthita Trikoṇāsana*, you can see three lines or the borders of the body in a straight line yet forming three right-angled triangles.

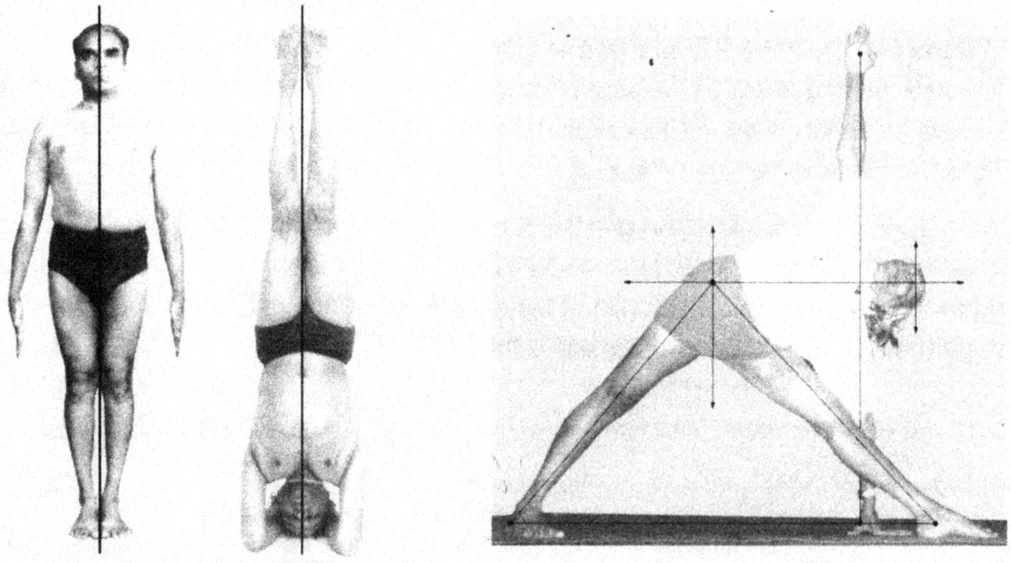

Tāḍāsana Śīrṣāsana Utthita Trikoṇāsana

Plate n. 17 – *Śīrṣāsana* as reverse *Tāḍāsana*, and the three triangles of *Utthita Trikoṇāsana*

I did not invent the word alignment, it is Lord Krishna, Yogeshvara (The Lord of Yoga) who has used the word alignment in Chapter 6.13 of the *Bhagavad Gītā*, *samam kāya śirogrīvam dhārayan acalam sthiraḥ*.[1] He has given a plumb line of the body to perform each *āsana* or an *āsana* to sit for *dhyāna*. These are the crown of the head, well of the throat and the perineum as plumb line. This means that each and every part of our body must be measured from the centre of the body and maintained in its bank. He uses the *samaṁkāya*. If one does the *āsana* with this guide of Lord Krishna there is no contortion, no distortion. The body does not go crooked, muscles do not get tilted. When one stands in *Tāḍāsana*, certain muscles work to bring stability. When one does *Śīrṣāsana* the very same muscles oscillate, causing change in the *āsana* though one says, "I am doing the *āsana* well". But are we keeping the body in that plumb line which is the centre of the right side and left side? This is what Lord Krishna demands. It is not that Mr. Iyengar demands precision. He says, *samatvam yoga ucyate*, (*B.G.*, II.48). Again, he says that there should be equanimity. Equanimity cannot happen without the techniques of alignment in body, senses, mind, intelligence and self. One can develop this in the art of adjustment in *āsana* which turns into auspicious action. Instead of attachment to *āsana* one has to become the *āsana*. In order to get that equanimity *(samatvam)* one needs *kuśalatā* or adequate skilfulness, *Yogaḥ karmasu kauśalam (B.G.*, II.50).[2] There should be skilfulness in action and that skilfulness of action cannot come unless one rubs with his mind and intelligence to gain alingment. This is actually *svādhyāya*.

There has to be a rub between body, organs of the senses, intelligence and the self. In order to rub one should be devoted. Devotion to the subject and *Īśvara*, a *sarvajña* (omniscient) is *Īśvara praṇidhāna*. Today the surrendering part is forgotten. This vital vehicle of yoga is superseded in commercialising the subject. The urge to yoga as *tapas* is disappearing. Ways of using *sādhanā* for *svādhyāya* have remained in the text books and not in practice. We treat the body as a master and follow according to its current.

We have lost the sense of balance and harmony. For example when you do *Uttānāsana*, you press one hand strongly but do not think of the other hand. Hence the mind is shifted to the stronger side. As the mind follows the right hand you never think of shifting the weight towards the left side in order to bring alignment and harmony. Give a thought through observation to correct the wrongs then alignment comes. Without right alignment you cannot get a composed state in body and mind. If this composed state is brought through observation action and

---

1 One has to hold the body straight and steady in line to the middle of the head, middle of the throat and the perineum in a plumb line.

2 Adequate skilfulness and concord without attachment and to maintain an undisturbed state of mind whether in success or failure is called *samatva* yoga.

alignment then automatically devotion *(bhakti)* sets in. When I say, "precision is God" this is what I mean - the precision of alignment at all levels is for me God.

The precision is that in which each and every part, every tissue and division in the muscles are retained and maintained in their positions. Hence one has to begin learning and knowing more about the body.

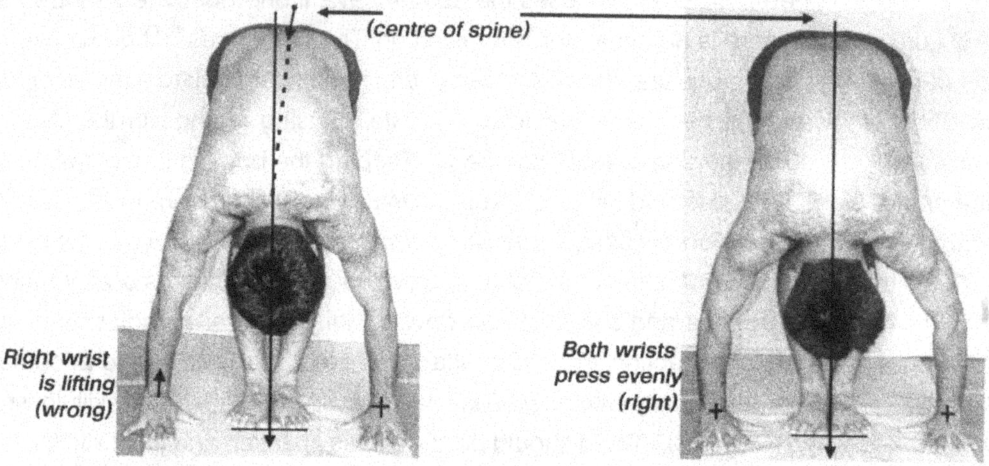

Plate n. 18 - *Uttānāsana*

We are made of *pañcabhūta* - five elements - earth, water, fire, air and ether. Bone is of the earth and air elements. The muscles are also of the earth element, but *medas* converts the earth nature of the muscles into the nature of *āp tattva* or water element. Then the one which makes the muscles to move or extend or contract is *tejas tattva.* The muscles touch the earth element, bone and the element of ether, the skin. Though the skin is of the air element, the exposure of the skin is *ākāśa tattva.* I am using the word which may confuse when I say that the skin belongs to the *ākāśa tattva* along with *vāyu tattva.* The skin is in contact with the *ākāśa tattva* as it is in contact with the macrocosm *(brahmāṇḍa)* or cosmic intelligence *(mahat tattva)* and *citta* is in contact with *cidākāśa* or microcosm *(piṇḍāṇḍa).* It means that *brahmāṇḍa* unites with *piṇḍāṇḍa* and viceversa.

The skin plays a great role in learning *āsana* and *prāṇāyāma.* The skin belongs to the element of ether/space. As the character of *vāyu,* being the sense of touch *(sparśa),* it is the skin that feels the touch. Apart from touch the skin is also stretchable. Space has the quality of expansion, contraction and power to create room, and what creates room belongs to the element of space. Based on this analogy, I say the skin belongs to the *ākāśa tattva* - the external sphere of space - the *mahadākaśa.* *Cit* belongs to the inner space. When you do the *āsana* you have to connect the inner space with the outer space and outer space with the inner space. Actually you are not doing the *āsana* as it should be done according to Patañjali.

When Patañjali speaks on *prāṇāyāma,* he explains *abhyantara-vṛtti, bāhya-vṛtti* and *stambha-vṛtti.* But it is for you to think as to how to interpret this in *āsana.* In *prāṇāyāma abhyantara* or *antara-vṛtti* is inhalation. In *āsana* it means going into the position by bringing the outer body close to the inner body. To remain in *āsana* in a non-disturbed state is *abhyantara-stambha vṛtti,* commonly known as *antara kumbhaka.* To release the *āsana* or to come out of *āsana* with a rhythm is *bāhya-vṛtti* in *āsana, bāhya-stambha-vṛtti* comes after exhalation. Coming out of the *āsana* and then to remain in a non-disturbed state is *bāhya-stambha-vṛtti.* In *kumbhaka* one should keep the body firm and the mind in a non-oscillating state. This firm body and non-oscillating mind *(stambha-vṛtti)* is *sthiratā.* This *sthiratā* of the *āsana* stands for *stambha vṛtti* of *prāṇāyāma.* In order to go advertently to the *āsana* is *antara-vṛtti,* and coming out from the *āsana* advertently is *bāhya-vṛtti.* This is how one has to know the connection between *āsana* and *prāṇāyāma.* Even *deśa, kāla* and *saṁkhyā* which are referred to in the context of *prāṇāyāma* are to be adopted in *āsana.* In *āsana* practice the body *(deśa)* is the field *(kṣetra).* The duration of stay in the *āsana* is *kāla* or *stambha-vṛtti.* As *saṁkhyā* stands for quality, staying in the *āsana* should be such that there must be beauty in the formation of the *āsana,* elegance, compactness and firmness. Even after you release from the *āsana,* the feel of that equanimity has to be continued even after the *āsana* practice. The right way of presentation of an *āsana* should be such that the right hand and leg or the left hand and leg should not vary in stretch, girth and weight. All dualities, deformities, differences and disparities in the various parts of the body have to be attended to and removed. The mind has to express its presence in each and every pore of the skin without oscillation or deviation. This is *saṁkhyā.*

How many of you use equal pressure while doing lateral movements of the trunk in *Marichyāsana* III? Do you use equal pressure in gripping or clasping? Do you observe that one hand holds firmly while the other hand remains loose? Yet you proudly say that you are doing *Marichyāsana* as it should be presented. It is the same with *Ardha Matsyendrāsana.* One hand is in *nidrāvasthā* while the other is in *jagṛtāvasthā.* As such how can you pride yourselves that you are stable in these *āsana?* You do *Marichyāsana* with the right hand entwining the left knee. The right arm-pit does not cover the entire knee and the tilt in the spine sinks the chest on one side and makes the spine narrow, instead of keeping the right and left side of the spinal column straight and parallel to each other without stooping. You do not see how many parts you disturb for the armpit to entwine the knee. Often you do these movements with parts distorting the entire structure at the base of the body. You have to work in order to bring the entire body as a whole to act in harmony between all its parts. Then only that action is considered as a benevolent action in the *āsana*. This is actual consecration of the *āsana*. If the action is distorted, how can that *āsana* be called benevolent? It is the same with *Ardha Matsyendrāsana*, *Pāśāsana* and *Paripūrṇa Matsyendrāsana*.

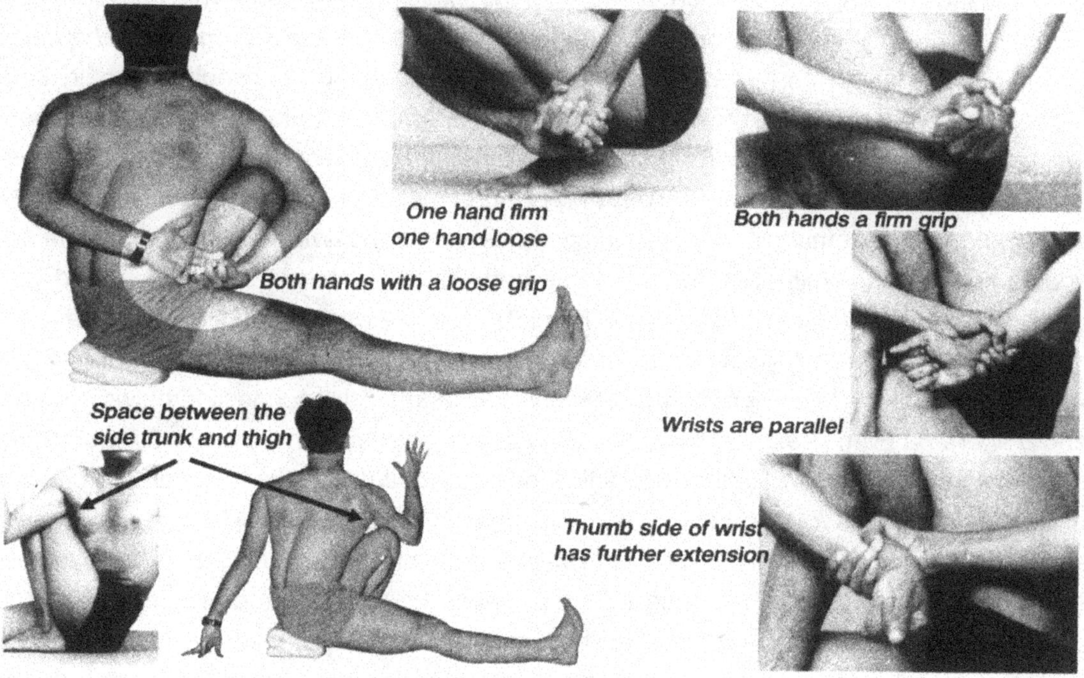

Plate n. 19 – The hands that grip in twisting *āsana*.

Take *Ardha Matsyendrāsana*. You sit exactly on the middle of the foot. The moment you take the hand up to clasp the knee you disturb the position of the buttocks and tilt them as the mind oscillates at that time. This oscillated mind disturbs the position of the body which in turn dislocates the intelligence and the state of the Self. Wrong presentation of *āsana* dislodges the position of intelligence, consciousness and the core.

Unfortunately many do not understand that they have non-deliberately moved and disturbed the needed establishment at the starting point itself. This unnoticed disturbance at the very source point brings disturbed and crooked movements, curving the mind, intelligence and consciousness along with the self. Some may do deliberately but do not give a thought to come back to the source point soon. Only you are sensitive to pain but never give a thought as to whether the body, senses, mind, intelligence and consciousness are rightly and properly established or not. You want to do the *āsana* to remain in a painless state without paying attention to the perfection of the *āsana*. You hate pain and love the painless state because of your attachment to the body. Protection of oneself is the cause for non-attention in presenting the right *āsana* which may become a cause to invite diseases later. In case I get pain, I take it as a boon and study where I went wrong. It awakens my intelligence and guides me informing me that somewhere I am wrong for this pain to occur. My five elements *(bhūta)* talk to me while doing the *āsana*. They communicate with me. They open my sensitivity and feelings and charge me to re-think from the bone to the skin making my energy and intelligence to communicate from the cells to the self and from the self to the cells in each *āsana* to bring *samatvam* in each and every part evenly from the centre. This is *tejas tattva*. My *tejas* wakes up my energy and awareness to move my body with attention. Wherever I feel the liveliness, I know the knowledge *(vidyā)* is there. Where I do not feel I take it to heart that, that part is filled with *avidyā* and *ajñāna* in that *āsana*. *Avidyā* means *ajñāna* and *ajñāna* means *avidyā*. Many of you do the *āsana* but do not know how to use *jñāna*. You are in the dark and therefore you are blank. Yet you pride yourself that you practise with perfection. What an irony! While doing the *āsana* you are aware a bit here and a bit there. You use *prajñāna* on the side you are active and show *ajñāna* where your body does not respond or send messages. Still you claim that you have done the *āsana* well. Do not count health, peace and lightness as the aim of yoga. These are all within the frame of the mind. Go beyond the mind whilst practising *āsana*.

Āsana is a balancing art. Like walking on a tight-rope it has to balance the senses, mind, intelligence, consciousness, conscience and the self to be in line with the body or viceversa. As the river with its tributaries runs within its two banks, the various tributaries of the *prakṛti* and the self are made to flow within the banks of the skin and consciousness without any deviation. When *prāṇa* and *prajñā* flow together in each *āsana* then dualities and deviations fade out. This is how the *āsana* have to be done.

Now, I hope you understand that you have to bring the *pañcabhūta*, *pañcaprāṇa* and *saptaprajñā* touching *(sparśa)* the muscle and the bone, the flesh and bone with the mind, mind with intelligence, intelligence with consciousness, and consciousness with the self.

People do brand me as an *āsana* man. But can they measure with all their intellect what *āsana* has taught me? It has taught me to understand and realise *viśeṣa*, *aviśeṣa*, *liṅgamātra*, *aliṅga* and *draṣṭā*. I remove the seed of defect *(doṣa bīja)* in my *sādhanā*. I watch my right side, left side. I watch whether I am in the centre. I treat all the ten directions of my body – east, west, south, north, north east, north west, south east, south west, *ūrdhva* (upward), *adhara* (downward) evenly while doing any *āsana*. I bring the energy *(prāṇa)* to spread in all the ten directions of the body and make the awareness *(prajñā)* to flow evenly concurring with energy *(prāṇa)*. I make the self travel in each *āsana* to occupy even the remotest part of my body measuring from the centre – the real SELF. I embank *(digbandha)* in all directions of my body for the self to rest in its abode in each *āsana* so that nothing enters in or goes out to disturb it. I make my body as a cave wherein I am alone and alive to everything.

When you do *Śīrṣāsana* again, watch what I said. You may re-work and re-adjust to experience what I have explained in each *āsana*. The earth element, the bone *(asthi)*, is the foundation in the body. If the foundation is strong not only do you get rid of problems but feed the bone-marrow by the muscles making them to move towards the bone. When you watch the diseased person you realise what I am talking about. These subtle actions cannot be described in technical terms. When the action is done with total awareness, prudence and insight, then the *āsana* happens. It is unfortunate that healthy people do not realise and the diseased do not understand. *Yogāsana* is not meant for curing diseases. It is not the main aim but a by-product of yoga. True that I am having remedial classes. I welcome them to induce them later towards the essence of yoga.

If a child does not do homework the mother says, "You finish your homework and I'll give you a chocolate or I'll give you what you like or whatever you want". This way the mother tempts the child to do homework. Yoga also needs to be introduced in that manner. People suffer. So I give them remedial classes like a chocolate relieving their pain so that they get interest to know more of yoga.

Unfortunately what is happening is that even healthy people take advantage and come for small petty pains and problems. They have tasted the chocolate of yoga which is health and peace, but they do not proceed further to taste the essence of yoga. This pains me because there is no real thirst for yoga in them. I see that even advanced students who have practised for thirty years or more have no devotion or dedication to go into the depth of the subject. Today people in large numbers attend yoga camps *(śibira)* which are run for a few days. Can anyone learn such a sacred art in a matter of days?

It is like a man searching for a lost ring under the streetlights when another person who sees him enquires what he is searching for. As he continues to search the crowd assembles inventing their own stories. Finally, one wise man makes his way to reach the first one who was searching for his ring which he lost in his backyard. The wise man asks him "Why are you searching here?" At which he replies that he has no light in his backyard and that is why he is searching here. This is exactly what happens in yoga camps *(yoga-śibira)*.

It is true that yoga helps one to get rid of imbalances but this is a limited aim in the field of yoga.

The moment birth takes place strains, sorrows, pain and joy are bound to be there. Only weak minds make big problems of such things. *Āsana* makes the mind come out from the pit of these impediments and builds up attention for steadiness in mind and intelligence to endure all shortcomings without becoming a victim of these pains and sorrows.

Do not practise for the pleasantness of the mind *(sukha)*. Remember *sukhānuśayi rāgaḥ*. Let not your aim to practise be restricted to removing pain. Let the aim in practice be to experience oneness in body, mind and self. Understand and reach that level where you remove differences between body and mind, mind and intelligence and intelligence and self. You have to experience this non-dualistic state. Continue *sādhanā* in order to remove the impurities and the essence of knowledge to radiate in glory, *yogāṅgānuṣṭhānāt aśuddhikṣaye jñānadīptiḥ āvivekakhyāteḥ* (*Y.S.*, II.28). Like the rays of the sun which cleanse the atmosphere, let your intellectual light through yoga remove the darkness that covers the intellect of the head and intelligence of the heart.

First of all you do not know how the body functions, how the *indriya* function, how the mind plays and how the intelligence oscillates. The body is called *pāñcabhautika śarīra*. Hence conquer these five *bhūta* so that the mind gets freed from the attachment of the body for you to proceed towards the higher and finer states of the consciousness. I have spoken in the earlier volumes about *citta*[1] and I want you all to re-read and remember them so that it becomes easy to understand while practising the *āsana*.

Whatever *āsana* you do, see that your intelligence *(prajñā)* is lighting each and every part of your body. The moment the light fades out you have to light again through attentive *sādhanā*.

Let me give you an example of how awareness unknowingly makes you inattentive. When you do *Śīrṣāsana* I have seen keeping your fingers advertently but the moment you place the head on the floor, the index finger goes far away from the pit. Is it not in-attention? This means that your mind moved according to the wind of your body. You forgot at once the positioning of the fingers and do not recollect how you joined your fingers. You do not know that the fingers got loose in the grip. So quick is the loss of memory *(smṛti-bhraṁśa)*. *Śīrṣāsana* is an inverted *āsana; Sarvāṅgāsana* is also an inverted *āsana*. How is it that you never observe how the grip of the muscles vary in touching the bone in *Śīrṣāsana* or in *Sarvāṅgāsana*? Do you know how the muscles of the legs move in *Śīrṣāsana* and how they move in *Sarvāṅgāsana?* Many of you just do *Śīrṣāsana* or *Sarvāṅgāsana*. You do not even know whether the posterior tailbone or the anterior tailbone is long. Here comes *antara-indriya-jñāna*. You have to awaken through the outer body, the inner body. It means that you have to move from *bāhyendriya*

---

[1] See *Aṣṭadaḷa Yogamālā*, vol. 1, p. 237, and vol. 2, p. 54.

towards *antaraṅga indriya.* The journey towards *antarāṅga* begins as the *bahirāṅga* touches the *antara indriya.* Do not get caught in *sukhānuśayi rāgaḥ.* If your attachment is to the knee then you are only on the knee. If it is painful, *duḥkhānuśayi dveṣaḥ,* then you begin to dislike the pain in the knee and get rid of it working on it at once. Watch your elbows while doing *Śīrṣāsana* though you place them accurately. The moment you go into *Śīrṣāsana* they shift. One elbow remains close to you while the other goes far away from you. The parts which are close to your mind play the role of *rāga.* As you do not pay any attention to the far away elbow, there is *dveṣa* though you do not mean it as *dveṣa.* You think your muscles are formed for it to go out, which you may think as *sukha* (attachment), but in it is a hidden *dveṣa* or hatred. So judge in *sādhanā* without love or hate, and cross these barriers.

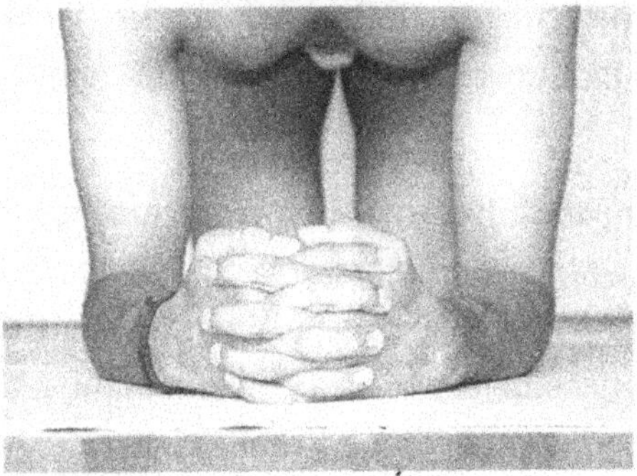

Interlocked fingers for Śirṣāsana

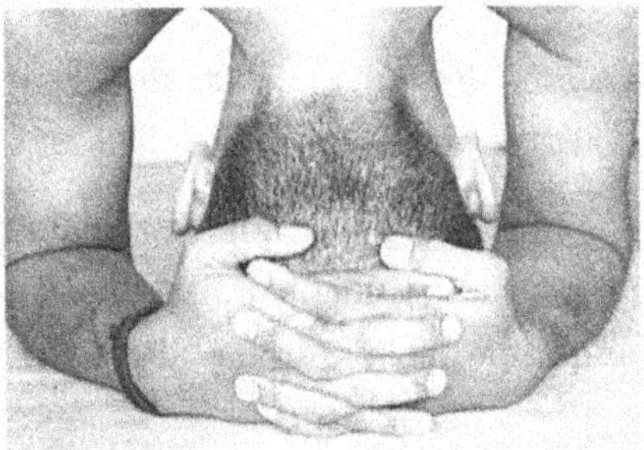

.... becomming loose while going to the āsana

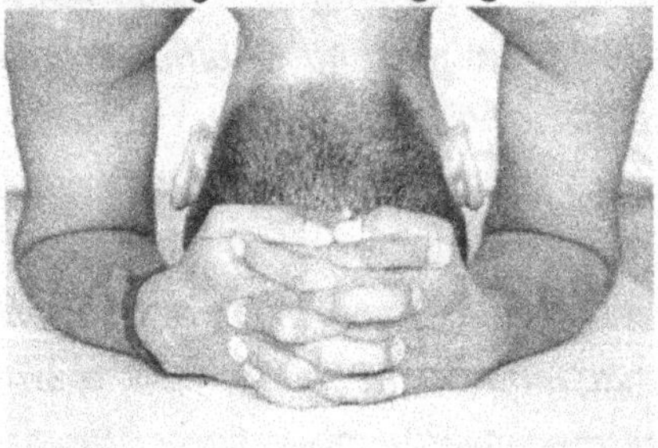

Established firmly without shaking in the āsana

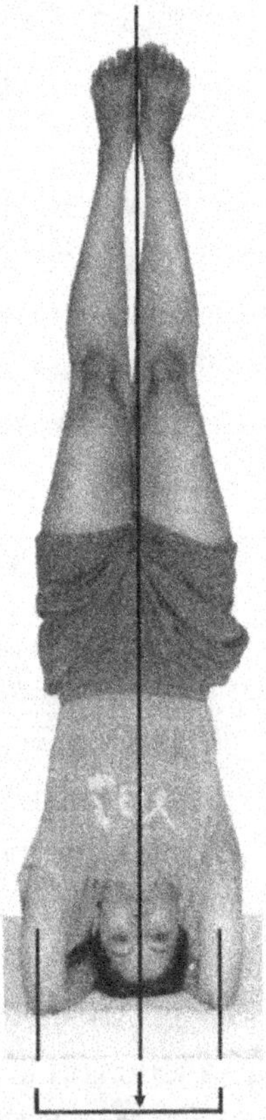

Elbows move going to the āsana

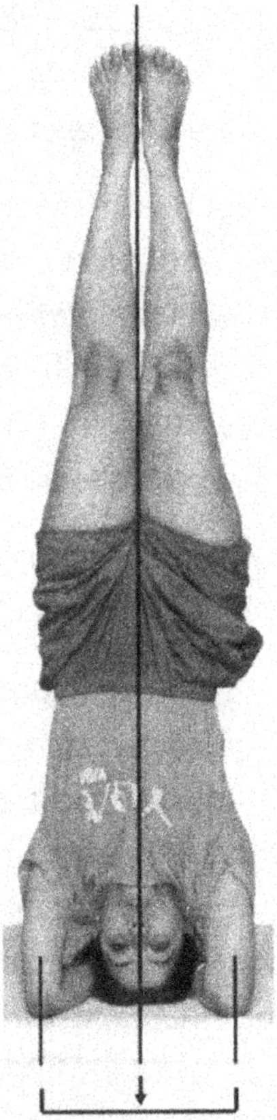

Remain an even distance from the centre line

Plate n. 20 – Tilt of interlock fingers and elbows in *Śīrṣāsana*

From now on do *Śīrṣāsana* and *Sarvāṅgāsana* observing all the things that I explained so far. Then I tell you that you experience auspiciousness and holiness in these *āsana*. If holes appear in your practices, remove the holes at once so that wholeness leads you towards holiness and auspiciousness. In perfect presentation of an *āsana* there is stability in body, mind, intelligence and consciousness. As such it becomes an auspicious moment. This is the true experience of *prayatna śaithilya ananta samāpattibhyām* (*Y.S.,* II.47).

I enlightened you in the field of yoga, especially on *āsana*. know your body is universal, your contents in the body are universal and yoga too is a universal subject. As *ātman* is impersonal, yoga also is impersonal. But only the mind expresses its individuality and in order to transform the individual mind into a universal mind, practise yoga to transform that mind towards universal entity.

ON *PRĀṆĀYĀMA*

Prāṇāyāma has become a fascinating subject these days because of its supply of oxygen. But *prāṇāyāma* is the most intricate subject and people are attracted without having any background of the subject. I do not know whether it has become a fashion without passion. It is like the blind leading the blind.

I don't know whether *prāṇāyāma's* new popularity is for the good or not but it is happening. When I started to teach *prāṇāyāma* in the classes I made everyone to do *Śavāsana* with relaxing techniques for a long time for quietening the mind and nerves so that they derive maximum benefit from *prāṇāyāma*.

Before *Śavāsana* I used to make them do certain *āsana* to bring elasticity in their lungs. I used to technically explain the qualitative effects of *dhyāna* in the language they could be understood in *Śavāsana*. Through these techniques I was quietening the brain and nerves for be fit for *prāṇāyāma* practice.

Actually, through these explanations for over twenty years the feed-back I got from them made me to undertake to write a book on *prāṇāyāma* – *Light on Prāṇāyāma*.[1]

Today *prāṇāyāma* is taught and practised without preparing the elasticity in the lungs, softness in the nerves and silence in the brain and mind. Practice of *prāṇāyāma* requires a great deal of enduring patience.

Even lots of people who approach our institute demand from us that we teach *prāṇāyāma* only and if we tell them that they have to undergo training in *āsana*, they quietly go away saying that they are only interested to learn *prāṇāyāma*.

They enquire as if *prāṇāyāma* is a buyable commodity like goods sold in the market place. They do not know the a, b, c or d of yoga and crazily ask us to teach *Kapālabhāti* or *Bhastrikā* or *Uḍḍiyāna* saying that they would like to awaken the *kuṇḍalinī* at once.

---

[1] Published by Harper Collins, London.

Even in television programmes these kinds of *prāṇāyāma* are taught where hundreds follow without observing the moral principles of *prāṇāyāma*.

First of all the moral or ethical principles of *prāṇāyāma* are to prepare the spine to be firm and mobile by removing the restrictions in the intercostal muscles of the ribs and lungs. They do not keep the brain as a witness to observe the lungs and chest. Yet people jump towards learning *prāṇāyāma*. They want the flower to bloom before the plant has grown.

In my time the custom was that *śiṣya* were staying with the *guru* for years and years and the *guru* was imparting the knowledge only when they realised the *śiṣya* were fit for subtle studies. They were postponing, mentioning that they were still raw in order to measure their patience. First the *guru* used to study the standard of the pupil to know when to give the knowledge. Then the *guru* decided what we were to do as *śiṣya*. Today it is reversed. The *guru* is available for the simple reason that he surrenders to the dictates of the students and is ready to teach them. Pupils choose on their own according to their tastes like flipping a coin.

The attention and caution that are needed for *prāṇāyāma* is not attended to at all.

Patañjali says, *sa tu dirghakāla nairantarya satkāra āsevito dṛdhabhumiḥ* (*Y.S.*, I.14) – years and years of practice make the foundation in yoga firm. Now a days diplomas are given after a crash course or a short course. Patañjali wants one to make the base of yoga firm and today each one jumps for the finer aspects of yoga; *prāṇāyāma* and *dhyāna*.

To construct a building, *bhūmi pūjā* takes place (*bhūmi* = soil, ground, land, *pūjā* = homage, worship, reverence, respects). Before construction work begins, the owner worships the Mother Earth for permission to dig. This *pūjā* is conducted on the north east side of the land paying homage with a sacrificial fire (*homa*) to commence the construction work. These days without the right foundation in the field of yoga, higher aspects of yoga are taught. I pray God to spare these innocent practitioners and save them.

In this present century the stress factor has become a great disease. Everyone is in the search of solution. Hence, meditation centres have sprung up for the de-stress factor. The tendency of the people is to take psychedelic drugs. They are purely sedative drugs whereas yoga is an intellectual and emotional but natural drug. Actually the biological and neurological relaxation is the true relaxation but not through psychological inducement though they help in relaxing and getting temporary relief. This biological and neural reaction comes under the five *bhūta* (the elements). The three elements, namely; *āp*, *tej* and *vāyu*, play havoc on individuals. If one can keep these three elements within the banks of *pṛthvī* and *ākāśa* then probably the word *stress* would not have come into the dictionary at all. The volcanoes, tsunami, hurricanes, conflagrations, earthquakes happen on account of disturbances of these elements. Similarly, in our bodies such things do happen and this means that the *pañcabhūta* are not maintaining their balance. Harmony and balance are needed to maintain their functions within the banks in order to make the life force play in the body harmoniously. That is why *yama, niyama* and *āsana* are introduced to control the movement of these three elements – *āp, tej* and *vāyu* using the earth element as the foundation and the *ākāśa* element as the distributing element. *Vāyu, tej* and *āp* are the foundation for the *tridoṣa (vāta, pitta, ślesma). Tridoṣa* is dependent upon these three elements. In modern terminology, cough and cold *(ślesma)* belong to *āp tattva,* while acidity, burning sensation, bloating feeling belong to *tejas tattva (pitta)* and neurological disharmony in the nervous system is to *vāyu (vāta)* element. Whether it is somatic, psycho-somatic or neurological, these three elements are the causes for these disturbances.

Coming to the stress factor, these sufferers are made to believe that *prāṇāyāma* and *dhyāna* are the panacea for such sufferings. This advice is nothing but bitter pills coated with sugar. Efforts and discipline are required to de-stress the stress factor. Many are under the impression that *prāṇāyāma* is the remedy for de-stress factor. In my early days I faced stress factors physically, economically, socially as well as mentally and being young I took chances and played with pros and cons or I may call it all tricks in yoga. Even to have a meal was not possible. I used to do *āsana* to kill hunger. My uncontrolled practice in the days of stress brought me sanity to build up a controlled practice and changed my restless attitude to a restful attitude. I used gross techniques of breathing also. However my inner conscience was prompting that what I am trying is not a right method. Surprisingly now this gross technique of *prāṇāyāma* has become popular. I did practise crazy methods like *Bhastrikā* and *Kapālabhāti* which affected my weak lungs. Instead of finding relief I was panting. At that time I realised that these *prāṇāyāma* were not refined *prāṇāyāma*. It is fine to do for a short time but doing beyond capacity disturbs one's nerves and brain. But this crazy method is raising its hood. Read what I have written in the preface of *Light on Prāṇāyāma*. This will give you an idea of what are the short lived effects and long lived effects of *prāṇāyāma*.

My diseased body could not accept these harsh *prāṇāyāma*. While teaching *āsana* I used to observe the breathing pattern of my students which were varying from person to person. I started seeing those differentiations; I started grouping the good ones on one side and bad ones on the other side and used their mistakes as guidelines to start afresh the *prāṇāyāma*. I began to see the zigzag flow, sometimes rough, sometimes smooth and at times shaky and at other times stable and exhilarating. From these various feelings, I began to construct a practice for as long as the movement of breath was smooth and exhilarating and stopped at once when restlessness and shakiness was felt.

Even today when I teach *prāṇāyāma* I make the students do *Śīrṣāsana, Adho Mukha Vṛksāsana, Sarvāṅgāsana, Dwi Pāda Viparīta Daṇḍāsana, Setu Bandha Sarvāṅgāsana, Supta Vīrāsana* to bring elasticity in the torso with *Śavāsana*.[1] When they are settled in quietness then I teach *prāṇāyāma*. This means I remove stress and strain to a great level so that they begin *prāṇāyāma* without stress in body, brain, nerves and mind. I transform change in these parts to feel the freshness because *prāṇāyāma* comes well and cools the nerves and psyche.

If *Śavāsana* is done without the above mentioned *āsana*, then those in *Śavāsana* may not relax the body nor the mind or the nerves. Instead of restfulness in body, mind and nerves only restlessness appears in body, brain, and mind. A dream in sleep may be a genuine dream. But in *Śavāsana* the mind acts as a devil's workshop. This is not what one wants in yoga.

Just *Śavāsana* has no effect on those who are in an oscillating state. *Śavāsana* is the study of quietening all vibrations but many beginners find it hard to close even their eyes.

In the 1930s it was a great task to convince people about the practice of yoga, particularly most of the people who were afraid to do *prāṇāyāma*.

Prāṇāyāma is a *bhakti mārga*. It is a devotional path. As *prāṇāyāma* practices are not so easy, I choose the simplest of the simplest method known as *Viloma prāṇāyāma* where inhalation is done with interruption and exhalation without interruption. This gave time for the lungs to rest in between. I used to take both way's, one with interrupted inhalation and smooth single exhalation and the other with interrupted exhalation with one smooth single inhalation. All were enjoying this method and took it as a base for other subtle *prāṇāyāma*. Actually in other *prāṇāyāma* if the inhalation is done at a stretch, they used to feel the strain in the lungs. Secondly, in many if the inhalation was long, exhalation was short and in some the opposite. If exhalation was long, inhalation used to be short. In *Viloma prāṇāyāma* there is *stambha-vṛtti* in each interrupted inhalation or *antara-vṛtti;* then *antara-vṛtti,* then *stambha-vṛtti* is followed. This way of practice were resting the tissues of the lungs whereas in other *prāṇāyāma* if the breath is drawn at one step they used to feel it is a strain.

Finally, these interruptions rest the fibres of the lungs so that the capacity of the lungs increases to take deep breath at one stretch later. The fear complex in students gets broken in *Viloma prāṇāyāma*.

I used to teach *Ardha Halāsana* and *Nirālamba Sarvāṅgāsana* with toes resting on the wall and *Bhastrikā* and *Kapālabhāti* for those whose nostrils were blocked. These days *Kapālabhāti* and *Bhastrikā* blastings have taken the major role in *prāṇāyāma* without judging one's lung capacities. Even in these blasts ears get blocked creating problems in hearing.

[1] Please see pl. n. 11 & 12, vol. 7, *Aṣṭadaḷa Yogamālā*.

As one understands the characteristic changes that occur in *āsana*, one has to feel the healthy changes taking place in *prāṇāyāma*. Before *prāṇāyāma* my advice would be to learn *Śīrṣāsana* and *Sarvāṅgāsana* and stay for some time regularly maintaining freshness in the lungs and spine as well as lightness in mind so that smooth breathing is done from the start to the finish. While doing these *āsana*, the moment they do not feel the freshness and lightness I ask them to come down. This way the body does not accept the strain, I stop that *āsana* and move to another to find whether that *āsana* freshens them or not. This way I followed in teaching *prāṇāyāma* also.

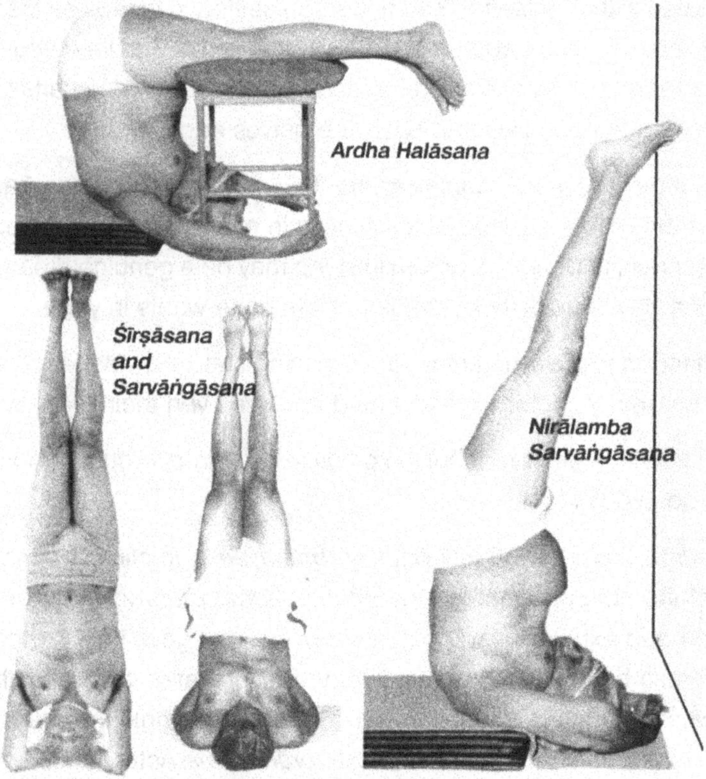

Plate n. 21 – *Ardha Halāsana* and *Nirālamba Sarvāṅgāsana*

As the texts say that *Kapālabhāti* and *Bhastrikā prāṇāyāma* awaken *kuṇḍalinī*, I started doing these. To begin with my lungs could take the blasts which were like metallic sounds. They were pleasing to start with but after some time were rough. Yet I continued and began feeling shakeyness in the body and tension in the head. This made me stop these *prāṇāyāma* the moment the original sound faded.

Many people are made to practise believing that their *kuṇḍalinī* power awakens. Please know that it awakens when one is pure in word, thought and deed. But I will only say that if *Bhastrikā* or *Kapālabhāti* is done for a short time they bring freshness like washing and stroking the brain.

The yoga texts do not say that only *Bhastrikā* awakens the *kuṇḍalinī*. They have also said that *kuṇḍalinī* awakens even in *Paśchimottānāsana*, *Mayurāsana*, *Paripūrṇa Matsyendrāsana* and so forth. Probably as these *āsana* are difficult to practise, many find easy ways like *Bhastrikā* and *Kapālabhāti* and introduce them. Often in *Bhastrikā* there are chances of micro damages

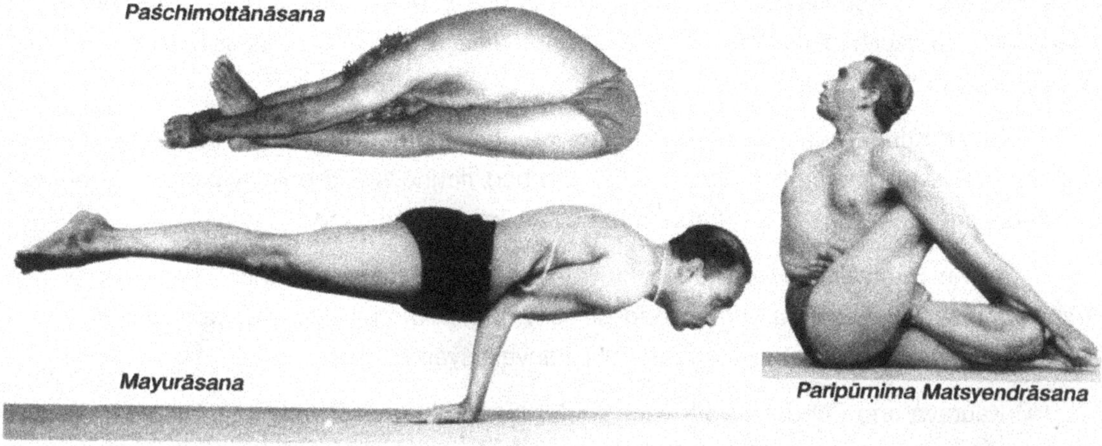

Plate n. 22 – *Āsana* recommended to awaken *kuṇḍalinī* by yoga texts

happening in the electrical nerves of the brain. People think and claim that their *kuṇḍalinī* has awakened. Probably the disturbances may make them believe that *Bhastrikā* has awakened their *kuṇḍalinī* in the nerves and brain cells.[1]

Though I do not like to interfere with those who teach, the question has been asked and as such I am expressing my views.

Yoga does not ask for 'blind faith'; it demands action first and faith only after it reveals its effect. I told you I was doing lots of things and tried several experiments on myself. I was restless and this restlessness made me feel as though I was insane. But persistent practice and right adjustments made me sane.

My advice is to be careful and cautious. Follow the *dharma* of yoga.

About *Uḍḍiyāna*. It is not easy to perform. Even the simplest of *bandha*, *Jālandhara bandha* (chinlock), is difficult. In *Uḍḍiyāna*, one exhales and sucks the abdominal organs to touch the spine without contracting the chest.

No doubt there is a sequence to learning *bandha*. There are three *bandha* used in *prāṇāyāma* namely, *Jālandhara bandha*, *Uḍḍiyāna bandha* and *Mūla bandha*.[2] Among these three *bandha* the first one is *Jālandhara*, then *Uḍḍiyāna* and afterwards *Mūla*. To perform *bandha*

---

[1] Read *Light on Prāṇāyama*, published by Harper Collins, London, chapter 10 – Hints and Cautions, and chapter 23 – *Bhastrikā* and *Kapālabhāti prāṇāyāma*.

[2] Please refer to the author's *Light on Prāṇāyāma*, Harper Collins, London, chapter 13, *Mudrās and Bandhās*.

the spinal muscles should be firm and the chest box strong. I have given the names of the *āsana* for the muscles of the torso to tone up and gain strength and firmness before going into *prāṇāyāma* practice.[1]

When Krishna was alive, Śiśupāla too was there. When Rāma was there, Ravaṇa was also there. At every stage of time both good and bad, richness and poverty existed. Good and evil, angel and devil were going hand in hand. It is happening even today.

When Hiraṇyakashyapu father of Prahlāda forced the educational institutes to utter *auṁ Hiraṇyakashyapaye namaḥ* instead of *auṁ namo Nārāyaṇāya,* Prahlāda opposed and stuck to the *mantra* of *Nārāyaṇa* and not of Hiraṇyakaśyapu.

Kaurava and Pāṇdava both were under the tutelage of Droṇācārya but their natures were exactly opposite. Lord Krishna in *Bhagavad Gītā* lists the divine or angelic qualities along with demonic and devilish qualities. This is the law of the world. It is for you to take what is good and leave what is not good. Know that discrimination is the key to learn. It is for the seekers to judge the teacher as the teacher judges his students in imparting knowledge.

Let your conscience known as *dharmendriya* be awakened through yoga so that you are guided on the correct path of yoga.

I had said that *prāṇāyāma* is a *bhakti mārga.* God exists in *parokṣa* (beyond the range of sight, imperceptible). As such He exists in the breath.

Inhalation is that wherein we draw in the breath as if God is in the breath. When we hold the breath we feel God occupying the entire torso without demarcating the body on the soul. In exhalation, the 'I' in us is made to surrender to the Lord in the form of out-breath. Hence, *prāṇāyāma* practice is *nādānusandhāna* where you connect the sound of the breath to the Universal Soul – God. Hence *prāṇāyāma* is a *bhakti mārga* in yoga.

---

[1] See pp. 172.

A THOUGHT ON *DHYĀNA*[*]

Today is *Patañjali Jayanti.* We do pray Lord Patañjali every day, but this day is a very significant day in our lives as it is the first day of *Dīpāvali. Dīpāvali* is the festival of lights which brings new hope and light. It is a custom in India to clean the house, paint the walls and decorate with the auspicious *rangāvali* in the front of the house. Then have a bath after anointing the body with sesame oil, wear new clothes, do the *pūjā* and go for the *darśana* of the Lord, meet friends and relatives and rejoice with them by forgetting all prejudices.

Today is also considered as *Dhanvaṁtari Jayanti.* We worship Lord Vishnu, who incarnated Himself as Lord Dhanvantari for the sake of mankind to enhance life with the nectar of medicines for health. These two incarnations happened at different times and it is a coincidence that they appeared on this earth choosing the *Dhanatrayodaśī* day of *Diwāli. Dhana* means wealth. Lord Vishnu presented medicines in the form of nectar of health and His couch – the Ādiśeṣa appeared with the science of yoga, grammar and medicine. It is not merely a coincidence but quite significant. Our bodies are filled with impurities *(mala).* The human race having the intellectual faculty can remove these *mala* through the study and practice of yoga and *āyurveda* and yoga with clean body and clear mind and intelligence.

In *āyurveda,* the *mala* is defined as *malīnikaraṇāt malaḥ* – the one which causes impurities is *mala.* The dirt, filth, dust, pollution, all come under *mala.* Often we refer to *mala* as the filth of the body. Any bodily excretion or secretion is *mala.* The faeces, urine and sweat are the *mala* of the body. Even the *sapta dhātu* – the seven ingredients also produce *mala* which pollutes the body. For instance phlegm is the *mala* of chyle *(rasa),* bile is the *mala* of blood *(rakta),* the mucus of the nose and wax of the ear are *mala* of the flesh *(māṁsa),* perspiration is the *mala* of fat *(meda),* nails and hair are the *mala* of bones *(asthi),* the rheum of the eyes are the *mala* of brain *(majjā),* the discharge from vagina is *mala* and there is *mala* in the semen *(śukra)* also.

---

[*] This lecture was given on the occassion of Patañjali Jayanti 2006, in the Ramāmaṇi Iyengar Memorial Yoga Institute, Pune, 2006.

In metallurgy, we study about refining each of the inorganic elements of the metals such as gold and iron which are found in ores. In order to get metals the mining of ores has to be done. The ores come with the mixture of stone, rock, mud and soil. One has to extract the pure metal from the ore. The metal is refined and purified by sieving, burning and watering. There are several methods of purifying the metals explained in modern chemistry. Similarly we have: *śarīra-mala, vāk-mala, indriya-mala, mano-mala, buddhi-mala, karma-mala, citta-mala* and so forth and we have to cleanse ourselves from the *mala*. As the ores are separated from metals, we too have to seperate and remove the *mala* and cleanse through judicious use of intellectual fire *(jñānāgni)* so that the inner gold, (the soul), shines forth like the sun when the sky is clear.

However, when we come to the point of our own existence we have defects *(mala)* in our body, senses of perception, organs of action, mind, intelligence, I-ness, consciousness and conscience. The embodied *ātman (jivātman)* called empirical soul is imprisoned in the mines of these impurities of nature. The *ātman* is always pure, unaffected, untouched, untainted and un-blemished because it is neutral and therefore there is no *ātma-mala*. All the experiences are known to the *ātman* but he being indifferent *(udāsīnan)*, he is unaffected by these experiences. The *ātman* or the Self exists but it does not interfere and hence the question of expression does not arise.

Puruṣa is mute and lame but knows everything. That is why Patañjali says in *Kaivalya Pāda, sadā jñātāḥ cittavṛttayaḥ tatprabhoḥ puruṣasya apariṇāmitvāt* (IV.18) – *Puruṣa* is ever illuminative and changeless. Being constant and master of the mind he always knows the moods and modes of the consciousness. The *prakṛti* gets polluted easily and not the *puruṣa*. *Prakṛti* is surrounded by the moss of *mala*. As *ātman* is surrounded by *prakṛti* filled with *mala*, it seems that the *ātman* too gets mixed up with *mala*. See *vṛtti sārūpyam itaratra (Y.S.*, I.4), which means that the Self identifies with the things of the consciousness and gets tangled in them.

We have to remove the *mala* of *prakṛti* so that it becomes free from *mala* so that the *ātman* too remains undistorted and unsullied. Therefore, today we are going to concentrate on this concept of *mala* as explained by Patañjali.

Basically we are filled with *śarīra-mala, vāk-mala* and *mano-mala*. In order to vanquish these *mala*, Patañjali has given us *āyurveda, vyākaraṇa* (grammar) and *yoga* respectively.

Śarīra-Mala

Āyurveda has discussed a lot about *śarīra-mala*. The aim of *āyurveda* is to keep *tridoṣa* (humours of the body) in a balanced state. Otherwise the body forms *mala* creating room for defects and diseases. The *śarīra-mala* is in the form of diseases which can be eradicated through medical treatment, the question is whether it is enough to eradicate the *śarīra-mala* by getting ourselves free from diseases. We, being dedicated practitioners of yoga need to give a thought on this aspect.

Āyurveda has given many details regarding the *dinacaryā* (daily routine) and *ṛtucaryā* (seasonal regimen). There are certain disciplines *(niyama)* to be followed on a daily basis as well as season-wise. It speaks much regarding the intake of food, drink, daily routine, the norms regarding clothes, entertainment, code of conduct, ethical restrictions, sensual and social behaviour to maintain sound health.

However we need to think that somewhere deep inside, the diseases *(śarīra-mala)* enter the body and mind and make man suffer with vitiated humours on account of our moods and actions *(karma)*. We normally attribute diseases, sufferings, pains, sorrows with fate or destiny, though they are *mala* of our own actions *(karma)*.

We possess this body on account of the imprints *(saṁskāra)* that we have imbibed through our previous lives, the actions of our *karma* cause that *śarīra-mala*. Therefore we need to know the purpose of utilising this body *(śarīra)* in a proper way. So that we eradicate or minimise our *citta-ṃala*, *śabda-mala* and *karma-mala*.

The purpose of existence of *śarīra*

First let us know what *śarīra* is. The word *śarīra* comes from two roots. The root *śri* means to support or a supporter. The root *śri* also means that which is easily destroyed or dissolved.

This clearly indicates that though the body decays and dies, it supports our living. We certainly cannot exist without body or live with a mere body. And we are born with a body which we cannot throw away. Clothes whether new or old can be discarded or given to others or they can be freshly made. It depends upon our will and wish. But the body cannot be discarded, exchanged, destroyed or newly made, though there is a purpose for its existence.

Āyurveda has certainly dealt with the body on its own terms and in its own sphere. The meaning of *āyurveda* literally is knowledge of life *(āyuḥ* – life, *veda* – knowledge). It means to lead an 'Artful Life'. It may teach you to lead an artful, well-managed, yet mundane life. It won't teach you how to lead a spiritual or *ādhyātmika* life. It may support to lead a spiritual life but it won't explain the practical approach.

If *āyurveda* ends with a perspective on life, the way to realise the gift of life begins with yoga. For ways of living the body is essentially required for progress. For this we need to know the purpose of this body and why it is a major instrument in life. *Āyurveda* declares that the healthy body is essential to follow and achieve the four aims of life, to carry on religious duty, the means to lead a family life, to have life's contentment and finally, to achieve freedom from the cycle of birth and death. This is known as *dharma, artha, kāma* and *mokṣa*.

Yoga factually helps one to move in this direction to earn these aims as it deals with the body, mind, senses, intelligence, I-ness and I-consciousness because all these envelop the soul. The final aim of yoga is to discover the soul. For this purpose, yoga plays a unique role on the practitioners.

Here I am not going into the details of the eight aspects of yoga as these days people do not want disciplined practice *(sādhanā)*. They only want to be inquisitive and want ready-made answers for their queries. No doubt inquisitiveness is the beginning of knowledge, yet, it leads only up to the point of gathering knowledge but does not give ways to experience it. The word 'yoga' has become attractive and mind gravitates towards 'yoga' because everybody is hungry and thirsty for peace. For example today you see "meditation for peace" advertised all over the world. Here let me pose a question; should it be "meditation for peace" or "peace for meditation"?

It is peace which is needed for meditation and not the other way round. Without knowing the qualities of turbulence and vibration of the consciousness, how can one leap or jump to *dhyāna? Dhyāna* is not meant just for peace of mind. In *Ardha Halāsana*,[1] you get peace of mind. But is that meditation? We have to question the precision of the language that is "meditation for peace" or "peace for meditation".

In order to know the purpose of *dhyāna* we have to turn ourselves towards Patañjali and his words. What is *dhyāna* and what is *jñāna?*

The tiers of knowledge

To know is knowledge. Knowledge comes in three grades: *jñāna, vijñāna* and *prajñāna*. *Jñāna* means general knowledge. *Vijñāna* means a special, specific and discriminatory knowledge *(viśeṣa jñāna)* and *prajñāna* means intuitive and luminous knowledge *(prakarṣa jñāna)*. It is experiential knowledge which no longer depends on outside sources or references to the past.

---

1 See plate n. 21, pp.172.

Jñāna is required for all to face the challenges of the world. After imbibing this knowledge, one has to test and experiment to be sure about it. Then one has to work attentively with practical means.

If someone says, "This tree has medicinal value for common cold", this statement has to be experimented with in order to find out whether it is real or not. This is *vijñāna*. Then comes the intensive, intuitive and luminous knowledge which is experienced by one not once but many times. This is called *prajñāna* or proven as totally right all the time. In other words to know the existence of *ātman* is *jñāna*, to know about the *ātman* compared to *anātman* is *viśeṣa jñāna* and to experience the *ātman* is *prajñāna*. We speak of attention and awareness. There is a vast difference between the state of attention and the state of awareness. *Jñāna* comes with attention; *vijñāna* comes with awareness. *Prajñāna* comes with attentive awareness. These two words, attentiveness and awareness have to enter the blood stream of each and every *sādhaka*. This attentiveness comes from intelligence *(buddhi)* and awareness comes from consciousness *(citta)*. When both are jointly executed, conscience *(antaḥkaraṇa)* takes the initative to guide the *sādhaka*. By attention you touch *dhāraṇā*, by awareness you touch *dhyāna* and by bringing unison of attention and awareness you experience *samādhi*. *Jñāna* leads towards *dhāraṇā*, *vijñāna* towards *dhyāna* and *prajñāna* towards *samādhi*.

Let us again go back to Patañjali so that we get further clarity regarding *jñāna*, *vijñāna* and *prajñāna*. While speaking of *prakṛti* in the *Sādhana Pāda* Patañjali clarifies why the body is given to us. He says, *sva svāmi śaktyoḥ svarūpopalabdhi hetuḥ saṁyogaḥ* (II.23) – the conjunction of the seen with the seer is for the seer to discover his own true nature.

There is a factual conjunction of nature's power *(sva-śakti)* and the Lord of nature *(svāmi-śakti)*. Their conjunction and power are definitely intended for knowing the *svāmi* – the soul. However their very purpose of union is forgotten. The *svāmi (ātman)* does not do any *karma*. When the *svāmi* and *sva (prakṛti)* are conjoined or united, the *karma* begins. The cause of their conjunction is forgotten because of ignorance or the lack of knowledge *(avidyā)*.

For instance every restaurant has several types of tasty food. Does it mean that we should go to a restaurant the moment we hear of tasty food? Then it is just for enjoyment *(bhoga)*. Even if we go we eat only when hungry. If we go to a restaurant to eat tasty food each time, this is misuse of our judgement. *Bhoga* or the experience of enjoyment cannot be used indiscriminately. Similarly, to misuse this conjunction of *sva* and *svāmi* leads one to a mistaken notion. Their conjunction is for two reasons. It is for enjoyment or emancipation. The ignorance in us indulges this union towards enjoyment whereas using the knowledge to trace the difference between *prakṛti* and *puruṣa* and understanding the difference between them and then conjoining them uplifts one to go for emancipation. We need to recognise ignorance and wisdom and sort out their conjunction from *bhogārtham* to *apavargārtham*. Enjoyment *(bhogārtham)* is no doubt an essential need in us. To survive we need food and water. To beget progeny, we follow *gṛhasthāśrama* and for this we need to get married. We use our senses, mind and intelligence to experience the world. Here the essentiality of the body is needed and it has to be used discriminately. Similarly the body is also needed for the sake of emancipation *(apavargārtham)*. We need the body to follow the discipline of morality like *brahmacarya* or *ahiṁsā*, to sit for *dhyāna*. The body along with senses and mind has a great potentiality. If we recognise its real essentiality and potentiality, it leads us to proceed toward emancipation. If we make the same source flow towards *bhoga* then the *mala* increases and gets stored and saturated. If we make it flow towards yoga, the *mala* diminishes.

Even in the practice of yoga if we say, "Oh! I am happy with what I am doing and what I am getting," then we are caught up in the net of *bhoga;* we are stuck there with no progression. We show no zeal to go any further and we are caught in the pleasures of yoga which store the *mala* of attachment and indulgence. At this point we need the *jñāna* to do *yoga sādhanā* but our 'self' misguides and misleads us as if we are doing yoga for health and happiness. We do not think of its ultimate aim, i.e., emancipation and freedom. Yoga is meant for *artha* and *kāma* as well as *dharma* and *mokṣa*. You stick to the first part conveniently but forget the second part. This is *avidyā*. The false knowledge regarding the conjunction leads towards want of knowledge. We need to know the very purpose of our existence whether it is for *bhogārtham* or *apavargārtham*. To know this *jñāna* is needed. But to select the purpose and guide the *jñāna* to proceed on the proper track towards *apavargārtham* is *vijñāna* whereas to train solely the *sva-śakti* and *svāmi-śakti* for *svarūpa upalabdhi* is *prajñāna*.

In short, to know the conjunction of *puruṣa* with *prakṛti* is to have the proper disposition of *puruṣa* and *prakṛti* for the purpose of *vijñāna*. To utilise it for the sole purpose of self-realisation is *prajñāna*.

Yoga *sādhanā* is essential for this body to remove the *śarīra-mala* in order to explore the Self. In order to remove *citta-mala* it is essential to remove first the *śarīra-mala*. To trace the reason for *mala*, we have to go to the fifth *sūtra* of the *Kaivalya Pāda; pravṛtti bhede prayojakaṁ cittam ekam anekeṣām* (IV.5) - it means that consciousness is one but it branches into many different types of activities and innumerable thought-waves. Thus the body which comes under the digestive system such as stomach, duodenum, small intestine, large intestine forms a group to effect digestion which is called *pakvāśaya;* similarly we have *cittāśaya* in us. *Citta* means consciousness and *āśaya* means the resting place, a receptacle or abode. Our *citta* along with its components - mind, intelligence and I-ness is one but it is a big storehouse of thoughts, words, their meanings with feelings along with intentions, involvements, modes of thinking and so on. *Cittāśaya* being the storehouse of all these factors, the stock of works and thoughts done by body, heart and mind remains stored in the form of merits and demerits but are unchecked as mental deposits with *pañcakleśa* and *pañcavṛtti.* These are safely stored in the *cittāśaya.* Though each individual has only one *citta,* its working style differs according to its tendency, instinct, inclination, propensity and motivation. These *saṁskāra* play a great role in presenting the *citta* in different facets which seem to appear as many though it is single. It sprouts and branches into many different types of thought waves creating room for merited or demerited actions.

Patañjali points out the *cittāśaya* and the transformations that occur in *citta* and assures us that we can re-create, re-construct and renew the *citta.* We can wipe out the old thoughts on a slate and write a new one on it. Since 'yoga' was not in vogue we were running after *bhoga-saṁskāra. Citta* inclined towards multi-faceted state. Now we have adopted yoga and we have to build *yoga-saṁskāra* to adapt to this new situation. We have to impress *citta* with the *saṁskāra* of *yama* so that *citta* does not gravitate towards *bhoga.* We have to discipline *citta* with *niyama.* We have to clean it in order to eradicate its duality with *āsana,* energise and invigorate with *prāṇāyāma* and re-channel, control and reverse the flow of it through *pratyāhāra.* Then we have to the power of *citta* for the sole purpose of having a hold on the goal with *dhāraṇā,* and then propel this fluency of *citta* centripetally towards *dhyāna. Citta* being of fluorescence we can compel it to absorb the rays of the *ātman* so that it is translucent with the soul. This is *samādhi.* If we do not want to use the word fluorescence call it illumination. Finally, it is the "Light on Soul", by the "Light of the Soul", for the "Light on Soul", or Light experiencing Light.

Coming back to *citta* the truth is that when purification in action *(karma-śuddhi)* happens, only then the purification in the consciousness *(citta-śuddhi)* takes place. In the context of yoga we say, *"ātman* proposes and *citta* disposes". In yoga we have to use discrimination *(viveka)* cautiously to understand the proposal of *ātman* and not to dispose it with *aviveka* – lack of discriminative faculty. Patañjali declares in *Sādhana Pāda* that we have to establish ourselves judiciously with devoted practice of all the eight aspects until the impurities diminish and wisdom dawns and surfaces consciously.[1]

These eight aspects are placed in an ascending order to result in *dhyāna* which is the seventh or the penultimate aspect close to *samādhi.*

---

[1] *yogāṅgānuṣṭhānāt aśuddhikṣaye jñānadīptiḥ āvivekakhyāteḥ* (*Y.S.,* II.28) – by the dedicated practice of the various aspects of yoga impurities are destroyed; the crown of wisdom radiates in glory.

Dhyāna

There are six *sūtra* allotted distinctly for *dhyāna* by Patañjali. The first one defines and beams *jñāna* of *dhyāna*. The second one throws light on the effect. The third indicates when to utilise *dhyāna* as a destructive weapon and the fourth for constructive usage. The third and fourth *sūtra* come under *vijñāna* while the fifth tenders the *citta* towards meditation. The sixth one comes under *prajñāna* as the fructification for emancipation.

Let me draw your attention on these *sūtra* with their definition for you to have a clear understanding.

The following two *sūtra* give the the outline for knowledge *(jñāna)* on *dhyāna: tatra pratyaya ekatānatā dhyānam (Y. S.,* III.2) – meditation or *dhyāna* means a steady continuous flow of attention directed towards the same point or region. Whereas *heyaṁ duḥkham anāgatam (Y. S.,* II.16) explains how one has to work to avoid the pains which are yet to come.

The next three *sūtra* is to explore through experimentation *(vijñāna)* on *dhyāna*. These are *dhyānaheyāḥ tadvṛttayaḥ (Y.S.,* II.11). It means that one has to learn to silence the fluctuations and afflictions of consciousness whether gross or subtle, through meditation, or *viṣayavati vā pravṛttiḥ utpannā manasaḥ sthiti nibandhani (Y.S.,* I.35), or to contemplate on an object that helps to maintain steadfast steadiness in mind; *yathābhimata dhyānāt vā (Y.S.,* I.39) or meditating on any desired object conducive for steadiness and gaining steadiness in the consciousness. The last *sūtra* indicates the ultimate transformation that occurs as *prajñāna: tatra dhyānajam anāśayam (Y.S.,* IV.6), this explains the actual state of *dhyāna* which is only possible for perfected beings who have stable and steady consciousnessses. This means that those who are free from latent impressions and influences experience the state of *dhyāna*.

Let us look into these *sūtra* to know in which way they lead us towards *jñāna, vijñāna* and *prajñāna* as well as preparation required for such transformation to occur.

If the question is what is *dhyāna* then the answer is only *pratyaya ekatānatā* and nothing else. *Pratyaya* means the content. The reservoir of consciousness is called *cittāśaya*. The contents of all the past and present experiences along with the contents of previous births are stored in the *citta*. It is the same thing like the garbage in the computer. The garbage from computer can be easily down loaded but not from the *citta*. In order to remove the garbage of *citta* we have to practise *aṣṭāṅga* yoga for *śarīra-śuddhi, manaḥ-śuddhi* and *citta-śuddhi*. However for *dhyāna* the *citta* which is disciplined with the practice of the earlier aspects from *yama* to *pratyāhāra* has to select the content (object) rightly. In *dhāraṇā* the selection is done and focussed attentively on that content. This content has to be a sacred and pure object which should not cause sensual attractions. We need to have strong faith and firm conviction in selecting a righteous thing. Then the object selected for *dhyāna* in *dhāraṇā* needs to be held uninterruptedly. One cannot waver or be choosy. The fickleness is not to be allowed to happen. This means that we have to be intensely aware of it. This continuous and intense awareness is called *ekatānatā* of *citta*.

This *sūtra* gives definition and technique of *dhyāna* and at the same time indicates that things like 'disturbance, fickleness' are not accepted or tolerated. *Ekatānatā* is a technical word. This *sūtra* gives us the feel and cognisance of *dhyāna* process.

Though *heyaṁ duḥkham anāgatam* (II.16) is not connected directly with *dhyāna*, I am referring to this here because it has an indirect bearing on *dhyāna*. Many of you are under the impression that *dhyāna* is meant for peace of mind. But Patañjali makes us aware of *karma* that cause disturbances and dislocate the state of being. Hence, he wants us to attend to this as *guṇa (sattva, rajas* and *tamas)* dominate our actions and they lead us towards mixed sorrows and pleasures. Therefore the sorrow or pain mixed with pleasure which is there and those which are yet to come has to be avoided. Those which are there have to be tolerated and endured and that which may be waiting to afflict is avoided. This is a thought given as a future provident fund.

Like the *cittāśaya*, the *karmāśaya* is also full of affliction and distress. *Karma* and the fruits of *karma* are closely connected. Our *karmāśaya* is filled with afflictions accumulated in the past, actions based on afflictions as well as fruition. It is *kleśa*, *kleśapūrvaka karma* and *kleśa-karma-pūrvaka vipāka*. These three types of actions may strangle and make us nervous or joyous. Here Patañjali makes us aware of, the cause of suffering with sorrow and calls it the philosophy of sorrow. He says that though it is true that everything leads towards sorrow yet he says there is a solution. He says, *pariṇāma tāpa saṁskāra duḥkhaiḥ guṇavṛtti virodhāt ca duḥkham eva sarvaṁ vivekinaḥ (Y.S.,* II.15) – the wise man knows that owing to the fluctuations, the qualities of nature and subliminal impressions, pleasant experiences are tinged with sorrows and therefore he keeps aloof from them. The following *sūtra* is *heyaṁ duḥkham anāgatam* – the pains which are yet to come can be and are to be avoided. What a relief, solace and assurance Patañjali has provided!

When we think or dream of our future we feel that it should be free from pains and sorrows. This is a common feeling in all of us and this is the reason why we always provide some provision for future. Patañjali too advises us to make such provisions. He advises us to minimise whatever garbage is stored in *karmāśaya* with the practice of *dhyāna*. *Dhyānaheyāḥ tadvṛttayaḥ (Y.S.,* II.11) – the fluctuations of consciousness created by gross and subtle afflictions are to be silenced through meditation.

In order to lessen the tsunami blow of *kleśa*, we have to practise *dhyāna*. When he uses the word *vṛtti* here instead of *kleśa*, he is indirectly informing us that the foundation for *vṛtti* are hidden in the *kleśa*. Modern science calls man a psychosomatic animal. The mental modifications take support from afflictions. Modifications cannot be restrained unless we discipline ourselves through yoga *saṁskāra*. Undoubtedly *dhyāna* is used as a weapon to lessen the intensity of *vṛtti*. In order to lessen the intensity of *vṛtti*, our *karma* have to be purified. Understanding this linkage between action and mental waves, we have to proceed with *dhyāna*.

Dhyāna needs early preparations. *Dhyāna* happens when all the previous six aspects of yoga are practised. The process of purification of *karma* occurs by practising *yama*, *niyama*, *āsana*, *prāṇāyāma*, *pratyāhāra* and *dhāraṇā*. This fear of suffering and wavering thoughts makes one to be aware of safeguards and protections. This is a kind of *jñāna* which opens the gate for *vijñāna*. Therefore, these two *sūtra* namely, *tatra pratyaya ekatānatā dhyānam* (III.2), and *heyaṁ duḥkhaṁ anāgatam* (II.16) give *jñāna* and the third *sūtra*, *dhyāna heyaḥ tadvṛttayah* (II.11) lead us towards *vijñāna*. As understanding of the general knowledge deepens, the freedom of will makes us move towards special knowledge where we choose the ultimate method of spreading the consciousness evenly. This process of spreading the consciousness evenly is called *citta prasādanam*. *Citta-prasādanam* also includes the *dhyāna* process which Patañjali indicates in two *sūtra* namely, *yathābhimata dhyānāt vā* (I.39) and *viṣayavati vā pravṛttiḥ utpannā manasaḥ sthiti nibandhani* (I.35). By contemplating on any desired object conducive to the consciousness or an object that helps to maintain steadiness in mind and consciousness so that one develops a meditative mood. *Citta-prasādanam* is a kind of *saṁskāra* through which we tend and nurture the inherent quality of meditation which is hidden in us.

Though I am going to explain about *citta-prasādanam* let me focus on these chosen six *sūtra* on *dhyāna*. The last *sūtra* on *dhyāna* which leads us from *vijñāna* to *prajñāna* is *tatra dhyānajamanāśayam* (IV.6). The *citta* is cleansed by *dhyānaja saṁskāra*. The meaning of *dhyānaja* means the one which is born of *dhyāna*. The subliminal imprints born out of meditation are known as *dhyānaja saṁskāra* which are of pure and perfect nature. No more do the past impressions influence the *citta*. *Dhyānaja citta* cannot store and does not store any past impressions. It is uninfluenced by actions or fruits. Therefore Patañjali says that the actions of a yogi are neither white nor black, or grey. Let us be sure as Patañjali assures that as the consciousness is charged with *dhyānaja saṁskāra*, the *citta* becomes the *prajñāna citta*. It is pure, intuitive and clear. It does not need any *pramāṇa*. It is not easily influenced by any kind of disturbances. It is a direct knowledge and a direct experience. It does not need any support or any logic or inference.[1] It is self-proven knowledge. In such a state, the *citta* conceives *ṛtaṁbharā prajñā*. This wisdom holds only the truth and nothing else.

These six *sūtra* on *dhyāna* make you understand how one progressively evolutes from *jñāna* to *vijñāna* and from *vijñāna* to *prajñāna*.

See how carefully Patañjali administers *dhyāna* as a dose for the attenuation of affliction. Then he leads us to avoid sorrows which are in store for the future with a single thought and action flowing towards *samādhi*.

n.	*Sūtra* ref.	*Sūtra*	Nature of *sūtra*	Category of knowledge
1	III.2	*tatra pratyaya ekatānatā dhyānam*	Technique	*Jñāna*
2	II.16	*heyaṁ duḥkham anāgatam*	Effect	*Jñāna*
3	II.11	*dhyānaheyāḥ tadvṛttayaḥ*	Utility purpose	*Vijñāna*
4	I.39	*yathābhimata dhyānāt vā*	Utility purpose	*Vijñāna*
5	I.35	*viṣayavati vā pravṛttiḥ utpannā manasaḥ sthiti nibandhani*	Utility purpose	*Vijñāna*
6	IV.6	*tatra dhyānajam anāśayam*	Fructification	*Prajñāna*

Table n. 2 – The progression of knowledge

After taking into account the *dhyāna sūtra* I am coming back to the *sūtra* on *citta-prasādanam*. *Citta-prasādanam* is a part in the process of *dhyāna* which brings not only steadiness of a favourable and graceful disposition of *citta* but also educates it for *ekatānatā*. Without the graceful disposition of the *citta*, it is not possible to achieve *adhyātma-prasādanam*. Hence, the importance for *citta-prasādanam* becomes the focal point for *dhyāna*.

Citta prasādanam

Patañjali has given several options and we have to choose according to our choice. People imagine meditation encapsulated in *citta-prasādanam* is something similar to that of a menu card presented by a waiter in a hotel. The waiter gives us the menu card to make our choices.

The relationship between Patañjali and ourselves is of a *guru* and *śiṣya*, the master and followers. *Guru* knows the weakness and standards of his *śiṣya*. Patañjali knows our weaknesses and our capacities. Therefore he gives varieties of methods for *citta-prasādanam*.

---

1 *śruta anumāna prajñābhyām anyaviṣayā viśeṣārthatvāt* (Y.S., I.49) – the wisdom that is gained through insight is beyond the knowledge gleaned from works, testimony or inference.

We have to study our own mind, behaviour, character, mental weaknesses, tendencies and the influencing ego, which are the causes of not only fluctuations but feebleness of *citta,* and then adopt accordingly. Know how each *sūtra* is a gift for us to correct ourselves as far as our behaviour, morality and discipline are concerned.

The first *sūtra* on *citta-prasādanam* really touches a raw nerve. It is, *maitrī karuṇā muditā upekṣāṇāṁ sukha duḥkha puṇya apuṇya viṣayāṇāṁ bhāvanātaḥ cittaprasādanam (Y.S.,* I.33), through the cultivation of friendliness, compassion, joy and indifference to pleasure and pain, virtue and vice respectively the consciousness becomes favourably disposed, serene and benevolent. This *sūtra* gives a quality of training to maintain steadiness in our emotional dispositions as we come in contact with other people. If someone is happy, we cannot tolerate his or her happiness. Hence, Patañjali asks to cultivate friendliness rather than criticising or belittling. This way the richness of our mind increases. If someone is in sorrow he says, show compassion rather than a feeling of superiority. It is not good to rejoice in someone's misery. When someone displays virtue, feel joy or gladness instead of distracting him from virtue and leading him towards vice. If anyone displays vice, advise him to cultivate what is good in life and then remain indifferent after showing the ways for progress. This is serenity in the consciousness.

Then he reminds us of the breath. The movements of breaths express the state of mind. Anger, sorrow, happiness and peace can be recognised by watching the movements, the stoppages, the places and the sound of breaths. We experience it very often. When we rush to class to reach in time, what are the movements of our breath, or when our money is lost, what is the state of mind and mood? When one is in agony, what is the state and status of the breath? When one is thinking seriously about something, how does one's breath move? Have we observed or noticed these things? He advises to calm down breaths and slow down movements so that the state of mind changes the system of respiration and brings some harmony between breath and mind. In that change of breath, the movement in the chest gets a rhythmic movement. The sound becomes melodious. This in turn brings calmness. Patañjali advises to suspend the breath or remain passive and pensive after exhalation. The quietness that comes after exhalation may take time as one has to get a correct rhythm in proper inhalation, inhalation-retention, exhalation and exhalation-retention. One needs to get the whole cycle of *pūraka, antara kuṁbhaka, recaka* and *bāhya kuṁbhaka* to be done properly so that the body gets accustomed to this *prāṇa vidhāraṇa* state. If the physiological body bears it and the psychological state does not get disturbed, then only the conscious body finds equanimity and stability. It is as hard as taming an untamed ferocious lion. The unrhythmic breath not only changes the rhythm but disturbs and shakes the body, mind and intelligence. Hence Patañjali asks us to tame the breath so that we cultivate the healthy disposition of consciousness. Patañjali asks us to use the breath as the object of contemplation. *Pracchardana vidhāraṇābhyāṁ vā prāṇasya* (I.34), he says by maintaining the pensive state felt at the time of soft and steady exhalation and during passive retention after exhalation, *citta-prasādanam* is experienced.

Then comes – *viṣayavati vā pravṛttiḥ utpannā manasaḥ sthiti nibandhani* (I.35) – or, by contemplating an object that helps to maintain steadiness of mind and consciousness.

The mind has the inherent tendency to gravitate towards the object of its liking. Again with the practice of yoga the *sādhaka* finds that he has developed the art of liking objects such as the idol of the Lord or nature or different colours of flowers and their fragrances which attract his attention. When the *yoga sādhanā* begins, the tendencies change gradually according to the *sādhaka's* moods *(pravṛtti)*. Under such a situation, when he contemplates on the objects of his likings the mind gets stabilised. Here Patañjali indirectly indicates that as the mind changes the liking changes and as the likings change, the tendencies change; as the tendencies change the objects of liking change. See the process of refinement. When this refinement comes the next two *sūtra* become meaningful, *viśokā vā jyotiṣmati* (I.36) and *vītarāga viṣayam vā cittam* (I.37).

Often we come in contact with people who are in a sad and unhappy state. Obviously their complaints are related to their bitter experiences in life. There are very few who keep themselves in a happy state. The happy-mindedness is rarely found compared to the sorrowfulness of the mind. Most people are more in a sorrowful state than in a happy state. Very few talk about their happy state and if they do talk at all, it is their ego which talks about this state. Often they express happy state in order to hide their sorrowful states. The sorrowless state of saints, great men or devotees differs from the common man. It is purely a blissful state and therefore helps one to calm down. Therefore Patañjali asks the *sādhaka* to contemplate either on the sorrowless state of saints or yogi or the luminous, effulgent light. This *jyotiṣmati*, effulgent light is not an external light but an internal light, the light of knowledge that shines in a saint, a yogi, a *muni* and a *ṛṣi*.

The great *ācārya* and the saints are people who are devoid of passions, desires, free from attachments and calm and quiet. The *sādhanā*, devotion and the way of living change our lives if we follow their ideal ways of living. All these give a kind of moral support, encouragement, confidence, solace and a feel of detachment to the petty objects of attraction. One can contemplate, think and reflect on such things and bring stability so that the mental disposition remains positive. Therefore Patañjali says, *vītarāga viṣayaṁ vā cittam* (I.37) – which means that by contemplating on enlightened sages who are free from desires and attachments, calm and tranquil, or by contemplating divine objects, one can have the embellished *citta*.

Then Patañjali asks us to watch the state of consciousness in sleep, dream and wakeful states. All of us have experienced good, undisturbed, deep and sound sleep. We also have sometimes dreams. Good thoughts or good feelings hidden in the sub-conscious mind or bad thoughts or painful experiences surface and come up in dreams. If we store such experiences as fearful experiences, they come up as dreams.

Therefore, we need to have *svapna-jñāna* and *nidrā-jñāna*. Similarly, we need to have the *jñāna* of wakeful state. We experience this state while doing *āsana* and *prāṇāyāma* in which we keep ourselves alert moment to moment. We have to learn to take a dip in the lake of yoga so that we think of yoga in all the three wakeful states whether, dreamy or sleepy. Patañjali tells us to contemplate on the dreamy and sleepy states in the *sūtra, svapna nidrā jñānālambanam vā* (I.38) – it means recollection or contemplation on the experiences of dream-filled or dreamless sleep during a watchful waking state.

Patañjali also advises us to choose the objects which are pleasing and conducive to our mind. We have to train ourselves to "indulge" in the activities connected to yogic *sādhanā* and not in the worldly affairs and enchanting objects.

As average practitioners we may try to choose the objects which are pleasing and desirable but may cause distractions later. Thus the process to know ourselves starts by thinking of our body - the skin, muscles, bones and so forth, then the senses of perception, mind, intelligence, ego, *citta* and finally the *ātman*. Through deductive logic, we get to know the disturbing factors as well as the soul which is steady, stable and undisturbed. This is a process to know the *prakṛti* to realise the soul. This is what, *yathābhimata dhyānāt vā* (I.39) conveys – by meditating on any desired object conducive to steadiness of consciousness, one can cleanse and embellish *citta*.

I have already explained in *Light on the Yoga Sūtras of Patañjali* that *sūtra* 33 to 39 and 41 of the *Samādhi Pāda*[1] which implicitly covers the eight aspects of yoga and the evolutes of *prakṛti* to get to know yogic knowledge *(jñāna)*, and get stabilised in it by experimenting *(vijñāna)* by using the blades of analysis *(vitarka)* and reasoning *(vicāra)* and then subjectively experiencing the real, the Soul *(prajñāna)*. When this state is reached, then all impurities from body *(śarira-mala)*, speech *(vāk-mala)*, impure action *(karma-mala)*, mind *(mano-mala)*, unripened knowledge *(jñāna mala)*, 'I'-maker or *ahaṁkāra-mala)* or *citta-mala* are cleansed, then the Self shines from its abode.

---

[1] See table n. 4: in the author's *Light on the Yoga Sūtras of Patañjali*, Harper Collins, London.

The two-faceted *saṁyoga*

Saṁyoga means conjunction of *sva-śakti* with *svāmi-śakti*. It may lead us in either direction because of our ignorance in understanding knowledge. We may even fall a prey to it. Due to *avidyā* the *saṁyoga* may lead towards *bhogārtham*. Our indulgence in worldly pleasures is due to want of knowledge. It is not the fault of *prakṛti;* it is not the fault of the body or the mind. It is the want of knowledge. The goal is forgotten by us.

The *sūtra* says, *tasya hetuḥ avidyā* (II.24) – lack of spiritual understanding *(avidyā)* is the cause of the false identification of the seer with the seen. This is the touchstone for our experience. Patañjali says, "This union is on account of *avidyā*". By experimental and experiential knowledge this *avidyā* has to be changed to *vidyā* (knowledge and wisdom). Then realise what that *saṁyoga* gives you.

Experiential wisdom has to be gained by a beginner through *yama, niyama, āsana* and *prāṇāyāma*. When these four aspects are practised with right approach, it makes the seed of *vidyā* sprout into a sapling.

People think of *āsana* only for physical health but do they question why a physical body was given to them? The physical body is meant to culture intelligence, consciousness and good thoughts to evolve. That is known as *sva-śakti* – power of the *prakṛti*. If *yama* and *niyama* have to be followed, read moral stories from the legendary *(purāṇa)* books to understand the ethical principles on life. Then *āsana* and *prāṇāyāma* play a direct role in training the body not only from the health point of view but also in developing the sensitivity in the mind to make the intelligence and consciousness sensitive. All these are within the frame of *sva-śakti* or *prakṛti-śakti*. And beyond these is *svāmi-śakti*. It is yoga *sādhanā* that brings conjunction between *sva-śakti* and *svāmi-śakti* through experimentations *(vijñāna)* in igniting one to experience the real meaning of conjunction. Experimentation results in feeling the experiences *(prajñāna)*. Then one should refine these experiences further and remove unwanted, non-supportive and misguiding memories. This process is called *smṛti pariśuddhi* (see *sūtra* I.43).[1] When this pure state of memory is built up then one reaches the state of *prajñāna*.

Therefore we need to know the *sva-rūpa* of *prakṛti* as well as the *svāmi-rūpa (puruṣa)*. This type of *jñāna* is very essential to feel the unalloyed Self. *Sva* means own. It is essential to know one's own state or one's own true form. We are not merely bodies or minds. We are much more than body and mind. We are a unique combination of body, senses, mind, intelligence,

---

[1] *smṛtipariśuddhau svarūpaśūnya iva arthamātranirbhāsā nirvitarkā* (I.43) – In *nirvitarkā samapatti*, the difference between memory and intellectual illumination is disclosed; memory is cleansed and consciousness shines without reflection.

consciousness, I-ness, conscience and self. This total form *(svarūpa)* of ours which has to be recognised by us, exists either in impure form *(mala-svarūpa)* or pure form *(śuddha-svarūpa)*. Unfortunately often it is in *mala-svarūpa*. Just as the ore is burnt to get pure gold, we need to convert *mala-svarūpa* into *śuddha-svarūpa* through the yogic *sādhanā* in the form of *tapas*.

Then we need to have *svarūpopalabdhi*. *Upalabdhi* means to obtain. We need to have discrimination in which form we have to obtain. Do we recognise *svarūpa* with *mala* or *nirmala?* If *vidyā* is ignited, we obtain *svarūpa* in pure form *(nirmala)* and if *avidyā* is retained we obtain *svarūpa* in the impure form *(mala)*. We need to obtain the *nirmala svarūpa* and therefore we need to understand the purpose of *saṁyoga*.

Here the practice of *aṣṭāṅga yoga* plays a major role. After this *svarūpopalabdhi*, we have to get *svarūpāvasthā*. The clear and refined filtering takes place between *sva-śakti* and *svāmi-śakti*. *Svāmi-śakti* is *ātman*. The *ātman* in its pure form untouched, untainted by *vṛtti*, dwells in its own true splendour. This is the *svarūpāvasthā* of *svāmi*. Patañjali mentions this in *Samādhi Pāda: tadā draṣṭuḥ svarūpe avasthānam* (I.3). The seer dwells in his own true splendour. Here we notice the *śuddha citta* as *svarūpamātra jyoti*. According to Vyāsa, it is the final stage of *saptadhā prajñā* where the *citta* is self-illumined as it has acquired the knowledge of the self. It is like the light of one's own form, one's visage or one's own sight. However in order to get the *svarūpāvasthā*, we pass through a state of *svarūpaśūnya* which comes through the early stage of *samādhi*. It is a state devoid of one's nature. What is this state? In this *samādhi*, there is an object outside the *ātman*. Therefore, the light of the soul is focussed on *citta* so that the enlightened *citta* shows the objects clearly to *ātman*. Since the light is thrown by the soul on *citta*, it is called *svarūpa mātra jyoti prajñā*. This is the first step of *samādhi*. This state is from *dhyāna* to *samādhi* in which the object we are meditating upon comes forth but the *ātman* remains in the background. On account of this one is in *svarūpaśūnya* state. From this point we proceed towards *svarūpāvasthā* state. In this state, the objects are dropped and only subject remains. The object that is referred here is non-soul or *anātman*. The subject is *ātman*. The last *sūtra* employs the term: *svarūpa pratiṣṭhā* and not *svarūpāvasthā*. In this state, one is absolutely and permanently in the state of *svarūpāvasthā*. The word *pratiṣṭhā* denotes permanency in *avasthā* as one is well established in his *svarūpa*. It is the consecration of the soul, the ultimate state of yogic *sādhanā*.

In short the journey from body to soul has stages, namely: *śuddha svarūpa* of *prakṛti*, *svarūpopalabdhi*, *svarūpa śūnyāvasthā*, *svarūpamātra jyoti prajñā*, *svarūpāvasthā* and *svarūpa pratiṣṭhāvasthā*.

To understand *sva-śakti* and *svāmi-śakti* is *jñāna*. Similarly the *sūtra, tadā draṣṭuḥ svarūpe avasthānam* (I.3) is giving informative knowledge and as such it is *jñāna*. However, knowing that these two *sva-śakti* and *svāmi-śakti* are required for the feel of *svarūpopalabdhi* and *svarūpa śūnya* state is *vijñāna*. Specifically at this stage the other *vṛtti* should not interfere as the *citta* is in total absorption *(ekatānatā)* with the object of meditation. Here only the knower, the knowledge and the knowing process exist in this state. This is *svarūpa mātra jyoti*. Then this leads one to the ultimate state of *svarūpa-pratiṣṭhā*. In this state not only all *mala* but *prajñāna* also drop out and nothing is left.

For self-education, self-experimentation, self-experience and self-realisation, the body, organs of action and senses of perception, mind and intelligence are the main instruments. When self-education and self-experimentation come to an end, then whatever we do, whether *āsana, prāṇāyāma* or *dhyāna*, all come under the purview of the Self and not through the body or the senses which are the instruments of the Self.

When we are practising, we experiment with the usage of our average knowledge that we gather from our teacher. In the beginning the teacher is our source of knowledge. Then we experiment on that knowledge to gain experiences. When the gathered knowledge and experimentation harmonises with experiences, then one sees the purity in the intellect of the head and the intelligence of the heart.

Jñāna is just ageneral knowledge which is devoid of experiment and experience. *Jñāna* conceives the concept not knowing whether the 'conceived concept' is correct through the instrument called 'intelligence'. Based on this assumption and presumption of intelligence the experiment begins through new light on experiences. At this stage *jñāna* becomes *vijñāna*. *Vijñāna* gives vision. Then the *vijñāna* is transformed to *prajñāna* through *darśana*. Patañjali calls yoga as *darśana* as yoga brings first hand wisdom in full view.

Sādhanā is experimentation for experience's sake. This has to be done with attention. By attentive practice the *sādhaka* develops certain faculties in the *sādhaka* through which he develops expansion of his intelligence which brings awareness in the consciousness for it to become absolute. In this awareness the *citta* no longer remains divided or compartmental. It becomes pervasive from the foot to the head in the body from all sides. This 'pervasiveness' is the *citta*. The intelligence of the consciousness spreads the beam of illuminative awareness in the *sādhaka's* life. This is *vedānta* or the end of the search for knowledge.

This *vedānta* of yoga comes after filtered experiences. Yoga ends with the experience of *svarūpa-pratiṣṭhā*. That is why I use the word *vedānta*. Understand what *vedānta* is! *Veda* means to know and *anta* means its end. When knowledge comes to an end and nothing remains to be known, that is *vedānta*. Technically the *Uttara-Mimāṁsā*, one of the six orthodox schools of thought is known as *vedānta*.[1] In *Uttara-Mimāṁsā* the gist of *veda* is read in the form of *Upaniṣad*. That is why it is called *vedānta*. Here, the practice of yoga leads us to reach the state of *prajñāna*. People call it science of yoga but they have no experience of *prajñāna*. They cast about guessing, "May be this, may be that". *Prajñāna* is a step beyond *vijñāna*. Don't be satisfied with experimentation only. There has to be maturity in experimentation. This means one has to experiment on the same topics again and again in order to get maturity and get to true essence of experience *(rasātmaka jñāna)*. Both experiment and experience has to end up in *vedānta*. The knowing process and the knowledge have to end. 'The knower' has to remain but not as a knower but in a pure existing state. The knower remains not as *jñātā* (knower) but as *sat* – the pure existence.

Let me give an example of *jñāna, vijñāna* and *prajñāna* in practice. *Śīrṣāsana* is nothing but *Tāḍāsana* upside down. But in *Tāḍāsana* the awareness is in the back of the leg, and that awareness is quite different to that of *Śīrṣāsana*. In *Śīrṣāsana* the most unthinkable area in the body is the skin at the bottom of the buttocks, bottom of the feet and the head of the front inner thighs. These areas are always out of reach for the senses and mind. Has one's *jñāna* ever reached that area? When one does *Tāḍāsana* there is an opening of his intelligence on the bottom of the feet, top of the legs and at the bottom of the buttocks whereas in *Śīrṣāsana* that intelligence does not penetrate as it penetrates in *Tāḍāsana*. This means that one does not experiment with his intelligence to find out what he is doing and where the body is going and what the intelligence does not see. In *Tāḍāsana*, the top of the back legs below the buttocks open. We feel the stretch of the skin there but in *Śīrṣāsana* we don't think of that part at all. Patañjali has used the word: *viparyaya jñāna*. This *jñāna* is similar to that knowledge that thinks the rope is a serpent though it is actually a rope.

Therefore, each one of us in *sādhanā* has to trace the dark, inattentive parts and bring the intelligence and consciousness to reach and touch these areas so that the *citta-prasādanam* is spread evenly covering the entire area of the body concurrently allowing the Self to travel and settle at every nook and corner of its frontier, the body. This means transformation of *citta-prasādanam* into *ātma-prasādanam*.

We should remain alert to differentiate *pratyakṣa jñāna* from *viparyaya jñāna*. For example, when we are in *Śīrṣāsana* we should not rest on our laurels but examine whether the various parts of the body have spread or contracted. Until the day comes when we realise that the rope was not a serpent but a rope, contracted muscles and skin below the buttocks may bite one day. Showing non-attention in these areas but taking it for granted that they are well attended is

[1] See *Aṣṭadaḷa Yogamālā*, vol. 7, p. 57.

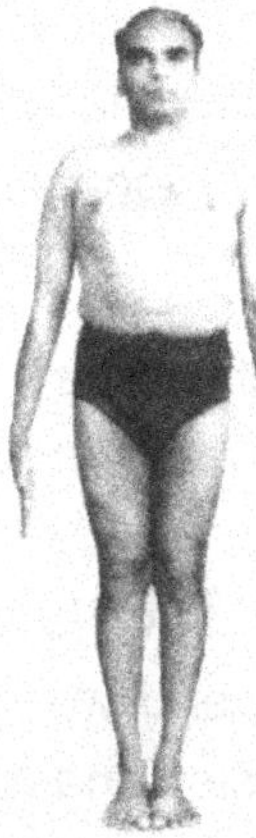

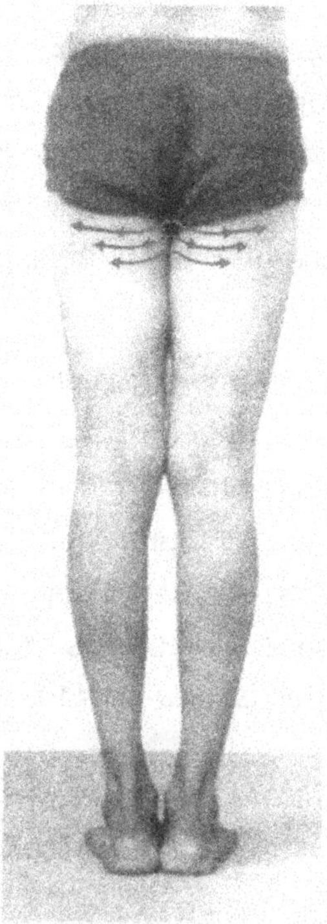

Tāḍāsana

The stretch of the skin at the top-back thigh is felt

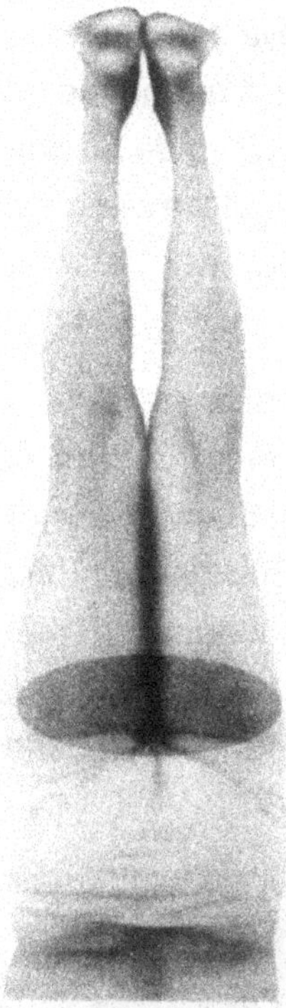

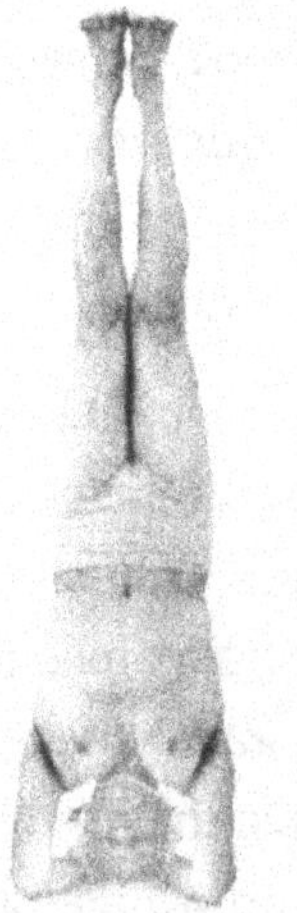

Śīrṣāsana

The same position reversed and the same area of the top-back thigh is not felt at all

Plate n. 23 – Awareness of the back leg in *Śīrṣāsana* and *Tāḍāsana*

viparyaya jñāna in *Śīrṣāsana*. This bite may begin to act to get rid of perverted understanding *(viparyaya jñāna)* into direct experience *(pratyakṣa jñāna)*.

If we take an interest in the back upper thigh we can incorporate what we have learned in *Tāḍāsana* in *Śīrṣāsana*. In *Śīrṣāsana*, we stretch the outer legs but forget the inner legs. In *Sarvāṅgāsana*, we stretch the inner legs and forget the outer legs. This is where we lose our *prajñāna*. Earlier I spoke about *āgama pramāṇa*, here I refer to *pratyakṣa pramāṇa* or direct perception. We are not using the enquiring mind while we are practising *Śīrṣāsana* or any other *āsana*.

Take *Sarvāṅgāsana*. If one watches the inner ankles, they remain above the outer ankles. In *Śīrṣāsana*, the outer ankles remain higher than the inner ankles. Is it not *avidyā* in *sādhanā?* Though we have knowledge and understanding in such matters, we are ignorant of our own transcendental knowledge. Patañjali advises to remove the veil which covers knowledge. He has said this in the context of *prāṇāyāma* but it is applicable to *āsana* also. Ultimately the practice of *aṣṭāṅga* yoga is for *jñāna dīpti*. Therefore, *tataḥ kṣiyate prakāśa āvaraṇam (Y.S.,* II.52) is applicable in *āsana* also. The veil covering the light of knowledge is removed for the wisdom to dawn. The light is covered by something which you do not know. This cover is *avidyā*. In cataract the lens of the eye becomes progressively opaque resulting in blurred vision; *avidyā* in the form of nescience and arrogance veils and covers the intelligence and the self. When we remove the cover of egoistic pride *(ahaṁkāra)* and ill-founded offensive arrogance *(durahaṁkāra* or *durābhimāna)*, the light of the self dawns. This light will serve to break the *tāmasic* and *rājasic* states of intelligence . This way the combined practice of all the eight aspects of yoga remove the veil.

The body is a place where we experiment with our intelligence in each *āsana* so that the vibration of what is seen and unseen, heard and unheard is felt in the body. When we stretch the ankle, we feel the vibration of the outer ankle but if our inner ankle is inactive it just remains as if in sleep. This way we miss many things in our practices. The life force is felt by vibration in *sādhanā*. By attending to the feel of vibration in order to adjust or extend, we will be able to remove impurities in body, mind and intelligence. If we see as well as listen and adjust, then we are spreading the consciousness evenly. This is *citta-prasādanam as well as ātma-prasādanam.*

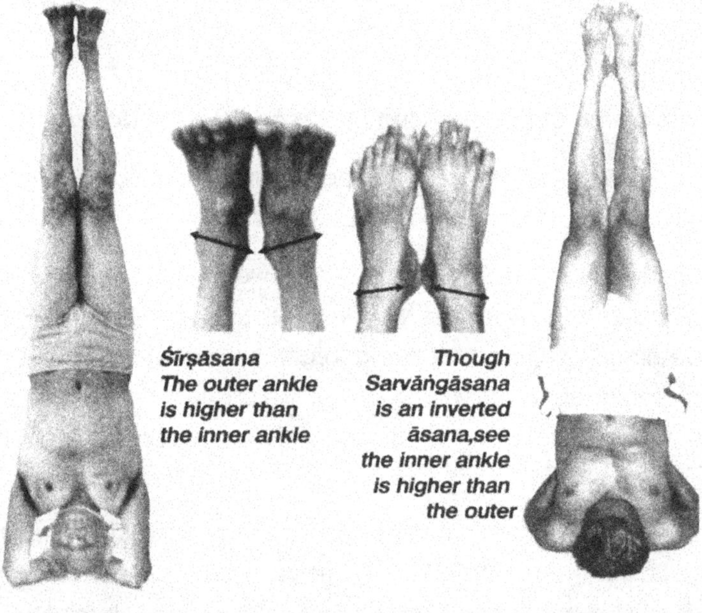
Śīrṣāsana
The outer ankle is higher than the inner ankle
Though Sarvāṅgāsana is an inverted āsana,see the inner ankle is higher than the outer

Plate n. 24 – Showing differences in the inner ankles of *Śīrṣāsana* and *Sarvāṅgāsana*

Even slight impure *guṇa* is referred to as *malīna*. For example Vibhiṣaṇa, brother of Rāvaṇa had *malīna sattva*. The moment he laid eyes on Rama, the covering on the *sattva* disappeared. He then became a *sāttvika puruṣa*.

When one does *dhyāna* one needs some support. It could be an object or the *praṇava, auṁ* which we saw earlier. The *citta* needs the support. In the class everybody is instructed to concentrate on something which makes one to get absorbed. Each one is supposed to have concentration on *bhūta* and *tanmātra.* Then why not concentrate on one's feet in *Śīrṣāsana* or tailbone in *Baddha Koṇāsana?* Is it not elemental? Has it not got *tanmātra?* Se e whether each part of the body is firm in its place and straight. Is the tailbone doing *Tāḍāsana* as it should be done? Is that not attention when one sees and feels such details?

Let us heed the words of Patañjali and strive to find out what each word conveys so that we can extract the knowledge from it. In *Samādhi Pāda,* Patañjali has given a clue while undergoing different stages of *samāpatti (samādhi).* He says that the objects selected for *samāpatti* could be words, five gross elements, five subtle elements, mind, intelligence, I-consciousness, consciousness and finally the *aliṅga* state of *prakṛti.* What do these convey? Is it not conveying to concentrate on our own *prakṛti?* Can we train ourselves to take the support of all these elements in *āsana* and *prāṇāyāma?* When the practice of *āsana* and *prāṇāyāma* reaches that subtlety, is it not *prajñāna* yoga?

Now, think over the two *sūtra* of Patañjali which are very familiar. One is *sthira sukham āsanam* (*Y.S.,* II.46) and the other is *atha yogānuśāsanam* (*Y.S.,* I.1). The first one is often translated as, "any comfortable *āsana*", and the second as, "the discipline of yoga". Watch the contradiction in translation. Why should Patañjali call the whole process of yoga an endeavour? If anything that is comfortable, why then *anuśāsanam?* What Patañjali means is that when we are doing the *āsana,* the *ananta* or the *ātmā* or the *puruṣa* has to surface and cover the body. It is not a question of the body feeling the soul, but the soul has to remove the veils that cover it for it to spread. This is *adhyātma prasādanam.* Let not the eternity of *ātman* remain merely at a verbal expression *(śabda).* In spite of its presence we feel its absence *(vastuśūnyatā).* The Soul exists as everyone says but we don't know since we do not see it! It is not a thing to see but it is to be felt. In *Bhagavad Gītā,* Lord Krishna says,

āścaryavat paśyati kaścid enam-āścaryavad vadati tathai'va cā'nyaḥ I

āścaryavac cai'nam anyaḥ śṛṇoti śrutvā'py enaṁ vada na cai'va kaścit II

(*B.G.* II.29)

Someone looks upon God – the Universal Soul – as marvellous; some speak of him as marvellous, some hear of him as marvellous; and some after hearing of Him shall not know.

Keeping these words of Sri Krishna, we have to do the *āsana* in such a way that the soul, infinity, *ananta* surfaces and effortlessly spreads into the body. Then *puruṣa* is felt everywhere.

When this all-pervasive experience is felt everywhere in the body, then it is called *prajñā-puruṣa*. It means that you have understood the meaning of the *puruṣa* which is 'This and Here'.

Patañjali has also used the terms *grahītṛ, grahaṇa* and *grāhya*. The seeker is the subject but acts as an object. Why is the seer seeking anything, being a seer? If you say, "I am seeking the Seer", then the Seer becomes seeker for the Seer. The same Seer acts as an object, instrument and subject. In the *āsana* the body should not be treated as an object, but as the Self and one should use that Self as an instrument to understand the entire structure of the body from the core. Then how can the Self *(grahītṛ)*, become instrument? Though it is not an instrument we feel it as an instrument. As a matter of fact the object *(grāhya)* and instrument *(grahaṇa)* act as instruments. If these two go to the background, obviously the *prakṛti* goes to background and the Self surfaces. Then one experiences the highest state of bliss.

Tomorrow is the festival of lights. Let yoga allow us to experience the festival of lights in our *āsana*. As *dīpa jyoti* or light removes darkness, let the *ātma jyoti* or the light of the soul, light in every cell of the body. Let the *ātma jyoti* burn our minds, intelligence and *citta*. See each day in practice, it should be a festival of light so that new light, new knowledge, new illumination arises in the *sādhanā*. Let everything be *prakāśamaya*. Let the *sattva guṇa* shine for *ātma jyoti* to reflect on it so that the feel of joy remains beyond measure.

As a beginner in yoga, one's *citta* is tainted, yet one experiences something different. This feeling is not connected to any object. If there is no motive in the *sādhanā* but to do as a *sādhaka*, we have to remain untainted as there are no motivators in the *sādhanā*. Let us enjoy doing *āsana*. Let us stop grumbling on pains. Then the light of illumination definitely dawns.

I wish all a happy *Dīpāvali*. Let the light of all lights, the very Self spread the light in you all, all the time. Let us not differentiate that this is body and that is mind. Let us treat the organs of action, senses of perception, mind, intelligence, muscles, joints, nerves, bones and everything as one and light the light of the Self. This is *prajñāna* which blazes brilliantly radiating the light of the Self. Let us celebrate *dīpāvali* of this *antaryāmin*.

I started with the topic of *mala* – the dirt, the impurities. Patañjali has given noble gifts in the form of yoga, *āyurveda* and grammar to remove the *mala*. The *āyurveda* and grammar undoubtedly remove the *mala* but yoga removes all the *trimala* of the body, speech and *citta*. Patañjali indicates in one single *sūtra, yogāṅgānuṣṭhānāt aśuddhikṣaye jñānadīptiḥ āvivekakhyāteḥ* (II.28) – by the dedicated practice of the various aspects of yoga, the impurities are destroyed: the crown of wisdom radiates in glory. Here the *aśuddhikṣaya* or destruction of impurities *(mala-nissaraṇam)* takes place and *jñāna dīpti* the light of *prajñāna* blazes.

Today being *Patañjali Jayanti, Dhanvantari Jayanti* and *Dhantrayodaśi,* let us rejoice on this very important day and may the Light of Yoga dwell in your hearts through the Light on Yoga as *dīpāvali* each day.

YOGA: A SAVIOUR IN WOMEN'S LIFE

I have often been bombarded with questions such as: can woman practise yoga? Does its practice differ for men and women? How will it affect the feminine body and mind? Can a married woman practise yoga? Is it essential for a woman to become a *sannyāsini* to practise yoga?

Though I have answered these questions concerning yogic practice for women over and over again, fear and ignorance persist even today in many minds. Doubts may persist but it is heartening to say that more and more women are practising yoga and are drawn towards its divine values. Yoga is not only beneficial but a 'pinnacle' for women.

The spiritual path is open whether one is a man or a woman. Therefore both have the same urge to know the origin of existence, the soul *(puruṣa)* and God *(puruṣa viśeṣa* or *Īśvara).*

The search to know *puruṣa* or *Īśvara* and to realise the Self and God depends on four paths namely, *karma, jñāna, bhakti* and yoga. These four paths are so closely interwoven that one cannot separate one from the other. If one path is explicit the others get implied indirectly though the ultimate goal is the realisation of the Self. Only an effort to start on any one of these paths (*karma, jñāna, bhakti* and yoga) is to be determined and practised according to one's mental frame as all paths lead towards the vision of the Self *(ātma-darśana)* and later towards the vision of God *(Paramātma darśana).*

Yoga is for all

God created men and women equal. Yoga too was created by Him. Yoga too does not differentiate or shun or exclude anyone by gender, colour or class. Both men and women are endowed with body, mind and intellect but are caught in the web of immature intelligence and mental upheavals. The instincts of both are drawn towards the aspiration for worldly pleasures and make them forget the very purpose of their life which is unalloyed bliss. This unalloyed bliss is nothing but consecration of the Self or the Soul *(svarūpa pratiṣṭhā)* and the aim of yoga is to experience this state.

Yoga is a way of life and its universal principles are applicable to both men and women with equal proportion without excuses or exemptions. All can follow thoroughly its principles without doubts and fears. Only its benefits depend upon his / her way of approach, capacity, strength, vigour, determination, will-power, enthusiasm and range of efforts in practice.

Nature (*prakṛti*) and Soul *(Puruṣa)*

Whether one is a man or a woman, nature *(prakṛti)* and the soul *(puruṣa)* exist in all. As far as nature's structure and evolution are concerned there is no difference. They are present in all creations.

Nature's evolution includes the five elements (earth, water, fire, air, ether or space) and the five infrastructures of elements known as *tanmātra* (smell, taste, shape, touch, sound), the five senses of perception (eyes, ears, nose, tongue, skin), the five organs of action (hands, legs, mouth, genital and excretory organs), mind, intelligence, ego and consciousness.

Mental Fluctuations

The fluctuations and modifications in all of us arise from the fabric of mind. These fluctuations and modifications may be painful or pleasurable, sorrowful or joyful. Yogic practice *(abhyāsa)* and renunciation *(vairāgya)* develop desirelessness and dispassionateness towards the fruits of actions and free one from dualities of pain and pleasure leading one to experience the hidden unalloyed bliss. To experience this unalloyed bliss one needs to practise yoga to control the senses and gain poise in body and peace in mind.

In the early days women had all the rights and opportunities to practise for the realisation of the soul. They were recognised as having every right to practise the four paths of *karma, jñāna, bhakti* and *yoga* in order to experience the establishment of the soul.

The names of such *yogini* may be found in the *Upaniṣad* and the *Purāṇa* or the stories of past legendary figures. During the *Vedic* period they used to have equal opportunities. Owing to invasions after invasions by outsiders, protection of women became an urgent necessity in order to save their honour and dignity. On account of these abnormal situations and circumstances restrictions got imposed on the woman's way of life, both in education and movement in society.

Today ideas such as equal rights and globalism are taking root all over the world. The intention and philosophy behind yoga have remained globally applicable and relevant from the time of their inception.

Men and women have the same fluctuations in thoughts and reflections, diseases, sorrows and obstacles. Only their approaches differ from each other because of their inherent natural disposition *(svabhāva).* Though both are endowed with intellect and emotions, man's intellect grows vertically filled with pride and ego whereas woman's intelligence develops horizontally with compassion and sympathy. If women are gifted with instinctive and intuitive feelings, men work with their analytical head. If women are endowed with emotional intelligence and devotional qualities, men are endowed with intellectual deliberation. Man disregards his emotional feelings and tries to resolve the emotional weather by means of his intellect which is usually founded in the pride of "I" ("I" decide, "I" know) rather than the reason and logic (*tarka*) of an objective mind. Women however, instinctively bring to bear their emotional intelligence to solve emotional upheavals.

Yoga helps both men and women to develop intellect in the head and intelligence in the heart to lead a balanced life maintaining harmony, balance and concord not only at home but in the community and society as well.

Though the principles, methodology, aims and obstacles are not different for men and women, the way of approach to practising yoga differs according to constitution and circumstance. A woman has a devotional mind and because of this her practice becomes a dedicated practice. This brings emotional stability which maintains her intellectual balance between head and heart as well as between things and thoughts. A man does everything analytically with his head but with a barren heart. If he practises yoga regularly, his barren heart may change towards fertility.

The heart is the seat of devotion, desirelessness and wisdom. Man thinks first before dedicating himself while woman dedicates first and thinks later.

In my experience of teaching yoga for men and women, women bear things bravely while men take time to accept. But persistent practice of yoga builds up balance and pacifies their intellect of the head whilst nourishing the intelligence of the heart *(buddhi-prasādana* and *citta-prasādana)* to live in harmony.

The spiritual path needs a good combination of feminine energy *(straiṇa-śakti)* and masculine energy *(puruṣa-śakti).* We, in yogic terminology call them as *iḍā nāḍī* or *candra nāḍī* and *piṅgalā nāḍī* or *sūrya nāḍī.* If *iḍā nāḍī* or the *candra nāḍī* is feminine, cooling, quiet, passive, *sūrya nāḍī* or *piṅgalā nāḍī* is masculine hot, active and energetic. In the Chinese system they call *iḍā* and *piṅgalā* as *yin* and *yang*. These energies need to be balanced so that the energy enters the *suṣumnā nāḍī* which is in between *iḍā* and *piṅgalā*. Women need to balance the *prakṛti-śakti* or *straiṇa-śakti* and men the *puruṣa-śakti* in order to enter *ātma-śakti*. *Yoga sādhanā* helps to unite this *prakṛti-śakti* with *puruṣa-śakti*.[1]

Though woman is vulnerable physically and needs protection, she should not be treated as an object of enjoyment. Man should not abuse his protective role with immoral or brutal acts. Know that the term *brahmacarya* holds good equally for man as well as woman and as such, is it not the duty of a man to protect the sanctity of a woman?

Brahmacarya does not mean that he / she has to live in celibacy. But he / she can get married and support each other to move towards the spiritual kingdom.

There is a good number of women who remained as *brahmacāriṇi*. For example Gārgi, Sulabhā, Śabari remained as recluses while some like Maitreyi, Kauślyā, Sītā, Anasuyā, though married, practised yoga and reached the pinnacle of yoga. Goṇikā transferred her knowledge to Patañjali. Pārvati taught yoga to many women. Akkamhādevi, Aṇḍāl, Śāradāmani were saints. In this way many women were educated in spiritual knowledge. Many were considered as guru. Even *ṛṣi-patni* (wife of a *ṛṣi*) were considered equal to a *guru*.

Yajñavalkya's second wife Kātyāyani took care of her husband's pupils while Maitreyi, his first wife, was involved in her spiritual quest.

No doubt, a woman is sensitive to emotions like love, affection, kindness, friendliness, service, compassion and humility and at the same time she is inherently strong within. Hence she can utilise these qualities for her spiritual progress with faith and will power.

Often these qualities are exploited to make a woman accept servitude. She has to learn to maintain her own identity and dignity by thinking that she is in no way inferior to a man. It is a kind of self respect which she needs to develop. There are quite a few examples where women came on the battlefield to face the enemy directly. But man has the natural tendency to pride himself and likes to possess the rights over women.

Many a time, woman is blamed for alluring man. Who knows, it may be other way also. Hence, Patañjali cautions that the celestial beings may tempt a *yogi* or a *yogini* and they should not fall a victim to such temptations.[2]

---

1 *sattva puruṣayoḥ śuddhi sāmye kaivalyam iti* (*Y.S.*, III.56) – when the purity of intelligence equals the purity of the soul, the *yogi* has reached *kaivalya*, perfection in yoga.

2 *sthānyupanimantraṇe saṅgasmayākaraṇaṁ punaraniṣṭa prasaṅgāt* (*Y.S.*, III.52) – when approached by celestial beings, there should be neither attachment nor surprise for undesirable connections can occur again.

There are six essential sources of wealth for spiritual progress. These are passionlessness *(śama)*, self-restraint *(dama)*, enduring power *(titikṣā)*, resistance towards luxury *(uparati)*, faith *(śraddhā)* and satisfaction *(samādhāna)* which need to be utilised wisely. Women have these required qualities whereas men have to struggle to acquire them.

Brahmā the creator, Vishnu the organiser and Shiva the destroyer have their consorts Saraswati, Lakṣmi and Pārvati. Sarasvati being the *vāṇi*, the organ of speech, she is the *śakti* of Brahmā. Hence, *jñāna* pours from his mouth. Secondly Sarasvati, is the first feminine creation of Brahmā who accepts her as his wife as she is the ocean of knowledge. Lord Vishnu holds his consort Lakṣmi, the goddess of wealth in his chest, for its distribution. Lord Shiva holds his consort Pārvarti, the goddess of power, strength and valour for the destruction of evils. God is one but He forms himself as *trimūrti*, Brahmā, Vishnu and Shiva with their consorts Sarasvati, Lakṣmi and Pārvati. The Goddess Sarasvati is the omniscient knowledge, Lakṣmi, the omnipresent ever existing, non-perishing wealth, and Pārvati, omnipotent eternal power. God showed His three forms, Brahmā, Vishnu and Shiva as Generator, Organiser and Destroyer.

Yoga has a philosophy of precept and practice. If philosophy is male *(pauruṣatva)*, the *sādhanā* is female *(strainatva)*. Precept and practice co-exist in order to keep the balance. It is said that yoga was taught by Shiva to Pārvati because she was his *ardhāṅginī*. *Ardha* means half, *aṅga* means body. Being his wife he shared his yogic knowledge with her. This is enough indication to show that husband and wife have to walk together in life as well as in the path of yoga in order to protect and guide the other for their evolution and upliftment in spiritual growth. This exchange of yogic knowledge from Shiva to Pārvati means that yoga is meant for both men and women.

Puruṣa is considered as 'He' and *prakṛti* is considered to be 'She'. This power of evolution according to yoga is recognised as *prasava dharmiṇi*. This *prasava* is known to us as the evolutory method.

Citta is considered feminine with two facets namely, mundane thoughts *(saṁsāra)* or spiritual thoughts *(kalyāṇa)*. If *citta* is filled with virtue it gets magnetised *(prāgbhāraṁ)* towards *kaivalya* and if it is caught in mundane or worldly thoughts, it gets magnetised *(prāgbhāraṁ)* towards sensual attributes *(saṁsāra)*. When *citta* is magnetised towards the Self, the divine power *(kuṇḍalinī) śakti* ascends and gets united with *puruṣa-śakti* or *śiva śakti*.

As far as the principles of *yoga sādhanā* are concerned, they are applicable to both in accomplishing *citta prasādanam* and *adhyātma prasādanam*.

Though there is no difference gender-wise in *yoga-anuṣṭhāna*, the difference is in a woman's *dehadharma* or *manodharma*. Her body and mind have significant characteristics which she has to learn to respect and adopt the *sādhanā* according to her *dehadharma* and *manodharma*.

I said earlier that women have emotional intelligence while men have their intellectual calibre. On account of this, a woman thinks on the emotional level while man shows his intellectual pride without emotional feelings. Man is empowered with analysis and reasoning *(vitarka, vicāra)* whereas a woman is endowed with friendliness and compassion *(maitrī, karuṇā)*. The blending of these four factors of men and women build a right foundation through yoga for a happy married life.

Man appears to be strong physically but a woman is strong mentally as well as neurologically. If something happens to a man he becomes restless and shakes the whole house but a woman does not even say what she is suffering from. Man cannot relax easily as a woman does. This is the only difference I see because her nerves withstand the burden while a man cannot bear even the mildest pain. A woman can endure the physical, physiological, neurological, mental and emotional problems with patience but a man loses his patience all at once.

Today yoga is termed as power yoga, sex yoga, hot yoga and so forth. For example, the balancing *āsana (Bhuja Tolāsana)* are called power yoga. *Light on Yoga* is filled with balancing *āsana*, but I never named them as power yoga. In my presentation there is grace and not muscular exhibitionism. I have taught balancing *āsana* to women for years but I never made them 'masculine'.

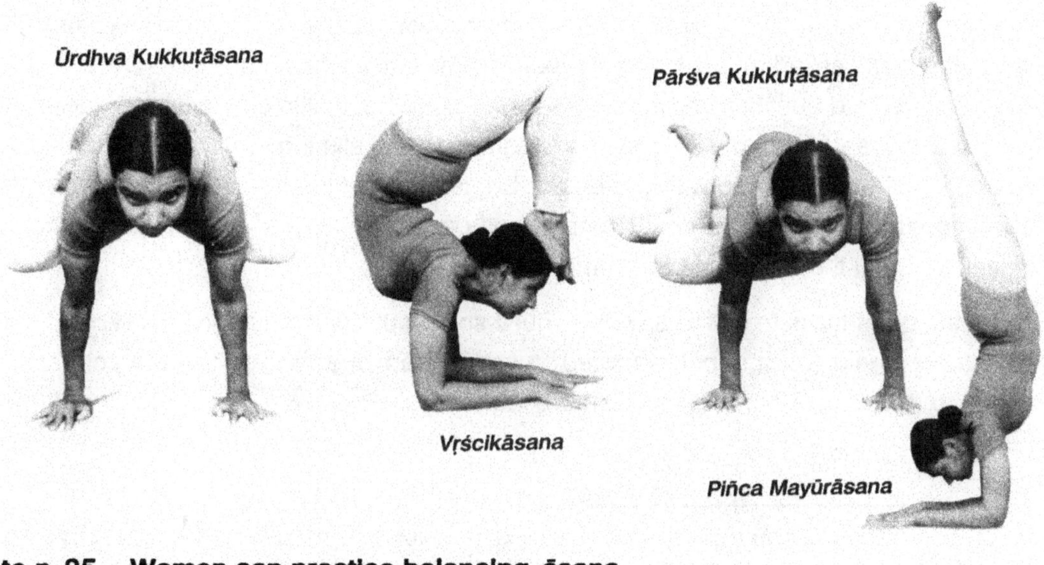
Ūrdhva Kukkuṭāsana
Pārśva Kukkuṭāsana
Vṛścikāsana
Piñca Mayūrāsana

Plate n. 25 – Women can practice balancing *āsana*

Women have a broad pelvic girdle for child bearing. Normally they use the vital abdominal organs instead of arms in balancing *āsana*. Hence I say that it is not advisable to do the balancing acts by using wrong means, but they can do them without straining the organic body. They need prudent care and skill.

Now books of *kāma* yoga are available in the market as if yoga is a *kāma sūtra*. Yoga is not a *bhoga śāstra* but a *mokṣa śāstra*. Let not women be caught with such sensual books. So let men and women treat yoga with the nobility that it demands. Secondly *āsana* and *prāṇāyāma* are not competitive but non-violent movements facilitating evolution on physical, mental and spiritual levels.

Women are self-sacrificing by nature. Women as householders face lots of physical and emotional stress. They have to maintain harmony at home. Hence, they come to yoga more than men. They take to yoga which brings them peace and poise. Men are a bit selfish and pay less attention to home and health. Having taught yoga more to women than men, I say with joy that they are more enlightened than men in understanding the value of life both intellectually and emotionally.

Some time back I was asked to explain the benefit of yoga to a group of nuns with Geeta's demonstration. Being nuns, they lead the life like our *sannyāsini*. I showed them what *āsana* and *prāṇāyāma* they should do to keep themselves in physical, mental and emotional control and I am happy that many of them are practising yoga.

I was asked in the class an absurd question by men who were observing a class where women were more in numbers. The question was, "Do women practise yoga to lure men?" I laughingly asked men who were attending the class whether they are coming to lure women! Such stupid questions arise because the colour of the skin changes, their faces glow with *tejas*. If you read this glow as glamorous, attractive and alluring it is the weakness of your mind and it has nothing to do with allurement. So get yourself to change mentally rather than building up such thoughts. No doubt yoga brings perfection, beauty of form, grace, strength, compactness, and the brilliance of a diamond.[1]

Man plays tricks to entice a woman but if she rebuffs with courage he will be afraid to approach her again. Yoga is not practised to lure a man or a woman. On the contrary it is practised to maintain self-respect and inner beauty.

---

1 *rūpa lāvaṇya bala vajra saṁhananatvāni kāyasampat* (*Y.S.*, III.47) – perfection of the body consists of beauty of form, grace, strength, compactness, and the hardness and brilliance of a diamond.

Purpose in a woman's life

Let women understand the purpose of their life. The childhood state of girls is almost identical to that of boys. So it is inexcusable when we hear that girls are abused by men, whether they be a father, uncle, brother or cousin. Often a question is raised whether yoga is meant for women. My answer will be that whether one is a woman or a man, yoga is essential from childhood itself. Perhaps I was the first one to introduce yoga in schools in the thirties when the subject was unknown. When the children complete six and enter seven, it is an ideal age to begin *āsana* as fun.

In olden days both girls and boys were initiated *brahmopadeśa*. They were trained to chant the *gāyatri mantra*. They were sent to the *āśrama* of *ṛṣi*, *muni* or a *yogi* for higher education. They were educated in all branches of knowledge whether it is *veda*, yoga, art, military training, language, grammar, commerce, agriculture and so forth.

Today apart from modern education, the seed of *saṁskāra* has to be sown at a tender age to culture the mind for purity and clarity.

As this chapter is on "Yoga: a saviour in a women's life", it is important to know that women undergo four important stages in their life. These are menstruation, pregnancy, delivery and menopause.

When girls reach the adolescent stage they become aware of their gender and begin to recognise their individualities. Their lives change and transform gradually towards sensuality as well as sexuality. At this point of time they need protection and right understanding of the value of life. They should be taught what self control is and what it means so that they should not fall a pray to temptations and attractions towards the opposite sex. I have raised funds on many occasions to help unmarried mothers in Africa and I know how much they are afflicted by unstable or troubled minds. In order to educate them to maintain self-respect and a certain amount of discipline, I was keen on introducing yoga in schools as I was a pioneer in co-educating boys and girls, men and women in yoga since 1937. However, this is still not happening. Swami Rāmadāsa had said long back in *Marāthi*, "action not words". It means the value of morality is not yet understood.

Menstruation

Menstruation, which begins between the ages of ten to fifteen and continues until forty-five to fifty-five is an important phase in women's lives. They mature earlier than males. At this time physiological and psychological changes take place in them.

At this time physical strength, physiological functioning, sensitivity of mind in dealing with complex emotional changes, development in metabolism, stabilising and maintaining the hormonal balance as well as strong will-power to build up moral conduct and character are important.

The right practice of *āsana* and *prāṇāyāma* is essential to deal with the above points in comfort.

Symptomatic menstrual disorders may occur, such as hygienic negligence, stress factors, occupational hazards, under-development, fears, frustrations, neurosis, glandular deficiency, malnutrition, anaemia, exhaustion, fibroids, cysts, inflammation of ovaries, fallopian tubes or womb, maldevelopment of uterus, displaced uterus, painful or absence of menstruation, irregular, scanty, short or prolonged heavy bleeding or clinical disorders caused through nephritis, diphtheria, tumours or strain on the nervous system. These disorders can be avoided or minimised.

For problems like amenorrhoea, dysmenorrhoea, menorrhagia, metrorrhagia, hypomenorrhoea, oligomenorrhoea, polymenorrhoea, leucorrhoea, pre-menstrual tension and so forth, there are corrective practices of *āsana* and *prāṇāyāma* which have to be practised regularly with proper sequence so that these defects are avoided, minimised or cured.

I am not giving the details of *āsana* or *prāṇāyāma* here as these practices have to be attended by practical means and with regard to the student's intellectual capability and emotional conditioning.

As children they can start from the age of seven and practise as many *āsana* as possible. At a young age, a child's head is longer than its clasped arms, therefore they need not be taught *Śīrṣāsana.* The moment their arms get longer then there is no harm in them doing *Śīrṣāsana.* They need to learn the standing *āsana* first for toning the muscles. Then they are taught a few *āsana* which are like *Sūrya namaskāra* but slightly variant to the conventional way of doing *Sūrya namaskāra.* Afterwards simple lateral anterior and posterior movements are taught.

By the time the girls face their first menstruation they should be able to do the basic inversions, namely, *Śīrṣāsana, Sarvāṅgāsana, Halāsana* and *Setu Bandha Sarvāṅgāsana,* a few forward bends and twists which benefit them greatly in regularising menstrual disorders. During menstruations they should avoid inversions. As the menstrual period ends they can practise inversions to feel normalcy in physical, physiological and psychological states.

Prāṇāyāma like *Ujjāyi, Viloma, Bhrāmari* and short time *Antara Kuṁbhaka* can be started from the age of fifteen or sixteen. Do *Bhastrikā* only when one is affected by a cold as it opens the sinus blockage. But do it for a very short time.[1] Those who suffer from a splitting head-ache before menstruation should practise *Ardha Halāsana* with legs resting on stool, *Viparīta Karaṇī, Setu Bandha Sarvāṅgāsana, Paśchimottānāsana* using bolster or pillows for the head to rest. This eradicates head aches bringing calmness in the nervous system and mind.

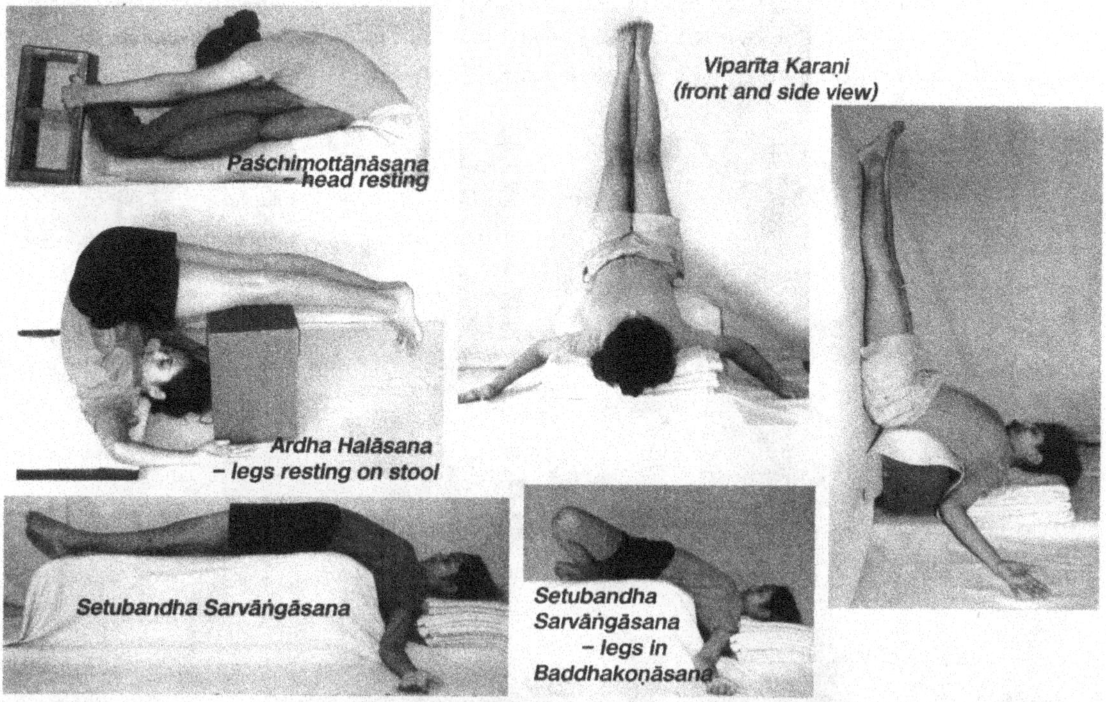

Plate n. 26 – *Āsana* for splitting head-ache before menstruation

Girls are now getting well educated in the field of their choice. As such, the present day life makes both mind and body race. This fast life affects their bodies and minds with the factor of stress, depression, dehydration, nervous tension, irregular menses, fibroids, cysts and infertility. On account of these unnatural situations for girls and women in particular, yoga acts as a god-given boon provided they practise it regularly at least thirty to forty minutes a day.

Gṛhasthāśrama

It is essential for both a wouldbe wife or husband to adopt yoga for healthy progeny. In Indian culture married life is known as *gṛhasthāśrama.* It is not meant merely to lead a married life but to maintain a healthy sexual life with purity and sanctity.

[1] For cautions, refer to the author's *Light on Prāṇāyāma* by Harper Collins, London.

Conception, pregnancy and delivery are the important events in married life.

These days conception has become a matter of choice in life by adopting un-natural means to postpone conception. Even in delayed conception, one can easily maintain a healthy state of life with hormonal balance by practising *āsana* like *Śīrṣāsana* and *Sarvāṅgāsana* with their cycles,[1] forward bendings and a few lateral *āsana* or twists. These *āsana* act as anterior massage and soothes the reproductive organs, while *Ūrdhva Dhanurāsana*, *Viparīta Daṇḍāsana*, strengthen and activate the ovarian glands, uterus, and fallopian tubes by increased blood supply for healthy pregnancy as well as normal delivery ensue.

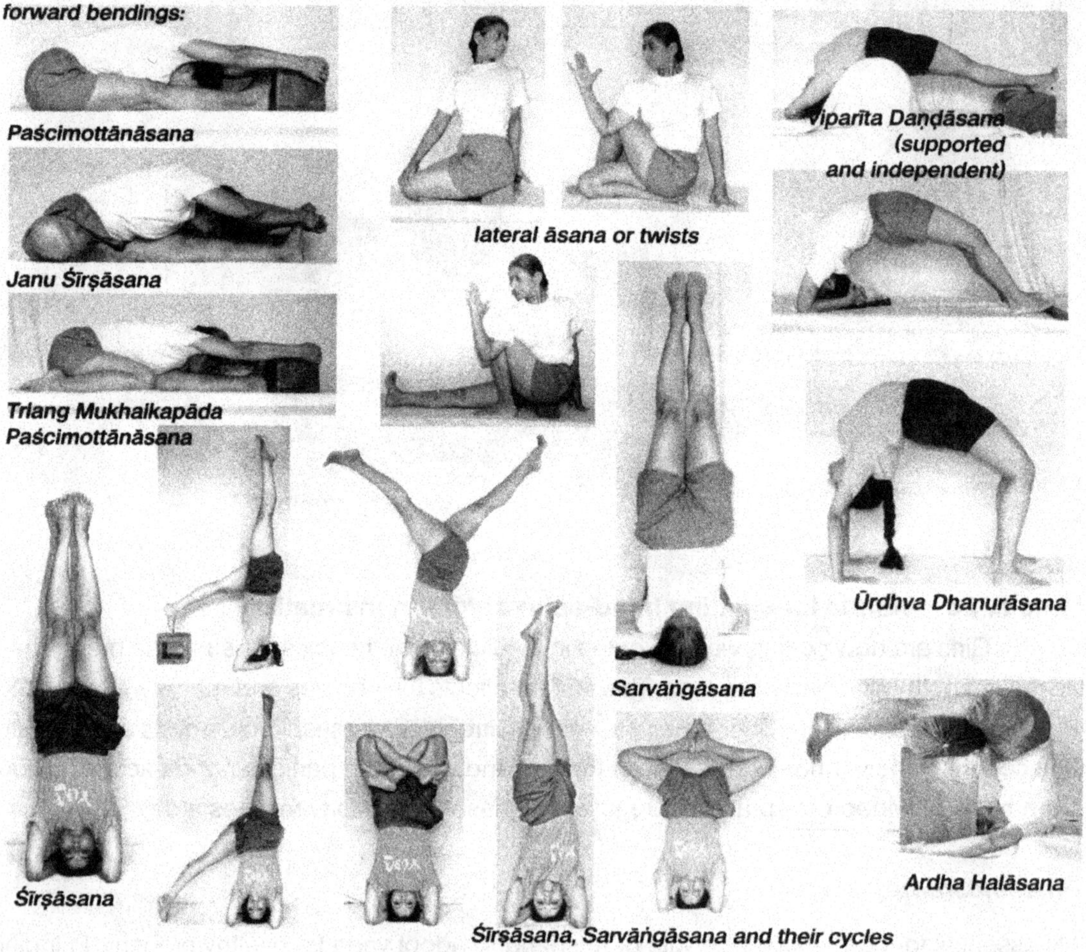
forward bendings:
Paścimottānāsana
Janu Śīrṣāsana
Triang Mukhaikapāda Paścimottānāsana
lateral āsana or twists
Viparīta Daṇḍāsana (supported and independent)
Ūrdhva Dhanurāsana
Sarvāṅgāsana
Ardha Halāsana
Śīrṣāsana
Śīrṣāsana, Sarvāṅgāsana and their cycles

Plate n. 27 – *Āsana* for hormonal balance

---

[1] See *Yoga - A Gem for Women*, by Geeta S. Iyengar, Allied Publishers, New Delhi and the author's *Light on Yoga*, Harper Collins, London.

However while doing backbendings, women with flexible lumbar area have to take precaution. They should learn to extend without contracting the lumbar area by maintaining softness in the abdominal organs by spreading them sideways. Do not hold the muscles of the abdomen or the throat hard or narrow while doing these *āsana*. By this they will avoid constricting the growth of the foetus. See that by wrong practice or by over-exertion one does not hinder healthy growth.

I have taught women who could not conceive and where doctors had declared that this was impossible. I have treated problems like hormonal imbalances, displaced or reclined or retroverted uterus, vaginal infections, blocked fallopian tubes, amenorrhoea and so forth. Often I have insisted the couple attend the classes regularly.

I am delighted to say that these women conceived and had healthy children as well as grand-children. For a yoga teacher it requires great skill to teach such women as the teacher has to see the extension, expansion and elongation to stimulate the exact required regions for proper activation.

Some women have anxieties regarding practising *āsana* thinking that they may cause gynaecological problems. On the contrary these *āsana* help to strengthen the spinal muscles and abdomen. Only those who are hyper-tense, short tempered or weak in lungs are advised not to do the standing *āsana*. In certain cases we make them do these *āsana* between the wall and the trestle in front to create courage and confidence to strengthen the spinal muscles.

Utthita Trikoṇāsana

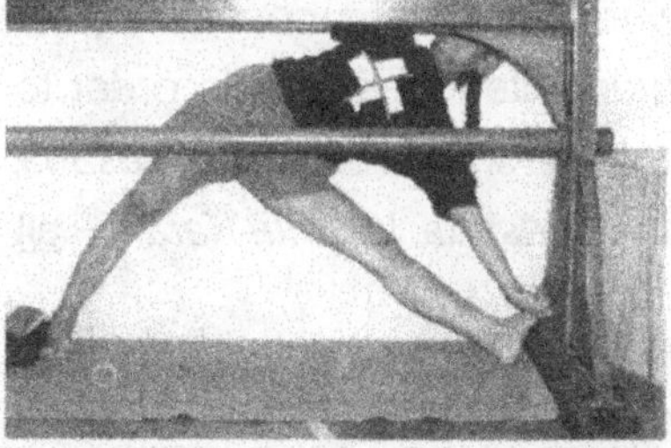

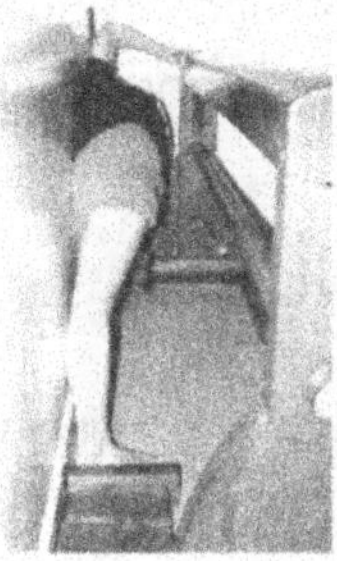

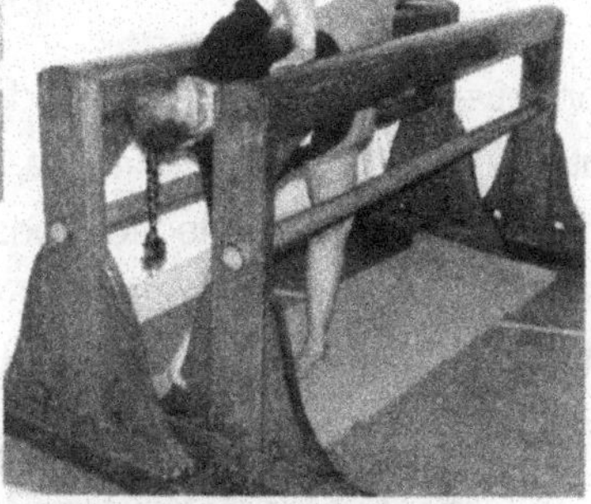

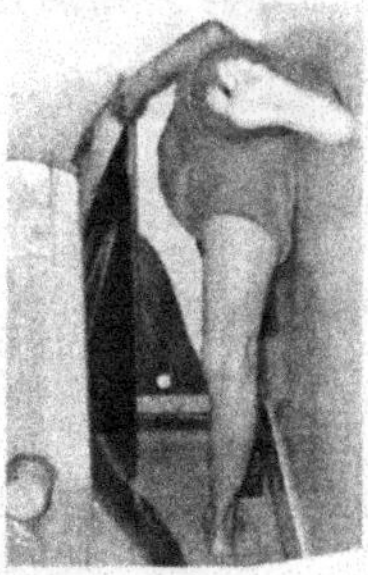

Ardha Chandrāsana

Plate n. 28 – Standing *āsana* between the wall and trestle

I have already mentioned about the balancing *āsana* which may hinder conception due to the hardening of the abdominal organs. Even a wrong way of doing backbends may hinder conception.

Many women perform drastic actions like *Uḍḍiyāna* and *Nauli* to reduce fat around the abdomen to appear trim.

My advice and warning to them is not to indulge in *Nauli* and *Bhastrikā*. Sometimes sucking the abdominal organs with intervals *(Uḍḍīyāna)* is not bad. They have to stop these practices the moment they know they have conceived.[1]

Suppose you have a small rose sapling in the garden, what happens if you uproot that sapling and replant it at a different place each day? The sapling perishes and dies. The same thing happens to the internal organs through *Nauli* or its revolving movements. This is the reason why the original texts have said that these are to be practised by those whose humours *(tridoṣa)* are abnormally in the state of imbalance *(H.Y.P.,* II.21). *Yogi* like Yājñavalkya are not in favour of *ṣaṭkarma* but prefer *prāṇāyāma. (H.Y.P.,* II.37).

Though I have said that *Uḍḍīyāna* is good as it contracts and massages the abdominal organs, they should know to do it correctly without constricting the thoracic cage. Before attempting *Uḍḍīyāna* my advice would be to practise first inversions where the natural and unintentional *uḍḍīyāna* takes place by which the abdominal organs are strengthened. Women are prone to many gynaecological problems and my advice would be that women should not attempt *Nauli* as it affects the system. About *Uḍḍīyāna* it can be tried periodically and never after conception. If they persist in practising they may invite gynaecological problems such as cyst or fibroids and conceiving becomes the problem. It is a hundred times better for women to practise *āsana* and *prāṇāyāma* which are non-injurious and safe. Let there be discrimination and prudence regarding its practical aspects and proper basic knowledge.

Pregnancy

After a woman conceives or misses her period not knowing whether she has conceived, her first duty is to protect herself from miscarriage. This happens very often for some. In order to prevent miscarriage or if she is habituated to repeated miscarriages she should stick to *Śīrṣāsana, Viparīta Daṇḍāsana, Sarvāṅgāsana, Halāsana, Setu Bandha Sarvāṅgāsana, Viparīta Karaṇi* – all supported so that the miscarriages are arrested.

[1] The proprietress of the Standard Oil Company from U.S.A., who was about fifty , practised *Nauli* for years and developed a stomach pit where the food used to accumulate without allowing it to move through the duodenum and alimentary canal. She tried all types of treatments but failed. Being a friend of Lord Yehudi Menuhin, she took his advice and invited me to the States to treat her through yoga. First, I watched her practices and stopped them all and concentrated in teaching *Śīrṣāsana* and *Sarvāṅgāsana* cycles. Within fifteen days, she recovered and the stomach pit disappeared and the floor of the stomach came to normal position. She lived up to the ripe old age of eighty-five without any problems.

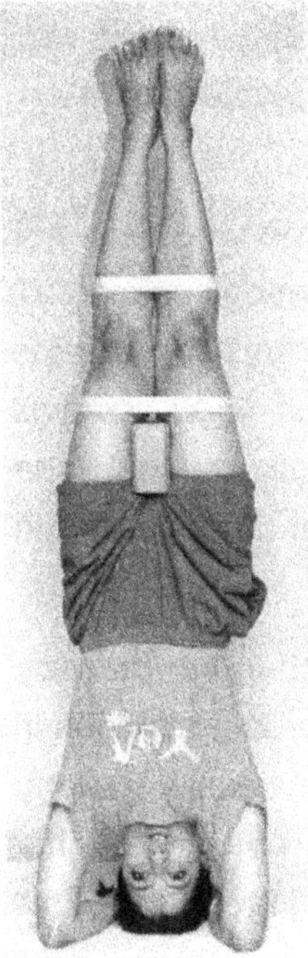

Śīrṣāsana

***Viparīta Daṇḍāsana* (supported)**

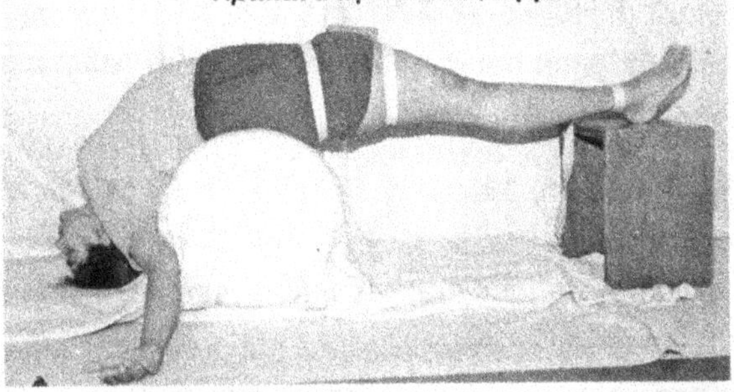

All *āsana* here are shown with the use of a brick tied with belts around the thighs and shins to create space for the baby to grow.

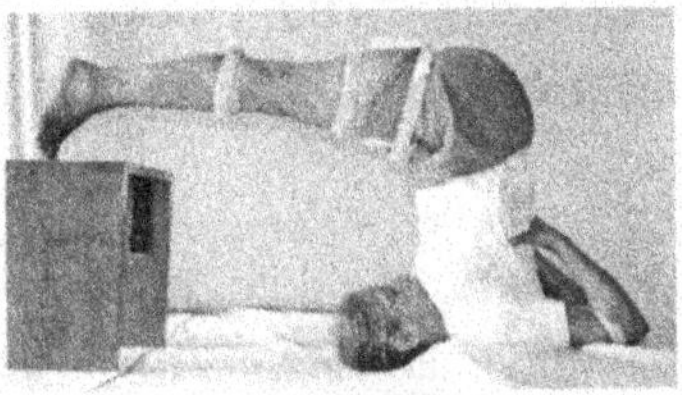

***Halāsana* (supported)**

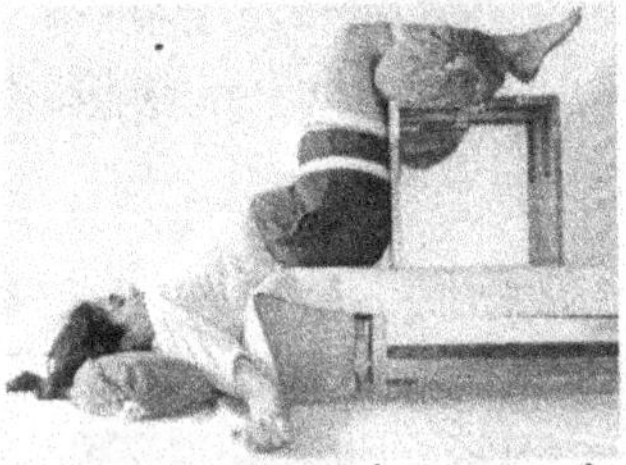

***Viparīta Karaṇi* (supported)**

Sarvāṅgāsana

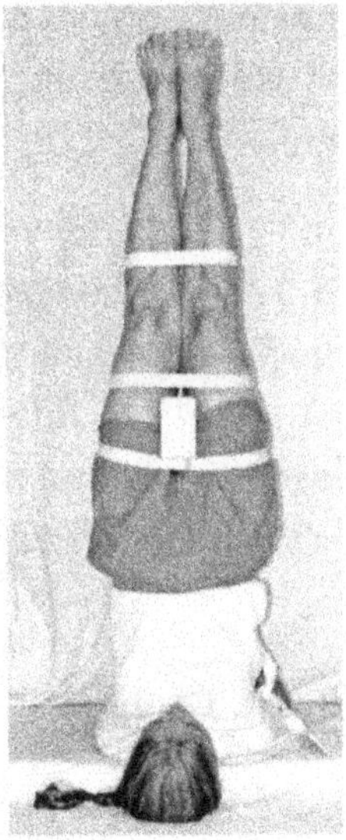

***Setubandha Sarvāṅgāsana* (supported)**

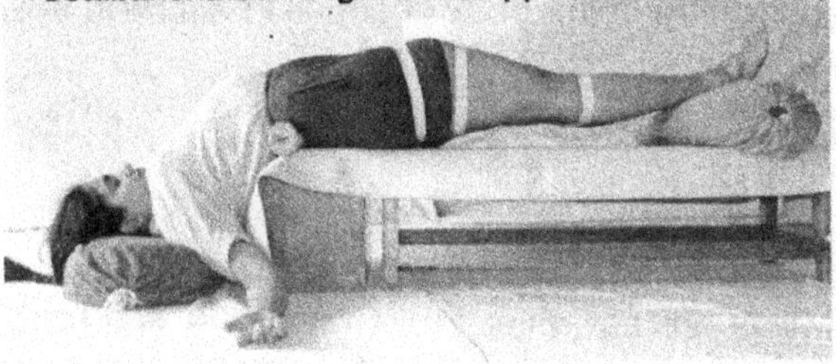

Plate n. 29 – *Āsana* when there is repeated miscarriage

However, I have taken hundreds of pregnant ladies making them do *āsana* and *prāṇāyāma* throughout pregnancy so that they create space for the baby to move and kick.

During pregnancy women normally are afraid or nervous to practise yoga. They cannot imagine standing on their heads during pregnancy. Let me assure them that these *āsana* are a boon for them. Daily practice of *āsana* and *prāṇāyāma* which are essential during pregnancy has to be done regularly. Then they maintain physical and mental health and also create good and auspicious *saṁskāra* in the baby while carrying. Yoga cannot be practised with suspicion or doubt. Then it harms both the mother and baby. Practice at the time of pregnancy establishes the "feel of contact" with the baby inside the body and showers good and auspicious thoughts with peaceful and untainted mind as its mother keeps her body healthy with relaxed nerves. Her digestive, circulatory, excretory systems function well and the glandular system undergoes a sea change in its hormonal functions. Besides these benefits, its practice will take care of keeping away diseases and infections and help in maintaining a good hygienic health with perfect immune system preparing her mind for an easy delivery without stress, tension, agitation, fear or anxiety.

I am happy to say that in my teaching career I taught so many women who were not conceiving owing to defects, deficiency, or incorrect functioning and subsequently conceived. Yoga protected and prevented those who had several miscarriages. Some who had no problems yet could not conceive after years of marriage got children after starting the *yoga sādhanā* together. I do not claim these achievements out of self pride but I emphatically say that yoga blessed those who practised accurately, honestly and religiously with faith and confidence in me.

If a pregnant woman is healthy then there are no restrictions as such in her practice. She can do the standing *āsana*, forward extension and sitting *āsana* paying proper attention in keeping the spinal muscles strong. She can do the inversions and backward extension as long as her breath runs normally and if any untoward feeling takes place, she can consult her teacher at once.[1] Only positioning of the body changes in *āsana* in advanced pregnancy. This holds good for *prāṇāyāma* also.

Some Cautions

However some prudent hints are essential. While practising *āsana* she should not hold the breath but breathe slowly and softly with a calm mind. She has to attend in keeping the spinal muscles well extended without wrong or crooked movements. She has to keep her chest well lifted without hardening the muscles but maintaining smooth, soft breathing. Never practise with laboured breath.

She should not do any type of vigorous exercises. She should avoid all the abdominal *āsana (udarākuncana āsana)* where compression, tightness and pressure take place. *Āsana* work on organic body like the glands, diaphragm, lungs, kidneys, bladder, uterus and hence they play an important role as they keep the abdominal organs without distension. A lively feeling has to be felt while practising to keep both mother and baby healthy.

The sequencing of practice changes as the pregnancy advances. In each trimester her programme needs changes according to growth. With this prudence, she can practise safely until the last day of pregnancy.

---

[1] Refer to *Yoga – A Gem for Women*, by Geeta S. Iyengar, published by Allied Publishers, New Delhi, India.

Prāṇāyāma

Prāṇāyāma at this stage is very important. She has to do *Śavāsana* by using two pillows to support the back with the buttocks on floor or it can be done with elevated chest and head in a comfortable sitting posture taking the support of wall, or sitting comfortably on the chair which keeps her spine erect without strain or collapse. As sitting on a chair gives a good lift, freedom in the pelvic area is felt for long deep breaths. I advise safe *prāṇāyāma* like *Ujjāyī* with or without short *Kuṁbhaka, Viloma, Bhrāmari* and digital *Pratiloma prāṇāyāma*. Never do *Kapālabhāti, Bhastrikā, Mūla bandha, Uḍḍiyāna bandha* or *Bāhya Kuṁbhaka*. However the passive, pensive *Bāhya Kuṁbhaka* for two or three seconds is good.[1]

Often pregnant women come and ask for yoga practice with back problems or loose motions. Though I help them on compassionate grounds it is not the right approach. If they take to yoga as a way of life earlier, then it is easy to teach as body and mind are toned to some extent. When pregnant women with problems approach for yogic practices, then methods and sequences are to be adjusted differently compared to those who attend the classes regularly before pregnancy. But those teachers who have no knowledge to teach pregnant women should not take risks at all.

Late marriages lead to late pregnancy which brings lots of problems like blood pressure, anaemia, diabetes, disproportionate weight gain, albumin in urine, toxaemia and so forth. Such problems can be handled through yoga with matured experience though it is a hard job. I have dealt with such problems when women have conceived at the age of forty and forty-five. Yet I want to advise to accept a child after marriage and then follow the means of birth control rather than giving a thought to have a child at a late age.

Before ending on pregnancy I would like to say that yoga acts as a boon to problems like morning sickness, weakness, dizziness, swelling, slowness, numbness in feet, pain, blood discharges, varicose veins, variations in blood pressure, backache, headache, leg pain, heaviness in the lower abdomen, acidity, poor digestion, constipation, blurred vision, water retention and frequent urination. Though I cannot claim emphatically yet I say that I have succeeded to bring foetus to natural position when it was in abnormal position or when the baby does not come to normal position before delivery.[2]

---

[1] For the details, refer to the author's *Light on Prāṇāyāma* and *Yoga – A Gem for Women*, by Geeta S. Iyengar.
[2] See pl. n. 34, vol. 5, *Aṣṭadaḷa Yogamālā*.

Delivery

During delivery though one does not do the prescribed *āsana,* we make them do certain *āsana* to keep the pelvic muscles, uterine muscles and spinal muscles strong to deliver with minimum labour pain. Then the mother in labour faces the spasms of contraction and relaxation courageously and with a relaxed mind. If the caesarean operation is unavoidable or inevitable under certain circumstances yogic practice helps the abdominal and spinal muscles to rejuvenate soon.

Lactation

The quality of mother's milk is very important for the baby to get immunity and proper development. Though it is nectar for the infant, it is likely to happen that mother's milk may develop certain problems. In *Āyurveda* we call it *stanya doṣa. Stana* means breast. The breast-milk is called *stanya.* It can get affected by *vāta, pitta* or *kapha* according to their diminution or increase which happens due to wrong diet and bad mental condition. The mothers need to keep themselves calm, composed and balanced. They should not get unnecessarily tense, agitated

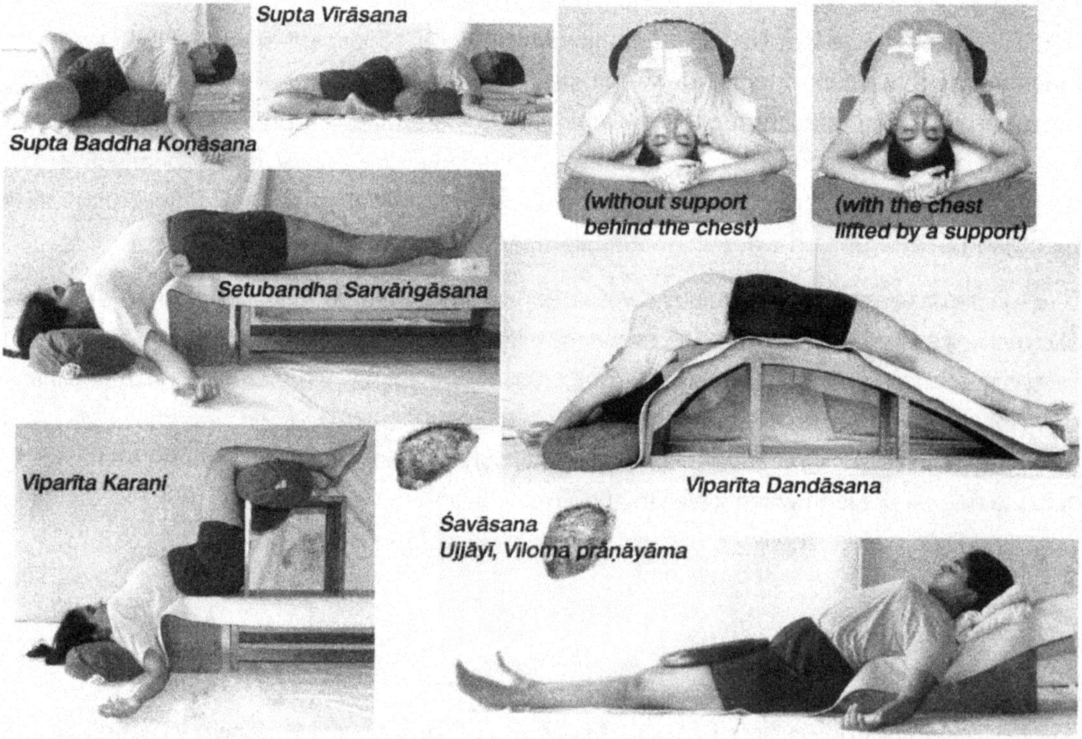

Plate n. 30 – *Āsana* for the young mother during lactation

or irritated. They should be free from fear, anger, greed, desires, unhappiness and sorrow. Even in these situations yoga proves to be "the mother" from which one can get solace. A good *Śavāsana, Ujjāyī, Viloma prāṇāyāma,* simple *āsana* such as *Supta Baddha Koṇāsana, Supta Vīrāsana, Viparīta Daṇḍāsana* or *Setu Bandha Sarvāṅgāsana* on bench, *Viparīta Karaṇī* help her to get back emotional stability, hormonal balance, rich milk, physical strength and nervous stability.

A month or two after delivery, she can start the practice of *āsana* and *prāṇāyāma* gradually in order to tone the spinal muscles and strengthen the abdominal organs.

Middle Age

Marriage, pregnancies, deliveries and bringing up children until the completion of education keep women busy and occupied. The responsibilities of children's education, sickness and looking after them through adolescence tell upon the mother's body and mind. Responsibilities and duties of house-keeping have a different kind of stress and load.

They in turn bring hordes of diseases such as indigestion, acidity, dyspepsia, ulcer, diarrhoea, constipation, hormonal imbalances, arthritis, rheumatism, circulatory disturbance, heavy breathing and cardiac problems.

If she continues practising *Ardha Nāvāsana, Paripūrṇa Nāvāsana, Jaṭhara Parivartanāsana (udara ākuncanā sthiti), Bharadvājāsana, Marichyāsana* III, *Ardha Matsyendrāsana (parivṛtta sthiti), Paśchimottānāsana, Jānu Śīrṣāsana (paśchima pratana sthiti),*

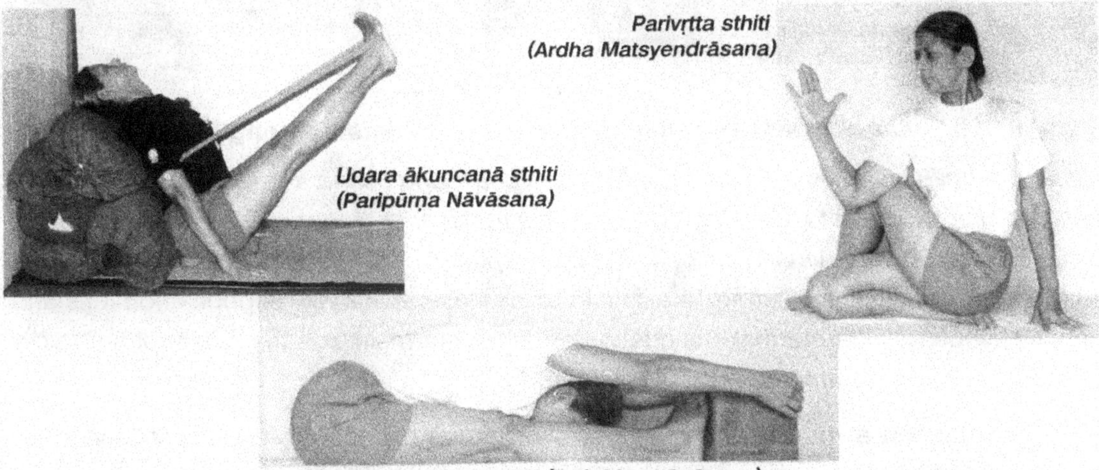

Paśchima pratana sthiti (Paśchimottānāsana)

Plate n. 31a – *Āsana* practice during midde age to maintain strength and health

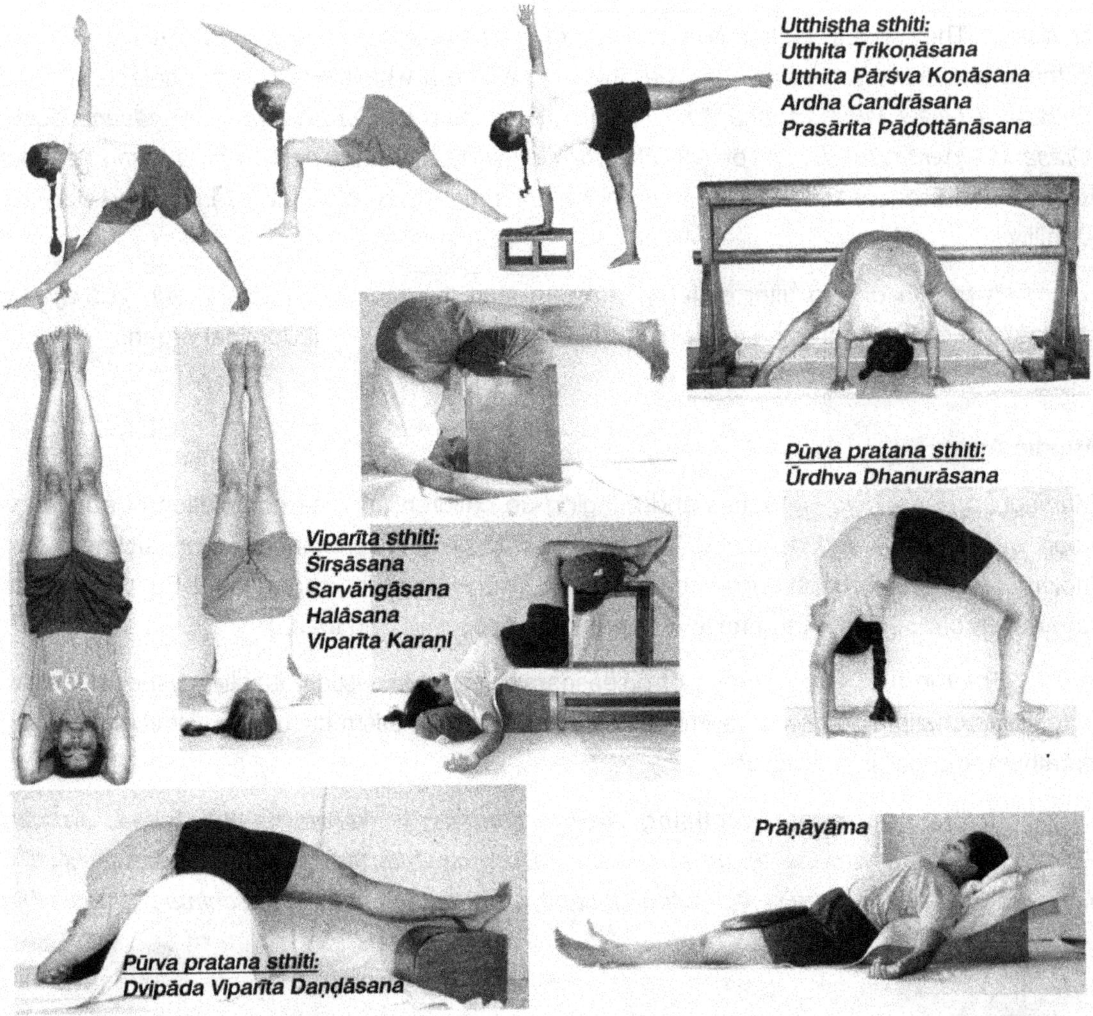
Utthiṣṭha sthiti:
Utthita Trikoṇāsana
Utthita Pārśva Koṇāsana
Ardha Candrāsana
Prasārita Pādottānāsana
Pūrva pratana sthiti:
Ūrdhva Dhanurāsana
Viparīta sthiti:
Śīrṣāsana
Sarvāṅgāsana
Halāsana
Viparīta Karaṇi
Prāṇāyāma
Pūrva pratana sthiti:
Dvipāda Viparīta Daṇḍāsana

Plate n. 31b – *Āsana* practice during midde age to maintain strength and health

Utthita Trikoṇāsana, Utthita Pārśva Koṇāsana, Ardha Candrāsana, Prasārita Pādottānāsana (uttiṣṭha sthiti), Śīrṣāsana, Sarvāṅgāsana, Halāsana, Viparīta Karaṇi, (viparīta sthiti), Ūrdhva Dhanurāsana, Dvipāda Viparīta Daṇḍāsana (pūrva pratana sthiti) along with *Prāṇāyāma*, her mind will remain quiet and strong. She should do all these *āsana* with support and props and not independently. She not only attends to her health but maintains the health of her family members to live in joy and happiness.

Excess flow at the time of menstruation or irregular periods, anxiety, fear of conception or use of contraceptives or forcefully creating hardness and tightness in the lower abdominal organs to maintain a youthful, attractive figure, brings disturbance of hormonal secretions, cysts and tumours in the uterus. So they have to learn to keep the uterine area soft and natural while doing the *āsana*. In backward extensions *(pūrva pratana sthiti)*, pay attention in extending and expanding the lower back and at the same time elevating the spinal column.

They should be aware of back pain and gripping abdominal pain that occur at the time of menstruation. At that time they have to practise soothing *āsana* so that tension, gripping abdominal pain, stiff back are removed and relaxation is brought in at the affected areas.

Menopause

Women of middle age going towards menopause have to understand certain facts of what happens to them. At that time fat accumulates around their waist. They want to reduce their fat. Taking drastic steps for reduction means inviting loss of vital energy and cardiac problems. Vigorous movements for fat reduction cause a hike in blood pressure, throbbing headache or heavy bleeding, fibroids, cysts, bulkiness of uterus and endometriosis.

Often she faces irregularities in menstruation. Sometimes the bleeding is less and scanty and sometimes the bleeding is continuous. All these happen due to the hormonal imbalances and at the same time for stopping menstruation.

Before the cessation of menstruation, it is called pre-menopausal state and after it ends, it is called the post-menopausal state.

After a major earthquake, tremors continue till the earth settles. It is the same with menopause or cardiac attack.

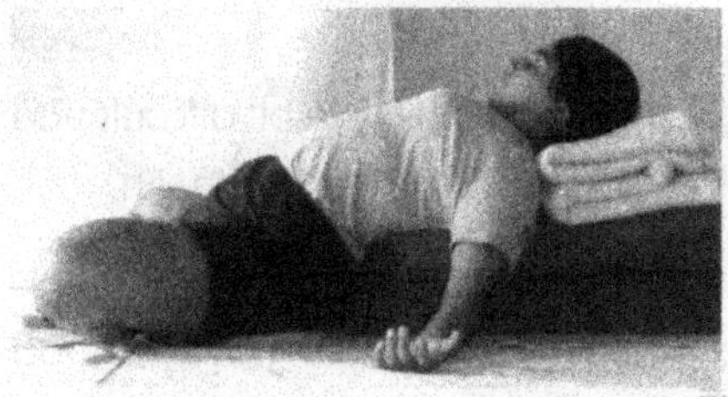

Supine āsana:
Supta Baddhakoṇāsana
Supta Vīrāsana

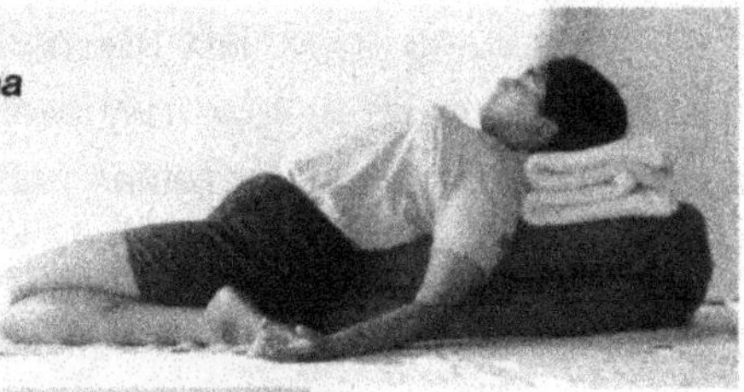

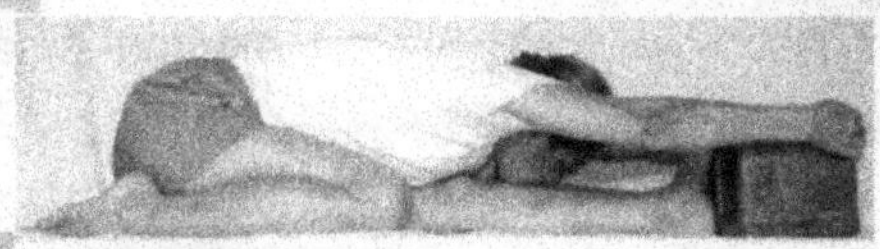

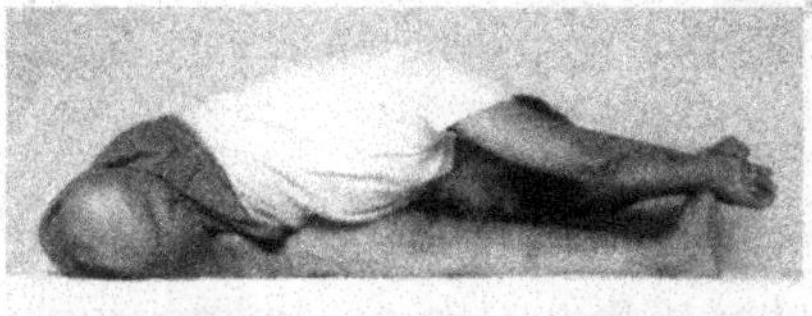

Forward extensions:
Janu Śīrṣāsana
Triang Mukhaikapāda in Paścimottānāsana
Paścimottānāsana

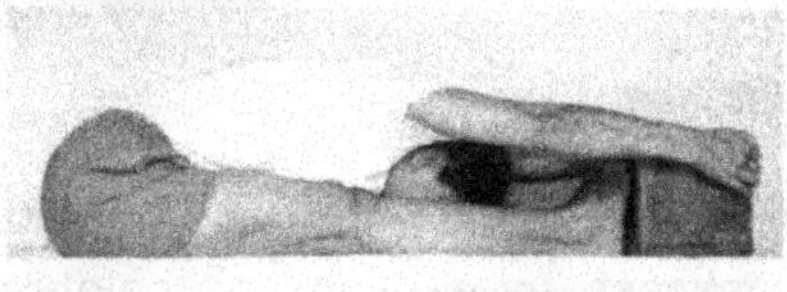

Plate n. 32a – *Āsana* to calm women's physical, physiological and psychological sheaths

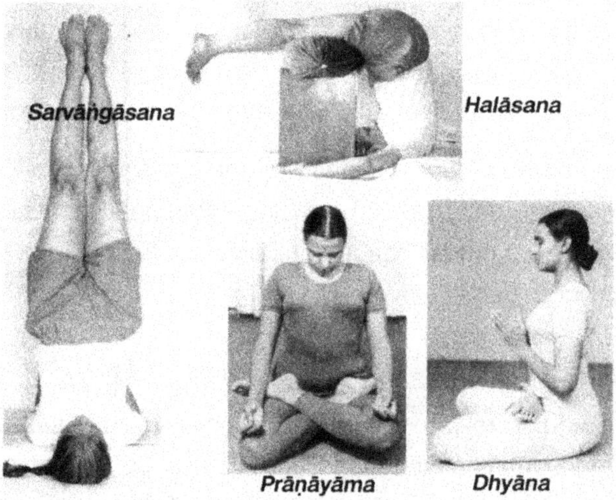

Plate n. 32b – *Āsana* to calm women's physical, physiological and psychological sheaths

The condition of a woman at the time of menopause is similar to what Patañjali says *duḥkha* (sorrowfulness), *daurmanasya* (depression or dejection) and *aṅgamejayatva* (nervous breakdown) and *śvāsa praśvāsa* (breathlessness). So she becomes either emotionally sensitive or gets irritated and disturbed over small issues. She becomes short tempered. In place of endurance, courage and self confidence; fear, anxiety, dissatisfaction, loss of self esteem and frustration can take place.

To face these mental disturbances she should practice supine *āsana,* forward extensions, *Sarvāṅgāsana, Halāsana, prāṇāyāma,* and *dhyāna* which help in calming her physical, physiological and psychological sheaths.

Years ago in the East, the mental stress and problems of menopause were considered a natural phenomenon. Now they have become a global problem. No doubt it is a bit difficult and a delicate situation but it is factual and hence women should not lose their heart and faith.

As such my advice for men is to pause and give time for women to recover. It is the best period of life for both of them to keep up the yogic practice in order to have a good understanding. Let men not forget that they too suffer in the same as women. Men should know that this period is for them andropause .

Old Age

At every stage of life not only women but men also face nervousness, fear, sickness and weakness. As we keep on celebrating each year birthday after birthday we are unknowingly reaching the doors of death. Yet we think that we are going to live eternally not knowing that the sword of uncertainty of life is hanging above our head. Many people have certain strange ideas that they have to divert their attention towards spirituality only at old age. Some think that they remain young for ever. Some others think that they should spend their old age by going to clubs, playing cards, golf and so forth.

Without proper preparation from youth, spiritual wisdom does not dawn in old age. Old age is a respectable age where one lives as an ideal example and guide the younger generation in the art of right living. However, they should think of treading on the path by balancing the philosophy of body with the philosophy of spiritual life. Adopting yoga at old age, though late, body and mind remain stable and steady without being dependent on others. If one starts yoga at an earlier age then death happens as a natural phenomenon. This means dying with serenity *(ātmānanda)* and majesty.

Often women may have to face hardships and live all alone if their husbands are bed-ridden or no more alive. One cannot jump to spiritual life at once. If their economic condition is a worry and helplessness taunts them, they have to sweat with labour to maintain themselves in old age. I have seen such men and women maintaining not only good health but mental balance by taking to yoga. I have seen their morale elevated and up-raised.

Sometime back, I was asked what is menopause and I said jokingly, "Men-O-Pause – men you pause". Everyone applauded. Menopause is a natural moment to switch over from the family responsibilities *(gṛhasthāśrama)* and to move towards *vānaprasthāśrama*. Though, I know many women are afraid of losing their husband's love and affection at the time of menopause, husbands also have to realise that they too may lose the affection from their wives at the time of andropause. At this stage the sex urge fades on its own. As such it is a common phenomenon for both men and women. Hence our saints showed the third order of *āśrama* after passing through *brahmacaryāśrama* and *gṛhasthāśrama*. This state – *vānaprasthāśrama* is the preparatory state to move towards *sannyāsāśrama* (*vānaprastha* means to stay in woods or forest close to the town without breaking the ties with the family).

Vānaprasthāśrama is a stage where one runs the family with non-attachment in learning the art of detachment by relinquishing or resigning from all worldly possessions and to turning one's mind towards spiritual knowledge, surrendering one's actions to the universal power – God. In this sense, *vānaprastha* is the touchstone for *sannyāsāśrama*.

Thus menopause is a natural stage in life that takes place for one to move closer to God.

Also I was questioned why there is no *sannyāsa āśrama* for women. It is not true that women have been banned from *sannyāsa*. In fact, she is a true *sannyāsini* as she does her duties without hankering for fruits and without wearing the saffron robes. Her motherhood itself is a great sacrifice, a great *yajña*. Hence, Manu says that where women are respected there is goodness around in abundance. Where women are not respected all goodness becomes waste with non-auspicious effect.

yatra naryastu pūjyante ramante tatra devataḥ I

yatretāstu na pūjyantesarvāsta trāphalāh kriyāh II

(*Manusmṛti* III.55)

FROM A *ŚIṢYA* TO A *GURU*[*]

I salute my *guru* and the *guru* of all *guru* in yoga – *Vyāsa* and Patañjali. I pray that they grace you all so that you may delve into the depth of the subject. Through their grace I am facing you to speak and if my expressions fail to convince you I take the blame on myself.

Today is a day of great significance as *Vyāsa Pūrṇimā* is celebrated as *Gurupūrṇimā* Day. Patañjali begins his yogic aphorism with *atha yogānuśāsanam* (*Y.S.,* I.1) – the very word *anu* indicates the tradition *(paramparā). Śāsana* means discipline and the subject yoga has a discipline that has been followed from time immemorial by the sages and yogi of India. That is why we find this terminology *anuśāsanam* at the very start of the text. Today our minds are perverted to a very great extent so that we all say that we do not believe in tradition but in rationalism. But you and I cannot utter a word without the background of tradition. As such no one can call himself a rationalist without the back ground of tradition. The words are traditional *(paramparā)* coming from the time the world was created.

For example, milk cannot be called by any other name except as milk. If you say, no, it is rice flour or curds, well that is called perverted intelligence or *viparyaya*. Appraisal of the traditional words can be called rational. Still they are dependent upon traditional words.

So let us respect the traditional words and traditional work which is in vogue from creation. This is the reason why *guru paramparā* is celebrated each year. Let us pay respects to those who gave us that knowledge to evolve from the state where we are and who showed how we can proceed to reach the pinnacle of wisdom to understand what we are.

Vyāsa was the son of Parāśara, a great *muni* and his mother was *Satyavatī* a good looking, attractive fisherwoman. The Sage fell in love with this attractive fisherwoman whose body was smelling with unbearable odour. In order to share bed with her, Parāśara removed that smell from her body as he knew that the seed he was going to plant into her womb would give birth to a son who will become great as Vyāsa. Lord Krishna in the *Gītā*, says that Vyāsa is his incarnation *(aṁśa)* as Krishna Dvaipāyana, the best of all the *ṛṣi*.

[1] Talk given 2007, Pune, India.

Krishna means total darkness. Vyāsa's skin was as dark as charcoal, yet his head was brilliant like the full moon. As his brilliance was compared to the full moon, the *ṛṣi* of past ages began performing this day as *Gurupūrṇimā* or *Vyāsa Pūrṇimā*.

He is the one who arranged the *Veda*. He is the one who gave us the philosophy of life *(Vedānta)*, and he is the one who wrote the first commentary on the *Yoga Sūtra*. He is a king amongst all *ṛṣi* and we respect him in observing this day as this day coincides with his biorthday. We should be particulariy grateful to him for his commentary on the *Yoga Sūtra*. Probably we would not have understood Patañjali's *sūtra* at all without his commentary as they are terse and concise.

Today I had something to speak about but something happened. Mysteriously there was a letter on my table to explain the difference between a student and a *śiṣya* and a teacher and a *guru*. Of course it is an interesting question. But the second question surprised me more. It was, "How did you become a *guru?"* All my thoughts of today's talk changed and I thought of speaking on these two questions which we should know. No doubt, these are challenging questions to know whether you are *śiṣya* or not; whether I am a *guru* or not.

According to the dictionary, a student is one who likes to acquire knowledge from his teacher. I think ninety to ninety-nine percent of students are those who go to college and universities. A teacher or a professor who teaches there is a man qualified academically to transmit what he has learned through the study of books simplifying them to the standard of their students' intellectual calibre. The moment the pupil comes out of the school, college or university the contact between the teacher and the taught mostly fades out. Hence, he is called an *updhyāya* or *adhyāpaka*. Though the word *guru* is quite different, it is hard to find a *guru* as it is also hard to find a *śiṣya*.

Girati ajñānam iti – one who removes ignorance.

Guru is one who removes the weight-fullness of his *śiṣya's* brain and makes it weightless. This means that the *guru* removes *tamo* and *rajo guṇa*. The innate nature of *tamoguṇa* is heaviness and dullness. The *guru* helps in bringing light into his pupil's brain and makes him to grasp the ideas of what he says. That is why he is called a *guru*. Just now we heard the prayer that *guru* is Vishnu, *guru* is Brahmā and *guru* is *Maheshvara;* because he, as a *guru*, transmits knowledge, admonishes when the pupil goes wrong and destroys his ego. He protects his *śiṣya* though he admonishes. The *guru* has all the qualities of Brahmā – the creator, Vishnu – the protector, and Maheshvara – the destroyer of ignorance. These *Trimurthi* (God in three forms) are nothing but Universal Soul or *Puruṣa Viśeṣa Īśvara*. The *guru* destroys the *śiṣya's* bad thoughts, creates new food for thought, and organises life as *anuśāsana* or discipline.

Now let me speak of a *śiṣya*. You and I are practitioners of yoga. We are *abhyāsin* according to Patañjali. He says *abhyāsa vairāgyābhyāṁ tannirodhaḥ, tatra sthitau yatnaḥ abhyāsaḥ* (*Y.S.*, I.12, I.13). Here he explains to a yoga student as a beginner, what *abhyāsa* is. A *guru* does not treat a beginner as a *śiṣya* but as a student. That is why the word *abhyāsa* has come at the very start of the textbook. A *śiṣya* is he who knows the *sādhanā*. As we are all students of yoga, we should know what *yoga sādhanā* is. To become a *sādhaka* you should have tremendous background of what yogic *sādhanā* is. As long as one does not know the background of *sādhanā*, one is not called a *sādhaka* but an *abhyāsin* or a practitioner.

Patañjali has divided the practitioners into four categories as: *mṛdu, madhya, adhimātra* and *tīvra* (*Y.S.*, I.21&22). Similarly, *Haṭhayoga Pradīpikā, Śiva Saṁhitā* explain four types of students. The first one is *ārambhaka*, a beginner. Then comes *ghaṭāvasthā* – to understand the body fully. When he begins to understand the body well, then the real *sādhanā* begins. At this time he becomes a *śiṣya*. Mild and average practitioners who show interest once in a while, are not considered as *sādhaka* as many people do to gain health. Some come for curiosity's sake. The very word *mṛdu* shows that they just like to scratch their structural or peripheral bodies through yoga as *ārambhaka*.

In the *Haṭhayoga Pradīpikā* a *sādhaka* becomes a *śiṣya* when he understands how to dominate his body through his intelligence. This is termed as *paricayāvasthā*. It means that I have to acquaint my intelligence (which is the mind) to be in close touch with my body and my self. At this stage, the *śiṣya sevā* in *sādhanā* begins and not before. He is just an *abhyāsin* till then. From this you can gauge whether you are a student or a *śiṣya*.

Many of you have been practising for a long time, yet I see that your intelligence follows the body while doing the *āsana* without questioning the intelligence to judge the action and flow of energy in the body. Make the intelligence to observe carefully dividing into two parts from the centre of the body and feel its evenness in stretch and expansion of the various limbs and the smoothness and rhythm in each part. Even if one practises for three hours without applying one's intelligence, then one remains an *abhyāsin* and not a *śiṣya*. *Paricayāvasthā* is when the mind introduces each and every part of the body to the intelligence. When intelligence observes and touches *(sparśa)* each and every part of the body without interruption, then the self along with the intelligence engulf the body. If this sensation enters within then you have entered the gates of *śiṣyatva*. Till then you are outside the gate of *śiṣyatva*. The seed of *śiṣya* is inside the body but many of you are still outside the gate of the inner body. The moment the judgment from the intelligence dictates and corrects the movements in each and every *āsana* and in each breath of *prāṇāyāma*, it means the association of the intelligence with the body has taken place. From this point, the transformation of mind into intelligence has taken place. This mind changing into intelligence is integration *(saṁyama).* When this happens, then he becomes a true *śiṣya.* Till then he is in studentship. Having explained the difference between a student and a *śiṣya,* it is for you now to gauge yourself whether you are a *śiṣya* or an *abhyāsin* of yoga.

The second question was, "How did I become a *guru?"* Well it may be interesting to many as many do not know where and when I was addressed as a *guru.*

I started yoga as a practitioner, an *abhyāsin.* I don't want to go into my early life which you all know. When I started practising my *guru* must have thought that one day I might be able to demonstrate. As my practice went on he asked me to demonstrate whenever he used to address the public in yoga. From practitioner I became a demonstrator. As a professor has an instructor and a demonstrator in colleges and universities, my *Gurujī* upgraded me from a demonstrator to become an instructor by asking me to take classes at the *yogaśāla* and on tours. Then he sent me to Pune as an instructor. The word instructor means one who instructs according to his boss! My *guru,* T. Krishnamāchārya, who was my professor and from whom I got and professed the knowledge, upgraded me as an instructor under his supervision.

I remained as an instructor in Pune instructing yoga for several years. As I was not well equipped with the subject, I used to approach my master when problems came which I found difficult to correct. Once or twice he guided me and then told me to work out from my own intelligence and practice. I thought I might get some encouragement from him to work out and practise independently for the problems that arise from teaching. Sometimes I used to get brain storming cases. I used to write him letters where I could not find solutions. Being young, it was too much for me to take the responsibilities of such problems of human beings like physical problems, physiological problems, and mental problems. As I was not yet a qualified teacher. I wrote to my guru to help me. The reply I got from him was that "if you do not know how to guide, you better send them to me". This was a great challenge to me. It meant either I had to find means to work on these problems or to say goodbye to being an instructor of yoga. Then I thought, why should I not take his strong words as an *āśīrvāda* or a grace from him and to use my own intellectual prudence to find ways by working on my own self to search for remedies.

I began working without his consultation making mistakes to start with. If I made a mistake on one person, then I was careful not to commit that same mistake when I handled another person. I used to muse on whether I could build up with new constructive ideas to teach better. This way I went on constructing new thoughts in my practice and developed a way to present the subject with liveliness. This new touch made people to call me a teacher.

From a practitioner I grew to become a demonstrator, then an instructor. After this, with experimentation I became a teacher.

When I was a teacher, the situation for yoga wasn't favourable at all. It was a herculean task to create interest in the subject. By the grace of Patañjali, it took years through demonstrations, teachings and remedial means to create that interest in yoga to gain popularity. Today the wind of yoga is flying high like the sands that reach the sky when the wind is strong. Now, yoga has become so popular that *guru* and *ācārya* have sprung up everywhere, whether they have the knowledge on the subject or not. But at my time it was the most ridiculed subject in my own mother land. The idea in the minds of the people then was that yoga was for those who had lost their head, or had some misunderstandings with their parents or who walk on fire, swallow flaming match sticks and so on. This was the situation when my *guru* and myself were teaching yoga.

In those days, Poona was under Bombay Presidency with half of Karnataka, half of Andhra, half of Rajasthan, half of Gujarat and whole of Mahārāṣṭra. At that time there were only half a dozen yoga teachers in this presidency which may give you an idea of what popularity yoga had in those days in India.

When people started calling me to teach, my homework began. Then I thought I should be a true *śiṣya* to yoga and to my *guru*. My *guru*'s advice to scratch my head and plan to practise yoga opened my eyes to work with an inquisitive mind with intensity. Through this vigorous and rigorous practice, I became a real *śiṣya* at the feet of yoga after a period of seven to eight years. As the Educational Institutes of Pune terminated my services after three years I became a true *sādhaka*, a *śiṣya* of yoga. Then I started giving private classes taking diseased patients to help them through yoga. As the medical people were pleased to see their patients improving through yoga, they started sending their patients to me. It was a great challenge for me from medical doctors which made me work on myself to study how the fibres, tendons, muscles, bones and nervous systems work.

Just a few years ago I spoke about *pañcabhūta* and *āsana*. Today I read in papers that people speak on *pañcabhūta* and *pañcatanmātra* and how to balance them in the practice of *āsana*. This means that we have professors and students in yoga and not *guru* and *śiṣya*. In 1975 I started building up, studying the *pañcabhūta* with *pañcakośa* and began presenting through demonstrations how the elements have to function as well as to balance evenly in various *āsana* and in various *prāṇāyāma*.

When Patañjali speaks of *viśeṣa aviśeṣa liṅgamātra aliṅgāni guṇaparvāṇi* (*Y.S.*, II.19) - how to master the various principles of nature and how infinitesimal parts like cellular system should be under thorough control - *paramāṇu paramamahattvāntaḥ asya vaśīkāraḥ* (*Y.S.,* I.40), this gave me to study the balancing of the elements and their counterparts. While reading the commentary by Vyāsa, it struck me to work on it in my *sādhanā*. If Vyāsa had not commented, I wouldn't have understood these *sūtra* of Patañjali to use them in a practical way.

We all know the meaning of *yogaḥ cittavṛtti nirodha*. In *prāṇāyāma*, we find words like *stambha vṛttiḥ*. If *prāṇāyāma* is on *prāṇa-śakti*, the word *vṛtti* on *prāṇāyāma* struck me. Patañjali speaks of *bāhya-vṛtti, antara-vṛtti* and *stambha-vṛtti*. Retention *(kumbhaka)* or *stambha-vṛtti* makes the mind stable. Is not this *stambha-vṛtti* close to *cittavṛtti nirodhaḥ?* If it is *astambha-vṛtti*, it means fluctuations. From this word *stambha*, I learnt *nirodha* is not restraint of thought, but to keep the consciousness stable. If *prāṇāyāma* speaks of *bāhya abhyantara stambha vṛttiḥ* (*Y.S.,* II.50) *(bāhya-vṛtti - antara-vṛttiḥ - stambha-vṛtti)*, I thought of using these in *āsana* in order to understand where, when and which parts have to be used for *stambha-vṛtti, antara-vṛtti* and *bāhya-vṛtti*. You have seen many people talking to themselves internally. This is *antara-vṛttiḥ*. The lunatic speaks loudly on the street. It is *bahirvṛtti*. This made me think and re-assess those words to fit into all the aspects of yoga. For me, explanation of *bāhya-vṛtti, antara-vṛtti* and *stambha-vṛtti* taught in *prāṇāyāma* is nothing but *cittavṛtti nirodha*.

When we have to practise, we have to understand these words of Patañjali which act as guidelines to use the intelligence with right judgment. Do you use your intelligence while practising these three aspects of *prāṇāyāma* according to the needs of the *āsana* in adjusting the body? This idea of *prāṇāyāma* technique of Patañjali struck me when people in large numbers started coming to me with problems which were beyond my imagination. I worked on them so that they feel the effect of it soon. When the effect of success on ailments spread people began to call me *masterji*. People never used to call me even Mister. It took people decades to consider me from a demonstrator to *masterji*.

As a demonstrator, I was demonstrating and showing the quality of each *āsana*. Then, after years of gap, people began to call me *ustād*. From *masterji* I became an *ustād*. People call top musicians *ustād*. Probably I was the first person to receive this title from my pupils in the art of yoga. I was performing *āsana* like a musical scale with rhythm elegance and softness. People started telling that I move the body like a musical *rāga* with smooth flow in presentation and in teaching and probably this must have made them to call me an *ustād*.

Later I started working with incurable diseases to prove that yoga has great value. I am the only person in the world who emphatically says that I have cured many of the ailments through yogic *āsana* without introducing medicine or diet. Many diseases which were not cognisable by the medical science named such diseases as allergic. Today you go to any yogi, he gives you *āyurvedic* medicine along with yogic discipline. Even my guru was advocating *āyurvedic* medicine prepared by him for needed ailments. In my case I have treated only through yoga. I was demanding disciplined practice allowing them to live in their natural ways and hence I can claim to be a pure *śiṣya* of yoga because I did not mix other things in my practice or teaching. I stuck to yoga to prove that it has a great value and I share the credit of yoga becoming popular today in the world.

Through patients who came to learn for treatment, I learned of the the anatomy of the body as well as the anatomy of each *āsana* and began synchronising the anatomical movement of the *āsana* with the living anatomical structure of the human body.

We say we know the body, but when you do the *āsana* you realise that it is not easy to adjust the subjective anatomy in the living body. When I began using the technique of human anatomy balancing anatomical structure of each *āsana*, people called me a wizard or a *mantravādi*. The patients used to say that the moment I touch, something happens. So they began to spread that I have got something like incantation power and thought I was like a *mantravādi*.

Then saints and yogi, like Swami Śivananda, Swami Satyananda, Swami Dayananda, Swami Sachidananda, Swami Krishnananda, Swami Chidananda and many others began telling the yoga practitioners to show their practice to me and get my advice in their *sādhanā*. On account of their admiration, people began to call me an *yogācārya*. *Ācāra* means "one who practises without fail as per traditions"; *ācāra* also means a system, hence one who follows and practises the system regularly and establishes it by syncronising practices and precepts is called an *ācārya*.

When new ideas and thoughts began flashing through my intelligence, people could see refinement revealing in my practices. Seeing such transformations taking place in my *sādhanā* quantitatively as well as qualitatively people began calling me a *yoga guru*.

I feel this is pure destiny or the grace of God and *ṛṣi* which played the role of lifting me from a *śiṣya* to a *guru*. This change in people to see transformation in my *sādhanā* took more than fifty years.

Today any yoga teacher calls himself a *yogācārya* or a *yoga ṛṣi*.

In yoga, *śiṣya vṛtti* is very important. If anything new strikes me, I become a *śiṣya* at once and I work on it to get a permanent imprint. Often new things strike and transformation takes place in my *sādhanā*. I feel a *sādhaka* must have an inquisitive mind to search for what is missing in his practices.

Even if props are used, these props should prick the cellular system and intelligence to act and study with reflection to react at once and keep the imprints in mind to start afresh the next day with these imprints and wait and watch to receive subtle changes that take place as a seed for further enlightenment.

When Bhīṣma went to the battlefield, he had to lift his dropped eyebrows and tie them firmly with a cloth so that the eyebrows would not fall while fighting. People glorify the act of Bhīṣma in the battlefield who had tied a cloth around his eyebrows. When I innovated the props which give right direction to learn the *āsana* better, people called me by names. We give respect to Bhīṣma when he used a cloth as a prop to tie the dropped eyebrows to fight the war. Like Bhīṣma I am asking you to fight the war which goes on within you in your practices by using the props.

You all know about *Mahābhārata* and the battle that was fought between the cousins *Kaurava* and *Pāṇḍava*. The place where the war to fight evil for good *(dharma)* took place is *Kurukṣetra*, which is near Delhi. God has blessed us with head and heart. If head is *kurukṣetra*, the battlefield with things and thoughts, heart is *dharmakṣetra*, where one feels the sense of guilt if something wrong is done. The heart is the seat of righteous life. *Kurukṣetra* is the battlefield where conflicting thoughts directly or indirectly happen second to second. Stilling all the thoughts is done by the seat of the heart which is called *dharmakṣetra*. Hence the principles of yoga as *sādhaka* are meant to unite the intelligence of the head and the heart into a single steady state of intelligence.

Patañjali speaks of analysis, synthesis, bliss and the feeling of 'I' resting in the abode of head and of friendliness, compassion, gladness and indifference resting in the abode of heart. If one compares analysis with friendliness, synthesis with compassion, bliss with gladness, he shows the meeting place of head and heart which is in this third place *ānanda* and *muditā*. The bliss of the head and gladness of the heart come close to each other. Patañjali teaches us to show indifference *(udāsinatā)* to the cultured consciousness *(asmitā)* so that one moves to experience the seedless *(nirbīja)* divine state – that is the Self.

For me associating the intellect of the head with the intelligence of the heart is yoga. From *Yoga Sūtra* of I.17 and I.33,[1] I thought that the aim of yoga is to unite the intellect of the head with the intelligence of the heart and for me this union is yoga. So I started associating the intelligence of the head and heart throughout my *sādhanā*.

---

[1] *vitarka vicāra ānanda asmitārūpa anugamāt saṁprajñātaḥ* (I.17) – Practice and detachment develop four types of samādhi: self analysis, synthesis, bliss and the experience of pure being.
maitrī karuṇā muditā upekṣaṇāṁ sukha duḥhha puṇya apuṇya viṣayāṇāṁ bhavanātaḥ cittaprasādam (I.33) – through cultivation of friendliness, compassion, joy and indifference to pleasure and pain, virtue and vice respectively, the consciousness becomes favourably disposed, serene and benevolent.

Each *āsana* needs *śiṣya vṛtti* as each *āsana* beams different rays of light. Take *Tāḍāsana*. If the lower leg's skin moves inside, why does the skin on the top legs not move in at all? As a *śiṣya*, I never allowed my intelligence to follow blindly the dictates of the body. I wanted my intelligence to judge in each *āsana* each movement and action and dictate terms to the body to move and act as per its discretion. This is another stage of *śiṣya vṛtti* which begins in *adhimātra* state of a *sādhaka*. Until the practitioner *(sādhaka)* reaches the state of a cleanser (śodhana), a filterer *(śoṣana)* and the auspicious state reflecting crystaline brilliance *(śobhana)*, he is an *abhyasin*. In *sādhanā kriyā* be careful not to be strangled by *viparyaya vṛtti* or perverted movement in the limbs of the body or in the energy flow. The intelligence may not be able to get the imprints of such perverted motion and action on it in each *āsana*. Hence discretion in intelligence is needed to stop the perverted way of presentation in *āsana* and *prāṇāyāma*. This is direct (right) perception or *pramāṇa (pratyakṣa)* in presentation.

While practising *āsana* and *prāṇāyāma* it is essential to give thoughts to the five *vṛtti*, namely, intuitive perception, perverse and indecisive thinking, state of emptiness and imprints of actions and re-actions.

The first four aspects of *vṛtti (pramāṇa, viparyaya, vikalpa, nidrā)*, are for me the main *vṛtti*, while memory as imprint is subordinate to the four.

Some parts of the body may be attentive and active, some parts may be wrongly stretching, some parts may be vacillating and oscillating without any direction and some parts may be empty without the feel of existence. Some parts remain in an illuminative *sāttvic* state, some vibrating in a *rājasic* way by changing actions every now and then. Some parts remain dull and stupid in a *tāmasic* way.

A *sādhaka* has to watch each and every part in each stage of an *āsana* and in each stage of *prāṇāyāma* and learn to transmit the feel of that illumination to the other parts as if the light of intelligence spreads there. Similarly, the *sādhaka* has to be a scrutiniser, a cleaner as well as a corrector on all parts of the body by removing the erroneous action in the *sādhanā*.

When a *sādhaka* has reached the state of *śodhana* and *śoṣana* actions in *sādhanā* then he reaches the fourth stage, *tīvra sādhaka (śobhana)* in *tīvra sādhanā*. Here comes total absorption *(śamana)*, a state of tranquillity and sootheness where he reaches the state of termination of effort.

Then the *sādhanā* in *āsana* or *prāṇāyāma* becomes meditation. When all the sheaths of the body are connected by intelligence with the Self, then the *sādhaka* has reached a state where he becomes the *guru*. A *sādhaka* has to cross all the four stages of *sādhanā* to be called a *guru.* At that stage he is a *guru* because he maintains a devotee of the *sādhanā* for ever. He maintains *stambha-vṛtti* in all five sheaths.

Maintainence of *stambha-vṛtti* in each *āsana* and in each breath leads one to balance *pañcakośa, pañcabhūta* and the *pañcatanmātra.*

Our body is made of five *bhūta* namely; *pṛthvī, āp, tejas, vāyu* and *ākāśa,* and five *tanmātra; gandha, rasa, rūpa, sparśa* and *śabda as well as five sheaths (kośa); annamaya, prāṇamaya, manomaya, vijñānamaya* and *ānandamaya.*

For example, when one is doing *Trikoṇāsana, Śīrṣāsana, Viparīta Daṇḍāsana* or *Kapotāsana,* the bone is the *pṛthvī tattva.* Bone is the centre of the body. If the bones are firm then one can do the *āsana* as firmness is the character of *pṛthvī.* In *Trikoṇāsana,* when one turns the right foot to the right side, the left heel becomes light like air. Due to want of understanding one forgets to rest the heel firmly on the floor. Also, if he notices, his left heel becomes small, right heel broad. Its toe-nail is in one direction, knee in another direction, while the thigh faces in different directions. Similarly, the top and bottom of the shin bone and ankles, the muscles at the bottom, middle and top thigh or hip do not find the middle line, which is the bone? In the same way one does not attend to positioning the joints. As the muscles represent the element of *āp* (water), the bones follow the movements of the muscles instead of muscles moving close to the bones. This way of doing makes the legs take the shape of a deck chair. Then how can one call it *Trikoṇāsana* when the bones, joints and muscles are not made to balance the five elements evenly in a triangular shape?

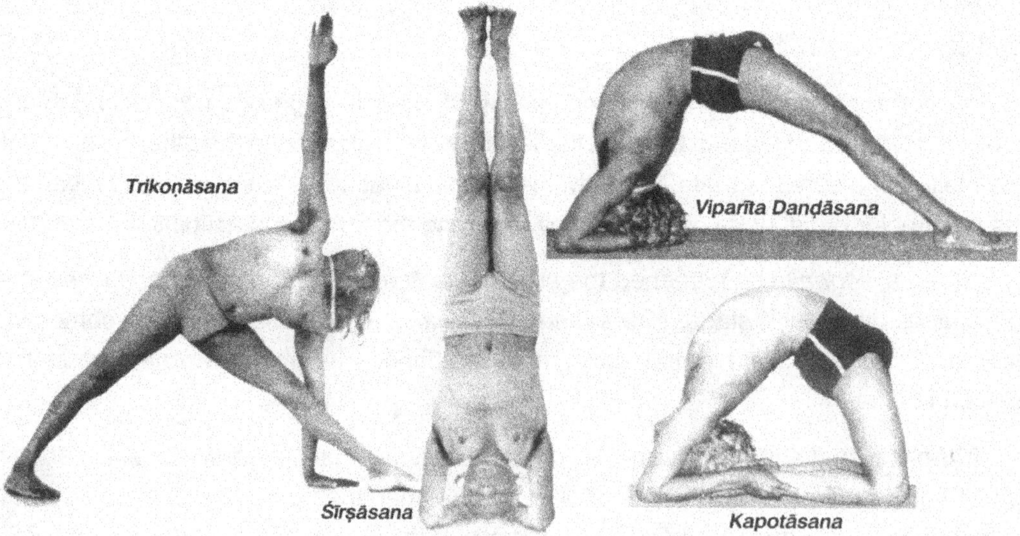

Plate n. 33 – Presentation of *Trikoṇāsana, Śīrṣāsana, Viparīta Daṇḍāsana* and *Kapotāsana*

Hence any small disturbance or disharmony has to be captured by the intelligence and the intelligence has to guide the five elements and five sheaths to find concord.

Muscles belong to *āp tattva*, bones to *pṛthvī tattva*, nervous system to *tejas tattva*, the touch of intelligence in contact with the other sheaths is *vāyu tattva*, and the skin, being the frontier of the body and self, acts as *ākāśa tattva*. Without the power of lengthening, broadening or shortening of the muscles, abduction, adduction and circumduction are impossible. This indicates that the skin is *ākāśa tattva*. *Ākāśa* means space which has the power to contract or expand. This contraction, expansion or circumferential action produces increased or decreased vibration according to the construction of the *āsana*. Hence skin is *ākāśa tattva*. All the five *bhūta*, five *tanmātra* have to run concurrently in this *pāñcabhautika śarīra*. For this, handling of *ākāśa tattva* or the skin and the self is very important.

Though one starts with the discipline of yoga with *pṛthvī tattva*, one has to use *ākāśa tattva* to reach the *adhimātra* state. Then one reaches precision in each *āsana*, *prāṇāyāma* or *dhyāna*.

Let this inner vision *(antara dṛṣṭi)*, and aim *(antara lakṣya)* through the eyes *(bahir dṛṣṭi)* look whether the *āsana* is architecturally maintained or not. This is how *pañcabhūta* and *pañcatanmātra* are observed to reach the level of *sthira sukham āsanam* (*Y.S.*, II.46).

In short the five elements, the five sheaths, the five *vāyu*, five atomic qualities of elements, mind, intelligence and consciousness should and must circumambulate the bones at each and every part of the body and then go close to the Self to circumambulate it. This is perfection in yoga or the union of body with the self and self with the Supreme Self.

Difference between a *guru* and a *śiṣya*

Bṛhaspati is a *guru*, a spiritual preceptor. Krishna was a *guru* to Arjuna. Droṇa was not called a *guru*. Droṇa was a preceptor, and never a *guru* though he had taught hundreds of students. Krishna alone is called *yogeśvara*, and no other.

Let us pay our respects to the guru of all, *Yogeśvara* – Lord Krishna. May his blessings be on us all so that we move from studentship of yoga towards the mastery of yoga with the vision of the soul – the *Ātman*.

THE WAYS OF RE-CONDITIONING THE *CITTA**

Children of yoga. As fellow travellers in the path of spiritual quest you have first-hand knowledge of building up from the basics of yoga all these years to savour the essence of its value from my teachings.

I am nearing ninety and the responsibilities on you is bound to be definitely high as the younger generation are attracted to yoga with interest. Life being dynamic and ever moving, changes take place in the younger blood. In old age this ever moving dynamism comes to a stand still to a great extent. People like me have to keep this ever moving life as stable as far as possible by maintaining the *sādhanā* that was undertaken at an early age to its utmost. In old age unfortunately, the mind being mercurial appears to become solid.

Yogic philosophy is not just about ignorance and knowledge, but for moving from ignorance to knowledge and from knowledge to wisdom with a non-corrupt simple, innocent mind. Enlightenment in yoga comes at a right time when one is at a peak state of *sādhanā* after years of endeavours. Then one has to learn to transform this toned intellectual growth, understanding and earned knowledge into wisdom. I concentrated especially on two petals of yoga namely, *āsana* and *prāṇāyāma* utilising the principles of *yama* and *niyama* as well as involving the other subtle petals, namely, *dhāraṇā* and *dhyāna*. As far as my experience goes these petals, *dhāraṇā* and *dhyāna*, cannot be taught because it is the *aiśvarya* or supreme ostentatious wealth of yoga. But the other basic aspects of yoga are to be followed for one to experience this opulent wealth of yoga.

Many of you may be practising but might not have seen the light that glows from yoga. Yet I am grateful that you all have begun practice though it may take a long time to reach this opulent power *(śakti)* of yoga. Whether the yogic light glows or not, let us all stick to our yogic *tapaścaryā* so that good *karma* is cultivated *(saṁskāra)* and l;ater renounced to reach the goal in this life or in the lives after.

---

* Talk given on December, 2007.

Do not mistake *tapaścaryā* which we often wrongly translate as austere rituals. The *tapaścaryā* is based on the of ethical pillars of *yama* and *niyama* with *śraddha* or faith to proceed towards the perception of the Self *(ātma sākṣātkāra).* Without cultivation of morality, spiritual experience may remain far off.

Tapas means to let the power of light *(śakti)* in the body, mind and intelligence to blaze forcefully and brilliantly to shine forth through the zeal in *sādhanā* so that it does not extinguish the will to stick to the *sādhanā*. *Tapas* is the fire of ascetic devotion towards the *sādhanā*. It is the fire from right action with attention, to brighten the infallible knowledge. However as a *sādhaka*, see the fire of *jñāna* bubbles and blazes in *sādhanā* like water boiling which goes on bubbling non-stop until it is removed from the fire.

Unfortunately the *sādhanā* in you all is still in a gross form. I think this is true to a great extent in many of you. You are not practising according to Patañjali's dictum; *tatra sthitau yatnaḥ abhyāsaḥ* (*Y.S.*, I.13). We are practising to remain just healthy and happy. But all of you have to change this form of thinking in *sādhanā* towards religious practices. Therefore, change your attitudes and practise with a devoted mind and heart. I have now crossed seventy-five years of teaching. Naturally to some extent, I feel disappointed and embarrassed. On this *Guru Purnīma* day I want all of you to make up your mind to change from casual practice and satisfaction towards attentive, stable and intense practice. The secret of success in this sacred yoga is that you should all be intense practitioners with total attentive awareness.

The colour of today's issue of *Yoga Rahasya*[1] is red. Red stands for *rajas* or vibrancy. This colour is significant for you all so that each of you keeps the candle of your intelligence burning like red flame till that flame changes soon into a luminous bright light. It is a fit colour for you all to make a declaration today to start your practices not only with steadfast effort to still the wandering mind but to remain stable in order to move towards intellectual and spiritual progress. This is the meaning that conveys not only from *Yoga Sūtra* I.13,[2] but also from the jacket of *Yoga Rahasya*.

You all see me practising repeatedly in front of you. I am practising to establish what I learned and also to adjust the subtle sensitivities that arise in my practices. In old age life force naturally declines. As such I like to be free from the obstacles and impediments that arises at this old age and I like to keep them at bay with a single-minded effort even now in my *sādhanā*.

---

1 Quarterly published magazine, published by Y.O.G. Mumbai.
2 *tatra sthitau yatnaḥ abhyāsaḥ* (Y.S., I.13).

I am saying this because I want you all to develop this tenacity as I have and practice with perseverance watching patiently for the changes to occur.

Tatpratiṣedhārtham ekatattva abhyāsaḥ (*Y.S.*, I.32). For me *pratiṣedhārtham* means the defects, disturbances and imbalances in my practices between the right and the left sides of the body between the mind and the body, between the mind and intelligence and between intelligence and the consciousness and the Self. I maintain and retain my practices so that no despair, sorrow, unsteadiness in body or mind appears in the frame of my intelligence or the self.

No doubt many of you are coming with a motive to get rid of your sufferings and ailments. Those of you who are practising for years and got rid of your sufferings and ailments should stop thinking on this base level but to proceed to find out the subtle hidden values of yoga that may dawn on you as you go on practising. You all see me practising without rhyme or reason. I also cannot explain to you why I am practising. I do it because I just live in it. It is not just pure love for the subject that makes me do that, but something inside me thrusts me to practise. I practise by keeping my mind afresh in me to trace the subtlest of the subtle dualities in case they appear between my body, intelligence and Self and bring back parity in them.

I practise with single pointed attention *(eka-tattva)*, not for integrating the cells of my body with my mind and intelligence but to integrate the Self to be precisely present everywhere in its frontier, the body.

I adapt friendliness and compassion according to the needs and conditions of my body and mind and bring co-ordination (if these two go in different directions), and practice with gladness with an unconditional intellect throughout the *sādhanā*. The moment I complete my *sādhanā* I remain indifferent towards the practices as I have finished my *sādhanā* for the day.

I want you all to take this method of my practice as a message and do your practices with fervour so that you all feel the presence of the Self. Patañjali gives very good advice for us as *sādhaka* to study the differences between body and mind and also the feel of the pleasantness on one side and unpleasantness on the other side; *vitarkabādhane pratipakṣabhāvanam* (*Y.S.*, II.33). Take the two words of this *sūtra: bādhana* and *bhāvanā*. *(Bādhana* means annoying or opposing and *bhāvanā* means felt feelings. It also means effectively one's well being or treating with respect). If *bādhana bhāvanā* is there, then there must be *abādhana bhāvana*. *Bādhana bhāvanā* means a conflicting feeling, *abādhana bhāvana* is a non-conflicting feeling. These words definitely help *sādhaka* like you to observe in your practices and study the conflicting or painful presentations with the non-conflicting or non-painful presentations.

This way compare and find ways and means to keep both sides free from *bādhana*. I hope you understand and study these terms well as you practise. Watch your mind whether it is observing the deviations and bringing harmony within the body and intelligence to position them accurately when presenting the *āsana*. Each one of you should be alert to watch the mind which may be conveying something different from the body. As such, watch your body and mind and observe from intelligence whether they are co-operating and co-ordinating to bring oneness in all the sheaths from the skin to the self.

See whether your practices convey the sense *bādhana bhāvanā* or *abādhaka bhāvanā*. If there is *bādhana bhāvanā*, then find out how to bring a coordinated action to experience the *abādhaka bhāvanā* and viceversa in both sides of the body as well as between the mind, intelligence and self. Hence, I consider this *sūtra* a wonderful *sūtra* which guides how to study in practice and find out means to bring unison within the five sheaths in you. Then you realise that the *pratiṣedhārtham* of the first chapter and *bādhana bhāvanā* and *abādhaka bhāvanā* of the second chapter signify a close relationship between the outer body and the inner body in guiding the practitioners to reach perfection in the *sādhanā*.

In your practice gauge this *bādhana bhāvanā*, the conflicting experiences with *abādhaka bhāvanā* or non conflicting experiences and then adopt the needed changes by filtering and re-filtering memory and experiences to reach an un-oscillating state of experiential wisdom. Patañjali re-establishes again in the third chapter the perfection in *sādhanā* saying that elements, senses, mind and consciousness transform from their potential states *(dharma)* towards refinement *(lakṣaṇa)* and zenith of refinement *(avasthā)* which is known as *dharma lakṣaṇa avasthā pariṇāma* (*Y.S.*, III.13). *Dharma* means characteristic quality in action, *lakṣaṇa* means qualitative change in action for the better whether it is *āsana* or *prāṇāyāma* or *dhyāna*. Maintain whatever was done yesterday with wide open intelligence. Then catch the non-progressive changes from the experience of the past actions and change them into new actions. Then the *sādhanā* becomes truly a mindful *sādhanā*.

Though life is dynamic, in some it remains in stasis and in others dynamic and stimulative. In old age, this stagnancy is the evident gap between the old generation and new generation. I belong to the old generation and by the grace of yoga I am still steady and stable to fit into this new generation. This credit goes to my yogic *sādhanā*. As I have kept up my practice in that advertant state I do not see any conflict between me and the new generation like you. Because my practice is kept afresh each day, the energy that flows in my life and in your life is like a flow of a river with fresh water gushing moment to moment.

As the fresh water gushes out the stagnated water, the new generation has to work on the foundation of the wisdom of the old generation in such a way that they add their new discoveries and share the knowledge for it to flow with a fresh approach in yoga by following *dharma lakṣaṇa avasthā parināma*.

The forces of the oscillating and vascillating consciousness and unstable mind act as obstacles (see *Y.S.,* I.30 and 31). Establish a state of non-dual conscious state in thinking and practice. If the format of yoga is its *dharma,* transformation of practice into a qualitive change is *lakṣaṇa.* Here, the practitioner eradicates the defects in his *sādhanā* and recharges the battery of his intelligence in order to reach the perfect state, or *avaṣthā* in *sādhanā.* Even the qualities of elements, chemistry of the body, senses of perception, mind, intelligence and consciousness change. Changes like these go on as one progressively practises with timings adjusting to the new methodologies that arise as one peels layer after layer the inner sheaths. The practice should be like peeling the onion till one reaches a state where no further peeling is possible. This is the seedless spot of the mind. Similarly in the yogic *sādhanā* each one has to reach that seedless state. This seedless state is the Soul or the core of our Being.

I have led you on several occasions from the various layers of the core of being, the *annamaya, prāṇamaya, manomaya, vijñānamaya* and *ānandamaya kośa.* Though many consider *ānandamaya kośa* as the core, it is beyond *ānandamaya kośa. For me cittamaya kośa* is *ānandamaya kośa.* One has to go beyond this *cittamaya kośa* to reach the core of the being. This core of being is an unbiased experiencing state where joy or bliss has no place. Therefore one has to penetrate far beyond *ānandamaya kośa* in the *sādhanā* to consecrate the Self *(svarūpa pratiṣṭhā).* One has to reach this state in the *sādhanā* so that each and every pore, every cell of the body feels the sense of the Self establishing itself everywhere. If each and everyone establishes the Self in each and every pore of the skin and each and every cell in their practice of *āsana* or *prāṇāyāma* or *dhyāna,* then this *sādhanā* definitely leads the *sādhaka* to live in the *ādhyātmic darśana* as *ātma-prasādanam.*

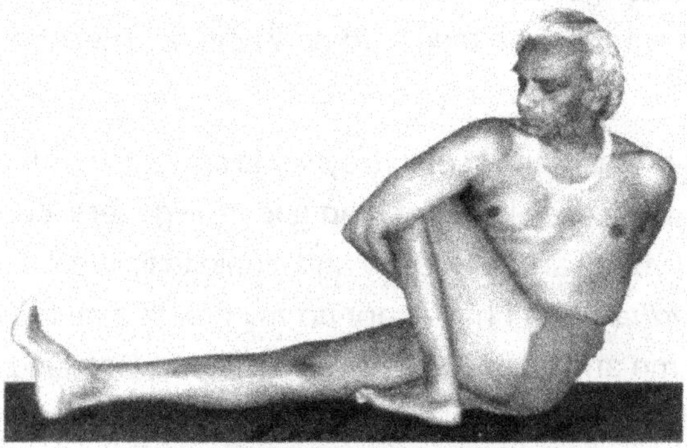

Plate n. 34 – *Marichyāsana* III

For example, if you are doing *Marichyāsana* on your bent right leg by bringing the left hand over the right, you establish your self in your left hand and forget your right hand. For this you have to use *pratiṣedārtham* as a stick to attend to the left hand that forgets. This way each one has to do *sādhanā* to remove such differences and rectify them. This way it becomes a real culture of body, mind, intelligence and consciousness. This culturing is *lakṣaṇa* or qualitative practice. Without qualitative thinking and acting one cannot change the chemistry of the elements, the behavioural pattern of the senses of perception and one's action nor transform the mind for the better. Therefore practise and work by using the intelligence judiciously.

If sitting in an *āsana* according to one's conditioning is *dharma*, if one gives a thought and thinks that one can do better, then I say one is following the right way. Learn to distribute the energy with even awareness on both the sides, lengthwise and widthwise in an *āsana* or in the in-breath and the out-breath, then this is considered as qualitative practice *(lakṣaṇa pariṇāma).*

Take *Trikoṇāsana*, which you all have done. Next time, while trying this *āsana*, observe the expansion of the touch or contact of the consciousness while performing on the right side. Observe the same on the left side and compare it to the right side. You find that consciousness touches differently on the right and on the left. Unfortunately we do not observe these differences. On one side you establish the consciousness with attention and awareness as if you are experiencing *svarūpa pratiṣṭhā* while on the other side, you do not observe the fading of *svarūpapratiṣṭhā*. There is a disparity in the presence of consciousness between the right and left sides. If one totally establishes the consciousness on one side and pays no attention on the other side, this is refraction in the *āsana*. This non-attention on the left side and attention on the right side is *bādhana bhāvana*. So you have to bring *pratipakṣabhāvanā* at once. To rectify such differences, the feeling *(bhāvanā)* has to be observed in practice and rectified at once in order to make the mind, intelligence and consciousness flow concurrently and evenly on both the sides of the body. This is *sthira sukha* in this *āsana*. Like this all *āsana* have to be performed by removing the disparities of all the principles of nature.

When one changes *Trikoṇāsana* to the left side, the *ātmā* shifts on to that side and remains non-attentive on the right side. So one has to develop sharpness and sensitivity to think and balance the intelligence and consciousness evenly on both the sides so that the *svarūpa* of *ātmā* is established at all places evenly. This is *āsana* in its right sense.

If one goes on practising without paying the needed attention in removing such imbalances, then that practice is a meaningless and unintelligent practice. My advice to all of you is to use your intelligence in order to recondition the disparities to reach a state of parity. Un-condition the old thoughts and re-condition with a new approach. This way of breaking old thoughts helps for re-adjustment in body which in turn reconditions intelligence. This conditioning, un-conditioning and re-conditioning goes on in any *āsana* till one reaches a state where no further adjustments and re-conditions are possible. This is the unconditional state of mind, intelligence and consciousness *(nirbīja)* where all conditions and views terminate and only the establishment of the immeasurable state of the Self is experienced in the *āsana*.

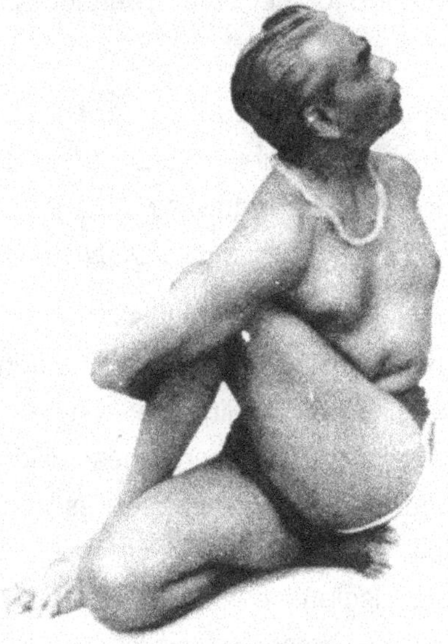

Plate n. 35 – *Ardha Matsyendrāsana*

Suppose if you have gripped the wrist in twists where one wrist turns in and the other turns out, then turn both wrists out. This creates a new sense of attention. This way of right adjustment must be the motive in the *sādhanā*.

In case you are doing *Ardha Matsyendrāsana* you are very strong on the thumb side of the wrist bone. As such the life force runs there, whereas your little finger remains dull and inactive. It means that half of the self is active working on half the hand while on the other half of the hand the self partially rests as if it is in a sleepy state. This means that in practice some parts are in a sleepy state in each and every *āsana*, some parts in a dreamy state while some parts in the wakeful state. Remember, *svapna nidrā jñāna ālambanaṁ vā* (*Y.S.*, I.38), you have to awaken the sleepy parts, charge the dreamy parts so that all parts of nature *(tattva)*, the elements of the body, their counterparts, mind, intelligence, ego and consciousness are evenly alert and balanced *(citta-prasādanam)*, so that the self not only witnesses but acts precisely to be present covering the entire body in all the *āsana*. This is *adhyātma-prasādanam*.

Yoga is an inward journey, hence all objective actions and *vṛtti* of the *citta* have to be converted into a subjective *vṛtti* and action. For this one has to give a thought on the right ideas given by our preceptors on yoga to follow them to link and integrate the twenty-four principles of nature in the *yogic-sādhanā*.

If a link in the chain is loose, the chain does not move smoothly. Similarly our preceptors did give us right knowledge. Probably the links on the subject must have lost its continuity due to a time gap between the first preceptor and other preceptors. So the way of practice is to think and findout ways to link those ideas projected from time immemorial though they continue with new thoughts and new ideas. These are like the waves which appear and wash off the old waves. In *sādhanā* the *guru* says to flush out the old thoughts without disturbing the basics in order to bring new thoughts and ideas so that the *sādhanā* gets qualified *(lakṣaṇa)* to reach the zenith in the *āsana (avasthā)*.

Culture develops when one begins to re-condition the old conditions to fit in to the present day's mental calibre. This conditioning, re-conditioning and un-conditioning moves like a perennial stream. That is why the sages say not this, not this, not that, not that. This thought of 'not this and not that' is not a pessimistic approach but an optimistic approach so that one does not get stagnated with fixed ideas or practices but proceeds to reach the exalted position where no room is found for re-conditioning. When no further re-conditioning is possible, it means that one has reached that permanent state of unconditional zenith.

The sages use the word 'not this, not this, not that' to keep us alert and aware of our endeavours. They support new thoughts, new feelings and when the filtered and re-filtered experiences come, all changes culminate as one cannot go beyond that steady and non-oscillating state. This is the *svarūpa pratiṣṭhā* state. When one's Self dwells in its own glory, it overshadows its agents (elements of *prakṛti*), then there is no room left for further readjustment. This is *avasthā*. If one gains this stable state, it is mastery in the *āsana* and maturity in *sādhaka's* intelligence. This state of *avasthā* or position stands the same whether it is in the practice of *āsana*, *prāṇāyāma*, *dhyāna* or the remaining aspects of yoga.

Though many of you are in the kindergarten of yoga, it does not matter, but it is for you to think to find out how to proceed to the higher standard from the present *sādhanā*.

Do not consider this as a public examination but as an examination of self-inquiry. I have to consider where I am and give a thought whether to remain where I am or should I transcend from that state. The moment you think of transcending, it means that you have cultured your body and you have cultured your mind and intelligence. Actually culturing is transcending from the state of the present mind to a new state of mind where new experiences set in by which *sādhanā* becomes intense and subtle. Till then it is a culture. When the culture is complete one gets civilized. There is no further function in operating the intellect or the intelligence and that is why Buddha, Christ or Zoroaster are called civilized people. You and I are not considered as civilized people as we are caught in greed *(lobha)*, anger *(krodha)*, delusion *(moha)*, pride *(mada)* and malice *(mātsarya)*. But a saint or a yogi is not caught in these disturbing thoughts and that's why they have pure knowledge living innocently in a simple unassuming life.

Having said so much, as *sādhaka*, we have to change *yatna* (persevering effort) into *prayatna* (well governed effort). This means *yatna* may be casual but *prayatna* means subjectively involving yourself with keen effort to study further by putting full effort from the peripheral body up to the core of the Self. So *prayatna* is to involve totally in a subjective way bringing right action with right thinking process. When right action and right thinking synchronise, then Patañjali says that one experiences *ananta samāpattibhyām* in the *āsana*. In that *ananta samāpatti* state one is in the state where the identity of 'I' just vanishes and *citi śakti (svarūpa pratiṣṭha)* gets established. This is how one has to practise according to Patañjali's definition of *āsana jaya*[1] and *ananta samāpatti*.

The capital 'I', in English alphabet and the running 'i' are wonderful letters to search one's intellect. The capital 'I' does not come in the middle, and the small 'i' appears very often in the middle.

The capital 'I' in each of us is the same from birth to death, but the small 'i' acts as a replica of the big 'I'. According to the *Yoga Sūtra*, the capital 'I' represents the *kūṭastha citta*. It represents the immeasurable, eternal, Universal state of the Self. This does not surface so easily and that's why we say the *ātmā* cannot surface so easily for everyone. This remains passive and pensive as a witness from birth to death. This real 'I' will not change but remains perpetually and universally the same *(kūṭastha)*. But the running "i" which assumes a false identity of the real 'I' deceives one as a deceptive true Self. This small 'i' causes problems in us as an impostor of the original Self. This running 'i' is a *hita śatru* (secret enemy). Yoga practises culture and transforms this secret enemy, the small 'i', to become a true friend of the real 'I'.

I hope you can distinguish between the big 'I' and the small 'i', which in philosophical language represent *puruṣa* as real *(kūṭastha citta)* and *ahaṁkāra* as its impostor *(pariṇama citta)*. This *pariṇāma citta*, the small 'i' changes according to moods, environment and mental weather. If the atmospheric weather is gloomy, the mind is gloomy. The same with the capital 'I' *(puruṣa)* when this capital 'I' changes into a running 'i' it gets carried or veiled with nescience *(avidyā)*. If the sun comes after the rains, the sky is bright and you also feel bright. This is what yogic practices bring in the practitioner.

The universe inside is known as the hidden consciousness *(kuṭastha citta)*. This remains uniformally steady and bright. But it is the transmission of the capital 'I' into small 'i' that creates problems for all of us in our day-to-day life. That's why I used the word un-conditioning in order to re-condition it. This reconditioning is the essential culture in the practice of yoga *sādhanā* so that one cannot decide this is it, because reconditioning may be still on. Like cause and effect, conditioning, re-conditioning, un-conditioning is a cycle. It is the rotational *sādhanā*. When this cycle stops there is no further motion at all both in the head and the heart.

---

[1] See *Aṣṭadaḷa Yogamālā*, vol. 2, pp.76-84.

If the big 'I' is the heart, the small 'i' is the brain. Hence the conflict goes on between the capital 'I' of the heart and the running 'i' of the brain or the head. Blending this small 'i' to the capital 'I' and then making both to fade out is the establishing or the core without a noun or pronoun.

For example, you stay in *Śīrṣāsana* for fifteen to twenty minutes and in *Sarvāṅgāsana* for half an hour. But I would like to ask you a question. Have any of you stood for even five minutes in *Tāḍāsana?* Not one. Why? The gravitational force is different in *Tāḍāsana* from *Śīrṣāsana*. Even the intellectual gravitation in *Tāḍāsana* which does not change changes in *Śīrṣāsana*. That is why one stays in *Śīrṣāsana* for a longer period than in *Tāḍāsana*. The centre of gravity is very stable in *Tāḍāsana* while it is not so in *Śīrṣāsana*. For example, stand for one minute stretching the skin of the bottom of the feet to touch the floor in *Tāḍāsana*. Then you experience a different *Tāḍāsana*. Understand that by culturing the bottom feet you begin to culture the mind bringing steadiness in intelligence like steady *Tāḍāsana*. Oscillation in *Tāḍāsana* is not *Tāḍāsana*, whereas one oscillates the body in *Śīrṣāsana* and it is the same in *Sarvāṅgāsana* or backbends. Therefore, I say any *āsana* is easier to perform than *Tāḍāsana*.

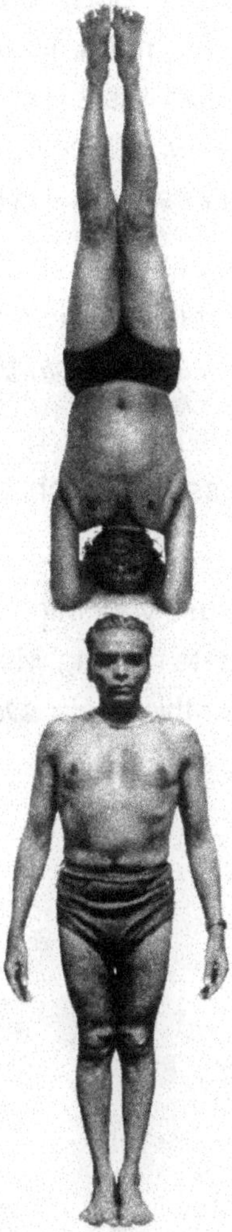

Plate n. 36 – *Tāḍāsana* and *Śīrṣāsana*

As one stands steadily in *Tāḍāsana*, one has to remain stable in *Śīrṣāsana* or any *āsana*. Then you realise that the culture of body and mind with intelligence has begun.

So begin to culture the body first from the feet and move on to culture the mind. When the culture of the body, mind and intelligence ends one has reached the state of divinity – an unconditional state of the Self.

From now on work how to culture your mind so that your small self changes into a real Self losing the identity of *ahaṁ*. From then on the Self takes the initiative in guiding to perform not only *āsana*, *prāṇāyāma* and *dhyāna* but all the eight aspects of yoga. This is how yoga *sādhanā* has to be done. This means that you have reached the level which is said to be impossible for thousands to reach. I say it is possible to reach this state by thousands if this level of practice is maintained with this state of heart.

I say that this is the message that I got from my practice which I love to share with you all. Practise with discretion and devotion. Practise measuring the alignment by adjusting the skeletal body. First try and begin to place the muscles evenly adjusting to remain close to the centre of the bones and joints as if the inner banks of the muscles touch equally with the bones and joints. Then measure the alignment of the mind latitudinally and longitudinally in each pore of your body in the *āsana* and *prāṇāyāma* whilst maintaining the healthy cellular system bringing closeness of the mind with the cells. The body has eight directions. These are north, south, east, west, northeast, northwest, southeast and southwest. While practising *āsana* or *prāṇāyāma* or sitting for *dhyāna*, measure the flow of energy and movement of intelligence to trace and cover the entire eight directions of your body, balancing the back and front of the body without any deviation or contortion. There should be no variation in balancing the mind, intelligence, consciousness and the Self. If this is judiciously followed then I say that it is *sthira sukham āsanam* or the characteristic of the *āsana* according to Patañjali. This is what I feel and this is what I measure while I practise. I distinctively work to characterise each *āsana*. That is why one sees elegance of each *āsana* in *Light on Yoga* and *The Art of Yoga*.[1]

As yoga graced me to practise with an accurate description defining each *āsana* to reach a distinctive mark *(lakṣaṇa)*, it helped me to reach that exalted state *(avasthā)* in each *āsana*.

This helped me to culture my conditioned consciousness, to reach a stable unconditioned state.

I wish and pray that all of you who have gathered here today to use your intelligence of the head and heart so that the head and heart co-operate and co-ordinate moving with unison to experience the infinite *puruṣa*, the Self in the finite body or *prakṛti*. For this yogic *sādhanā* is the means and yogic *sādhanā* is the end.

---

[1] Both published by Harper Collins, London.

CITTA-VṚTTI TO *CITI ŚAKTI*

Citta-vṛtti means thought oscillations and fluctuations or movements of the consciousness and *citi śakti* means the power of the Self.

If anyone asks, "What is yoga?" one answers immediately that it is the restraint of consciousness, *citta-vṛtti nirodha.* However *yogaḥ cittavṛtti nirodhaḥ* (*Y. S.,* I.2), puts us into the jigsaw puzzle, because the four words yoga, *citta, vṛtti* and *nirodha* have several dimensions.

Yoga means union or yoking; it also means going to the state of trance or *samādhi.* A neophyte gets puzzled because he finds it hard to grasp the connection between the word union and restraint of consciousness.

Citta is translated as consciousness which indicates liveliness and vibrancy. It is an energetic force *(caitanya śakti)* of life or animation as it evolves from the first principle of nature, *mahat* or cosmic energy.

As *citta* is part and parcel of the first principle of nature, namely *mahat,* I hope you understand and realise that with our average intellectual standard you cannot directly touch *citta* the moment you begin yoga. It is its *vṛtti* which we have to consider as *vṛtti* or fluctuations cause our actions and re-actions. The senses of perception and organs of action attract the mind which is a part of *citta* causing the fluctuations, modulations, modifications and so forth. Hence, we have to tackle first these eleven (five senses of perception, five organs of action and mind) before thinking of *citta-vṛtti nirodha* when we begin the *sādhanā.*

Citta has three components, mind *(manas),* intelligence *(buddhi)* and 'I'-ness or 'I'-maker *(ahaṁkāra)* having their own ways of expressions and behaviours. These three influence the consciousness according to the flow of *guṇa.* The *guṇa* are *sattva, rajas* and *tamas.* These *guṇa* are found in differing ratios and as such the fluctuation of *citta* functions differ quality-wise or standard-wise in each and everyone.

Vṛtti is another complex word. It is derived from the *Sanskṛt* root *vṛt* meaning, to rotate, to revolve, to turn, to roll. If we watch our thoughts carefully, these thoughts jump like monkeys.

As monkeys jump from one branch to another or from tree to tree, our thoughts jump like monkeys without rhyme or realm. Our thoughts keep on rotating around like in a game of musical chairs.

Vṛtti also means the mode of life according to our likings or mode of conduct or character. It also stands for the course of action. *Citta* and its *vṛtti* act accordingly. Therefore *vṛtti* have to be thought of in all perspectives.

Nirodha means restraint, control. *Ni* is a prefix which indicates negation or privation. *Rodha* is the act of stopping, checking, obstructing, impeding, preventing, suppressing. The root word for *rodha* is *rūḍha* which means to stop further growth.

Language, words, expressions, vision, analysis, synthesis, deliberation, experience, experimentation, format of actions, pros and cons, intellectualisation and memory have their own characters. Patañjali covers all these in *pañcavṛtti: pramāṇa* – valid and experienced knowledge, *viparyaya* – perverse or illusory knowledge, *vikalpa* – delusion or imagination, *nidrā* – sleep and *smṛti* – memory. *Vṛtti* are processes of intellectualization. In sleep there is nescience and absence of thought or thinking waves. As thoughts jump quickly from one object to another we miss the causes for fluctuations and modifications.

Citta being the composite of *manas, buddhi* and *ahaṁkāra,* with each one of them having their own way of playing in thought waves according to the influence of *sattva, rajas* and *tamas.* Emotions go with mind *(manas),* intelligence *(buddhi)* goes with deliberation and I'-maker *(ahaṁkāra)* with will power.

Though we understand *vṛtti* as explained theoretically by Patañjali, the process to arrest or stop its movements is not simple. *Vṛtti* influences man from time immemorial with his many lives, throughout . Even in this life mind, intelligence and I-consciousness influence *citta* based on *tridoṣa, pañcabhūta* and *pañcaprāṇa.* Also he is caught in the web of actions and re-actions. All these put together affect one's thinking process. Therefore, one needs to look at all these to relate with one's behaviour through one's own study or *svādhyāya* which is a part of *Pātañjala Yoga.* Let us understand the *vṛtti* and see how these affect one.

Mano-vṛtti

Let me take the fluctuations of the mind *(mano-vṛtti). Manovṛtti* means movements in mind. Mind is the exterior sheath of the consciousness *(citta),* its master is all-pervading *(vibhu).* It can reach and penetrate the smallest and the subtlest area of the body and react speedily. Body, mind, intelligence and consciousness have close connection with each other. But the mind *(manas)* lacks consistency and therefore lacks decisiveness. Its indecisiveness is in its nature. As it easily comes in contact with the senses of perception and the organs of action, it bosses over them. Hence, yogi and sages considered the mind to be the eleventh sense organ *(ekādaśendriya)* along with five *jñānendriya* and five *karmendriya*. As it moves like mercury, it is hard to grasp. Because of its quickness it seems as though it is coming in contact with all the *indriya* at a time, though it cannot. If the eyes are looking at an object, the mind follows the eyes and so does the self. The mind and the eyes are incapable of seeing without having the contact of the self. It flashes its energy on the mind to feel and eyes to see.

The mind is an external *indriya* and the cells too are *indriya*. Lord Krishna says, *tasmāt tvam indriyāṇyādau niyamya bharataṣabha* (*B.G.*, III.41). As cells and mind are made of food, they are *indriya*. The mind is made up of what we eat. The food we eat gets divided into three parts; one part as *sāra* nourishes the body, the other one as *kitta* is excreted, and the third nourishes the mind as *sattva*.

The food we eat plays a great role on our body, senses, organs of action, mind, intelligence, I-consciousness and *citta*. As we say, "One reaps as what he sews"; it is the same with food that forms the mind. As food comes under *triguṇa (sattva, rajas* and *tamas)*, the food we eat affects the mind accordingly and as per the quality of mind our disposition to work will be.

As the mind depends upon what we eat, its thinking process depends upon the quality of mind. If the intake of food is heavy, the mind becomes dull and slow. If the mind gets disturbed, it suffers with grief, sorrow and dejection. When one eats bitter, salty, sour and pungent food, the mind becomes '*rājasic*. If one eats uncooked, putrid, stale and polluted food his mind becomes dull, stupid and inert. It is *tāmasic*. If one eats *sāttvic* food which is juicy, succulent, substantial, unctuous, creamy, the mind too remains *sāttvic*.[1]

As the mind is the exterior layer of the consciousness, most of the time it is influenced by *rajas* and *tamas*. Therefore mental pain *(daurmanasya)* is possible even if there are simple diseases like fever, diarrhoea, constipation and so forth. It gets easily affected and oscillates

---

1 *āyuḥsattvabalārogya sukhaprītivivardhanāḥ* I *rasyāḥ snigdhāḥ sthirā hṛdyā āhārāḥ sāttvikapriyāḥ* II *(B.G.,* XVII.8) – the foods which promote life, vitality, strength, health, joy and cheerfulness, which are sweet, soft, nourishing and agreeable are dear to the "good".

Kaṭvamlalavaṇātyuṣṇa tīkṣnarūkṣavidāhinaḥ I *āhārā rājasasye 'ṣṭā duḥkhaśokāmayapradāḥ* II *(B.G.,* XVII.9) – the foods that are bitter, sour, saltish, very hot, pungent, harsh and burning, producing pain, grief and disease are liked by the "passionate".

Yātayāmaṁ gatarasaṁ pūti paryusitaṁ ca yat I *ucchiṣṭam api cā 'medhyaṁ bhojanam tāmasapriyam* II *(B.G.,* XVII.10) – that which is half cooked, insipid, putrid, stale, polluted and unclean is the food dear to men of *tamasic* disposition only".

and therefore remains indecisive. Yet it has the quality like attention, selection and rejection depending upon *sattva, rajas* and *tamas.*

There are characteristic behaviours of mind which are recognised as *mano-vṛtti.* The mind is fickle and therefore it plays tricks and does not remain trustworthy. If it approaches its subtle part (intelligence), then it helps to stop its fickleness to take decisions. Mind often gets caught in the dual state of 'this or that'; due to its own likings, attachments, and allurements.

Mind is perceptive to emotions more than to intellectual reasoning. Emotions are closely connected with motivations. There are several states of emotions like fear, terror, rage, anger, fury, apprehension, suspicion, scorn, contempt, disgust, abhorrence, loathing, remorse, shame, alarm, dread, horror, pity, gratitude, joy, delight, elation, and affection. One's behavioural responses come from such emotions which not only affect the physical body and organic body but also make man stable. If there is an emotional excitement, the heartbeat throbs, liver throws sugar into the blood, breathing goes fast. If the mind faces failure, it goes into pieces, while in victory it acts in jubilance.

Emotions mean *bhāvanā.* Normally *bhāvanā* are considered to be irrational due to want of reasoning. But the mind being based on *tejas tattva,* it can be shaped and cleansed.

For example emotions like love, affection, friendliness, compassion, kindness, forgiveness come from the *sāttvic guṇa* of the mind. Patañjali mentions this indirectly while explaining *prāṇāyāma.* Through *prāṇāyāma, sattva guṇa* surfaces and the mind becomes eligible for *dhāraṇā.*[1] All these *vṛtti* have to be stabilised for a steady mind.

Buddhi-vṛtti

Buddhi is intelligence. It stands for imparting knowledge, instruction. It has the decisive power. It thinks, exerts and analyses the facts. It does not get carried away easily with emotions but acts and inter-reacts with them thoughtfully and thoroughly. If one acts with motives like robbery, murder, threatening, rape, cheat or love affair, *buddhi* thinks destructively and hence it is a negative approach. If its thinking is destructive, it is filled with *rājasic* and *tāmasic* quality. In planning the course of action for professions like business, agriculture, military force, educational field and so forth, it can think constructively.

---

[1] *tataḥ kṣīyate prakāśa āvaraṇam* (*Y.S.,* II.52) – *Prāṇāyāma* removes the veil covering the light of knowledge and heralds the dawn of wisdom.
dhāraṇāsu ca yogyatā manasaḥ (*Y.S.,* II.53) – The mind also becomes fit for concentration.

Intelligence can be clear as well as clever. It does not depend upon the mind for thinking but it may depend on memory in order to process it. Mind too depends on memory. But *buddhi* deliberates the memory thoughtfully. Its *dharma* is to think rightly and judge accurately. Yet, sometimes it may end up in success or in failure. Infatuation or anger can obstruct its rays as the clouds stop the rays of sun falling on earth. Therefore it has to remain sharp and keep on unsheathing the sheaths that veil it. It should be close to faculty of judgement *(viveka)* and classifying things according to their proportion. If it leaves the friendship of conscience *(dharmendriya)* in its judgement and embraces the mind or the *ahaṁkāra*, its downfall is certain.

However if *buddhi* is caught in *kliṣṭa-vṛtti*, it is bound to fail in its decision and may lose its rationality. When it gets delirious it gets illusional, deranged, demented and may lead to insanity and hallucination. If it gets deranged it is hardly possible to find a cure.

Lord Krishna says that one has to develop the *vyavasāyātmikā buddhi*. The *buddhi* being sharp goes in all directions. It has a hunger for knowledge but mind can pull it towards its desires. *Buddhi* shows interest in many things and objects; therefore it can have innumerable aims. Because of its *kliṣṭa-vṛtti* we have to convert it into *akliṣṭa-vṛtti* by directing it towards the real. That is *vyavasāyātmikā buddhi*. It means settled determination, resolve, endeavour, strenuous effort and diligence.

It is said that knowledge *(vidyā)* can be acquired through books but *sāttvic buddhi* (*sāttvic* intelligence) is earned through the process of experience.

Ahaṁkāra-vṛtti

Ahaṁkāra or ego is the third aspect of *citta*. Its major role is to oppose or eclipse *buddhi*. It wants to impose itself as *ātman* (the very being).

However *ahaṁkāra* builds up will power. It has the power of *icchā śakti*. *Icchā* is motivity. It has the power of determination. It ignites hopes to proceed with will power. Yet its weaknesses are hypocrisy, superiority or inferiority complexes. It has the power to act as if it is highly intelligent and active. Pride is its nature. Its inherent behaviour is to show off.

The *ahaṁkāra* which is translated as I-consciousness or maker, is of two faceted, constructive and destructive. There could be the *sāttvic ahaṁkāra*, *rājasic* and *tāmasic ahaṁkāra*. Without having any substance, often we puff our ego even if we are empty inside and show off as if we know. This is *tāmasic ahaṁkāra*.

Rājasic ahaṁkāra is that which expresses itself as being superior than our actual state. Acting for selfish gains, use of muscle power to rule over others is *rājasic ahaṁkāra.* The intention to destroy by means of competition is also *rājasic,* and if the intention is to judge one's own capacity, it is *sāttvic.* When a person with honesty helps and uplifts others by using his power in right direction, then this becomes *sāttvic ahaṁkāra.*

It is very difficult to be intelligent and humble at the same time. When one is intelligent, the ego lifts its hood up. Though *buddhi* and *ahaṁkāra* co-exist, they compete with each other. The *ahaṁkāra* should not get elevated into vanity or pride. Very often those who are very intelligent behave arrogantly.

To take pride in action and intelligence is *kliṣṭa ahaṁkāra.* Even those who do *sādhanā, japa, bhakti,* worship or yoga take pride in what they are doing. This is the *ahaṁkāra-pravṛtti* and this acts as a great obstacle in reaching *viveka buddhi.*

This is how *citta* gets caught and gets imbalanced with the *vṛtti* or *pravṛtti* of *manas, buddhi* and *ahaṁkāra.* Let us now see how *vṛtti* are connected to our body *(śarīra).*

Śarīra-vṛtti

Basically the body has an inherent inclination towards plesant actions and their fruits *(karma bhoga-pravṛtti).*

Since the body is made of bones, muscles, five elements, it is often mistakenly concluded that it won't have any *vṛtti.* It is basically dependent on *tamoguṇa.* But the mind which is close to the body uses it for its own enjoyment and satisfaction. The serenity of mind needs to be acquired by educating it; otherwise the mind is primarily fickle, volatile in nature. This volatile mind remains close to the body like Siamese twins. As these two are woven together, science terms man as a psychosomatic animal. If the mind moves, the body moves and if the body moves the mind moves. If mind is restlessness, body becomes restlessness and if it is restful, the body too feels restfulness.

When we use the body to work or do something we often observe involuntary movements occurring. This is on account of the nervous system which connects body and mind to function. Even in a totally vegetative person or one who is in comatose state, body language expresses what the person wants to say. Sometimes unnecessary, unwanted and undue movements of the body occur unknowingly.

In *Śavāsana* when you are not supposed to disturb the body, the disturbance occurs. Often, such movements get unnoticed by the mind. Some form habits like shaking the legs, fingers, head or shrugging the shoulders. These are uncontrolled *vṛtti* of the body. To discipline these movements of the body is as difficult as controlling the fickle mind. Even if one claims that one is not moving or doing nothing, yet in reality one can see this happening. Not a single moment goes without a movement. The movement may just be physical or mental or intellectual. It is perpetual.

Though the mind is the origin for action orientation *(karma-pravṛtti)* and body responds to plesant orientation or *(bhoga-pravṛtti)* at once.

The mind shows its lordship over the body and uses it for its pleasures. This is *kliṣṭa-vṛtti* of *śarīra*. *Yoga sādhanā* is meant to change *kliṣṭa-vṛtti* into *akliṣṭa-vṛtti*. For this, practice of *āsana* is advocated in order to bring right actions, right efforts, proper placements, non-rigidity, firmness, non-stressfulness and stability.

Often imbalance in mind causes the body to pick up wrong actions involuntarily and unintentionally. However such wrong actions are possible with auto-mechanism from within. Practice of *āsana* and *prāṇāyāma* help to control such actions to experience the *akliṣṭa* state.

Patañjali mentionsthe effect of *dharmamegha samādhi (Y.S.,* IV.29). It means that from hereon the *sādhaka* does only non-painful *(akliṣṭa)* actions.

Pañcamahābhūta-vṛtti

Body is made up of five elements, *pṛthvī, āp, tej, vāyu* and *ākāśa*. These elements have five *tanmātra*, their subtle infrastructures. They are *gandha, rasa, rūpa, sparśa* and *śabda*. Stability, heaviness, solidity and grossness indicate earth element. Rough voice and grating sound in joints, heaviness, immobility, laziness, lack of motivation are their characteristic marks and make progress slow. Even the thinking process may slow down. However they enjoy the smell of food.

The *āp tattva* or water element is fluid, soft, insipid, vapid, sludgy, sticky and oily. People with more water element will be friendly, soft natured and stick to something which they would not easily give up. Sensitivity to tasty food is strong in them.

The *tejas* or fire element is hotness. Therefore, people of *tejas tattva* have good digestive power. They look fair. Their skin blushes when they are angry or laughing or in fright or embarrassment. They show brilliance, sharpness, braveness, fearlessness. They are attracted towards beauty, shape, and figure. Their imagination is strong but show impatience, intolerance, and less enduring power.

People of *vāyu tattva* have suppleness and flexibility. They feel strong, work hard and are touchy but relax soon. They hold on to what they want and their thinking appears logical.

People of *ākāśa tattva* have a big heart. They remain clean. They do not have double standards. They are straightforward and honest and mix easily with anyone. They listen to their inner voice and then act. Predominance of elements plays on persons according to their characteristics.

Each *mahābhūta* or its *tattva* is controlled by the *cakra*. For instance, *pṛthvī tattva* is governed by *mūlādhāra* and *svāḍhiṣṭhāna cakra* , *āp tattva* by *maṇipūraka, sūrya, manas* and *anāhata cakra, tejas tattva* by *viśuddhi cakra, vāyu tattva* is governed by *ājñā, soma* and *lalāṭa cakra, ākāśa tattva* by *sahasrāra cakra*. When *kuṇḍalinī* awakens, undoubtedly, the elements are conquered by the *sādhaka*. Until then the *bhūta* affect *citta* according to the fluctuations in the elemental balance.

For instance, persons born with the predominance of *pṛthvī tattva* will be slow; their senses of perception act slowly as their intelligence remains in a *tāmasic* state. They lack self-esteem. Lord Ganesha and Brahmā are presiding deities of the *mūlādhāra* and *svāḍhiṣṭhāna cakra* which belong to *pṛthvī tattva*.

Persons born with the predominance of *āp tattva* stick to some ideology or somebody they like and lose their individualism. They lack judgement and fall a prey easily to any fake *sādhu, svāmi* or *sannyāsi*. If the *āp tattva* is in a balanced state their sensitivity will be strong with right discrimination. They are sensitive to taste and friendly at a right time and at a right place. *Maṇipūraka, sūrya, manas* and *anāhata cakra* control *āp tattva*. They have fluent minds and catch on to the ideas and thoughts fast. *Tapas* and *svādhyāya* are easier for them. Lord Vishnu is the presiding deity of the *cakra* where *samāna vāyu* has its province. They have the sense of equilibrium, evenness and equanimity.

Persons born with the predominance of *tejas tattva* will be intelligent by nature. As fire burns impurities and cleanses everything, the *tejas tattva* brings purity in them. They lack patience and do not tolerate delay in work but are good in planning. *Viśuddhi cakra* and *samāna vāyu* govern this *tattva*. Rudra is its presiding deity.

Persons born with the predominance of *vāyu tattva* have strong inspiring power *(preraka śakti)*. They inspire thoughts. Mahatma Gandhi is an example of *vāyu tattva*. *Vāyu tattva* is governed by *ājñā, soma* and *lalāṭa*. *Prāṇa* will be close to this *tattva*. People of this *tattva* understand others' problems and feel for them. The presiding deity being the *ātma-devatā*, they work with conscience.

Persons with the predominance of *ākāśa tattva* have clarity in themselves. They have strong will power and tend to know the spiritual aspects of life. *Sahasrāra cakra* and *vyāna* govern this *tattva*. The presiding deity is *parambṛahma*.

Tridoṣa-vṛtti

The three humours of the body are *vāta*, *pitta* and *kapha*. These are known as *tridoṣa*. Though by birth they give certain constitution to each and every one, yet, one differs from another constitutionally since the ratio of *vāta*, *pitta* and *kapha* differs in each one. They affect the *vṛtti* of *citta* accordingly. *Haṭhayoga Pradīpikā* says that balance of *tridoṣa* is essential. When the *tridoṣa* get imbalanced, they not only affect the body but also play a great role in bringing about change in one's mental state.

The *vāta*, *pitta* and *kapha* affect the *śarīra-vṛtti*, *mano-vṛtti*, *buddhi-vṛtti* and *ahaṁkāra-vṛtti*. They dominate in their ways of thinking and action affecting either in *kleśa-vṛtti* or in *akleśa-vṛtti*. Therefore, it is good to know and understand the characteristics of *tridoṣa*.

For instance, a person of *vāta* shows lack in determination, lack of will power and indecisiveness. His fickleness and unsteadiness do not allow him to look with clarity.

Persons of *pitta* constitution are fiery by nature. They get angry soon and do not forgive easily. They are short-tempered, courageous, stubborn, friendly, brave, highly imaginative with sharp intelligence. They like to live with self-respect, self-esteem and at the same time show pride.

Persons of *śleṣma* or *kapha* constitution are quite intelligent, wise, tolerant, calm, promising, friendly with clear foresight, insight and strong memory.

This way, the life of each one is an admixture of *tamas*, *rajas* and *sattva* as well as *vāta*, *pitta* and *śleṣma*.

Pañcaprāṇa-vṛtti

Viśva cetanā śakti (God) causes *viśva caitanya śakti*. This becomes the source behind birth, life and death. When the ovum and sperm meet along with the *jīvātmā*, the *viśva caitanya śakti* enters to conceive the birth of the foetus. The very vibrations of *sattva, rajas* and *tamas* or *vāta, pitta* and *śleṣma* happen due to *viśva caitanya śakti,* whether these are in a balanced state *(sāmyāvasthā)* or in an imbalanced state *(asāmyāvasthā* or *viṣamāvasthā).* This *viśva caitanya śakti* becomes *vaiyaktika śakti* at the time of conception. This *vaiyaktika śakti* is recognised by five names, namely, *prāṇa, apāna, samāna, vyāna* and *udāna.*

These five *vāyu* contribute to the physiological functions of the body along with *pañcapitta.* The *pañcapitta* act as *ālocaka pitta* in eyes, *sādhaka pitta* in heart and brain, *ranjaka pitta* in blood, *pācaka pitta* in stomach and intestines, and *bhrājaka pitta* in skin. The *pañcakapha* act as *tarpaka kapha* in the head and eyes, *bodhaka kapha* in the tongue, *avalaṁbaka kapha* in the chest, heart, neck and shoulders, *kledaka kapha* in the stomach and duodenum and *saṁśleṣaka kapha* in the joints. These *kapha* have close connections with the mental, intellectual and spiritual body also.

Prāṇa and *citta* are closely interwoven. Their place *(sthāna)* is the crown of the head and heart. Yet it moves in the throat, chest and brain. *Prāṇa vāyu* supports, holds and sustains body as well as the power of intelligence, emotions, senses and action.

The *tarpaka kapha* of *prāṇa* keeps the brain calm and cool. It satiates and nourishes the brain. The *ālocaka pitta* along with *vyāna vāyu* helps the eyes to see and keeps them cool and lively. *Udāna* exists in throat and lungs. Its main function is exhalation which brings lightness in the body. It creates vibrations in the larynx to talk or sing. *Udāna* energises the fuel *(agni)* as *sādhaka pitta.* Its nature is to fulfil the wishes of the mind of the *sādhaka.* It gives *buddhibala (medhā śakti)* and *tapobala* (the power acquired with passion in *sādhanā*). The *avalaṁbaka kapha* which has its place in the heart connects the back of chest to the heart and supports the armpits and hands. In *āsana, prāṇāyāma, dhāraṇā* and *dhyāna* the torso which plays major roles is supported by *udāna vāyu, sādhakāgni* and *avalaṁbaka kapha.*

The *samāna sthāna* is in the stomach, duodenum and intestines. *Samāna vāyu* basically does the job of digestion. *Samāna vāyu* is recognised as *agni-sakhā* (friend of fire). It is the centre of *annamaya kośa. Samāna* means equal. *Prāṇa* exists in the head. *Apāna* exists below the navel. *Udāna* exists in the chest and *vyāna* moves in blood vessels and nerves. *Samāna* distributes equal energy to all these four *prāṇa* to keep them functioning. The *pañcaprāṇa* are fed by air and *samāna* balances water and food evenly. The *sthāna* of *ranjaka pitta* is in the liver, spleen, pancreas as *āmāśaya.* The blood is red because of it. *Samāna* works by igniting *pācaka pitta* and supports *ranjaka pitta* to have a balanced healthy state of life. This in turn brings the lustre and brightness in the skin as *bhrājaka pitta.*

The *apāna sthāna* is below the navel, which rules over excretory and reproductive system. *Apāna* is the base of our existence and dynamic life. The production of energy gets affected if *apāna* is affected. *Sādhaka pitta* with *udāna vāyu* instigates one to do the *sādhanā* whereas *apāna* provokes, elevates will power. If *apāna* fails, depression is certain. The *sādhaka pitta* helps in controlling wrong intentions.

Udāna instigates to do *tapas; apāna* gives energy; *samāna* balances, *vyāna* protects from downfall and *prāṇa* fructifies it.

Vyāna sthāna moves everywhere through the blood and nerves. The contraction and expansion of the muscles, blood vessels, peristaltic movements, blinking and motor nerves are under the control of *vyāna*. *Vyāna* cleanses the *śrotas, nāḍī, dhamani* and *śirā*. Whatever *kriyā* (function) are left by other *vāyu*, they are done by *vyāna*. When *vyāna* fails, the other *vāyu* and their functions get affected.

When *pañcaprāṇa* become feeble, they affect a person physically and mentally. We know the story of Śvetaketu (son) and Uddālaka (father) from *Chāndogya Upaniṣad*. The son comes to his father saying that he has learnt everything and whatever is to be learnt and known. Then the father realises that his ego has been puffed up. This reminds me the story of the frog and the buffalo. A baby frog sees the buffalo and tells mother frog that it saw a huge animal. The mother frog begins to puff her body asking the baby frog whether it was that big. The baby frog kept on replying "no" and mother frog continued to puff herself and finally dies. This is what the *pañcavāyu* do. Though it is a story, yet a lesson to human beings. The pretension puffs up the ego and finally affects the nervous system. The emotional upheavals, behavioural patterns change for the good or bad by the *pañcavāyu*. The story of Śvetaketu and Uddālaka is based on the fact that Śvetaketu becomes arrogant thinking that he knows everything and tells his father that he cannot understand what he has learnt. Then the father asked him how a tree grows from a seed. The boy had no answer. Then the father collects the seed of the tree and asks him to cut it to find what is inside it. He finds a tiny seed. He asks his son to peel it also. He goes on peeling one after the other and at the end says that he finds nothing. His father then opens his son's eyes saying from this nothing the tree has grown. By this Śvetaketu becomes his father's pupil. Accepting him as his pupil, the father keeps his son without food for fifteen days, later without water for fifteen days, and later to live with air. The son finally tells his father that he does not remember or recall anything as his intelligence and *prāṇa* fail to function. Then he was given food, later water with food and lastly ghee (clarified butter). Then he finds changes and says that food brings life in mind, water brought his energy back and *tej* (ghee), the power of speech.

The source of energy in all of us is in the *ātman* who is the Lord of *vāyu.* It is through *ātman* that the *pañcavāyu* remain intact keeping one healthy through right diet, clean water and balanced fat in food.

If we go against the principles of *yama* and *niyama,* the *tridoṣa, pañcavāyu, pañcapitta, pañcakapha* get affected disturbing *pañca-vṛtti* into *pañcakleśa.* The body-chemistry changes.

By *āsana* and *prāṇāyāma sādhanā* the *vaiyaktika śakti* is nourished by *viśva caitanya śakti.*[1] *Āsana* and *prāṇāyāma* practices bring *snāyu-vṛtti nirodha* and *prāṇa-vṛtti nirodha.* The *abhyantara, bāhya* and *stambha-vṛtti* of *prāṇa* bring changes in the behavioural pattern as well as the movements of cells *(snāyu)* of the body. They yield perfect balance in activity, vigour, valour, quietness, passivity, pensivity as well as clarity in intelligence and cleanse the memory.

Pañcakleśa-vṛtti

The *Yoga Sūtra* begins with the *vṛtti nirodha* in the first chapter and ends with the effect of *sādhanā* as *kleśa karma nivṛtti* in the fourth chapter. The question arises how this is possible. The answer is that *kleśa karma* vanishes with *dharmamegha samādhi* while *vṛtti nirodha* occurs with *savitarka, nirvitarka, savicāra, nirvicāra, ānanda* and *asmitā* state of *samāpatti* or transformation. Our *vṛtti* are built up according to *mano-vṛtti, buddhi-vṛtti, ahaṁkāra-vṛtti, śarīra-vṛtti, bhūta-vṛtti, tridoṣa-vṛtti, prāṇa-vṛtti* and *kleśa-vṛtti.* These will fade out gradually with different stages of *samāpatti.*

The *pañcakleśa* or five afflictions are *avidyā, asmitā, rāga, dveṣa* and *abhiniveśa.* These afflictions are instinctive, emotional as well as intellectual, and can affect the body, mind, intelligence and consciousness. The *vṛtti* of *śarīra* are affected by *tridoṣa, pañcabhūta* and *pañcaprāṇa* along with *sattva, rajas* and *tamas.* This is how the net or maze is formed for the *pañca-vṛtti* of *citta.*

Avidyā is the root cause of other four *kleśa. Avidyā* means want of knowledge or nescience. Normally, one does not accept ignorance easily. Just reading and writing is not *vidyā.* But to know the real meaning of life is *jñāna vidyā.* The real *ānanda* (happiness) is not in acquiring the objects of external world but to know the very core of our being. The real *ānanda* is *ātma-jñāna* (subjective) and not in *vastu-jñāna* (objective things).

Avidyā (nescience) brings chain of sorrows, vitiation in *doṣa,* mental disturbance and feebleness of *prāṇa-śakti.* For this we need to do good, virtuous and auspicious *karma* in order to accumulate good *saṁskāra. Aṣṭāṅga yoga* helps to achieve these *saṁskāra.*

---

[1] Please refer to *Aṣṭadaḷa Yogamālā,* vol. 2, pp 47, 108, 261, 274, 275, 276, 277, 279, 282, 283, 284, 285, 287, 313, 324 and vol 6, pp 224 and vol. 7, pp 161,162 – table.

Our approach should be to keep on doing good work and restrain ourselves from bad work. As time passes the true knowledge dawns. See what Lord Krishna says in *Bhagavad Gītā*, "Do *karma* without thinking of its fruits. Do the duty without hankering after fruits". *Karmaṇyevādhikāraste mā phaleṣu kadācana* (*B.G.*, II.47). Fruits *(vipāka)* tempt us to do *karma* again.

Behind every work there are hidden hopes of achieving something. Often people do *pūjā* (worship), *homa* (oblation), *yajña* (rituals) for the attainment of worldly and heavenly pleasures or through fear of going to hell. Each action is bound to leave its effect and it happens.

If the effect is transformation *(pariṇāma)*, fructification is *vipāka*. *Vipāka* means the ripening process. For instance, when we cook food, it is called *pāka*. *Paripāka* means essence. *Vipāka* means cooked. The prefix *vi* stands for *viśeṣa* – the specific quality. So the word *vipāka* indicates specifically cooked with essence. In this sense *vipāka karma* means the essence of *karma;* and *pariṇāma* means the change. The seed that transforms into root, tree, flower and fruit is *pariṇāma*. The effect of seed is fruit and the seed is again hidden in the fruit. However the transformation keeps on occurring from seed to fruit and fruit to seed. The essence of root, tree, flower and fruit is in the seed. In other words, the seed has already 'cooked' the tree with fruit from within. If the seed is of high standard, then its effect in the form of fruit will be of a high standard. This is *vipāka*. Therefore, if *karma* is good, *vipāka* too will be invariably good. If good and bad actions are mixed, then accordingly the results will be. In the same way, if we need to bring transformation, we have to do good *karma* for it to yield good result. The seed of birth and abode of *kleśa karma* is the body. *Kleśamūlaḥ karmāśayaḥ*. In order to change, Patañjali advises *anuṣṭhāna* in *aṣṭāṅga yoga*. Through the practice of *aṣṭāṅga yoga*, transformation *(pariṇāma)* occurs and as such the effect occurs in the body *(śarīra)*, organs of action *(karmendriya)*, senses of perception *(jñānendriya)*, energy *(prāṇa)*, elements *(bhūta)*, mind *(manas)*, intelligence *(buddhi)*, pride or ego *(ahaṁkāra)*, consciousness *(citta)* culminating with exalted intelligence *(viveka)*. Eventually, the *karma* are cleansed and purified, and therefore the *vipāka* too comes in pure and auspicious form.

Pañcakleśa are enclosed between *avidyā* and *abhiniveśa*. *Avidyā* is nescience and *abhiniveśa* is clinging to life. In between are pride *(asmitā)*, attachment *(rāga)* and aversion *(dveṣa)*. To tap these *kleśa*, conscience *(dharmendriya)* has to be tapped and awakened to cleanse and purify our *karma*. As a person with jaundice sees all objects yellow, our nescience, infatuation, attachment and jealousy make us to think wrong and act wrong. *Abhiniveśa* (attachment to life) makes us afraid to scrutinise the facts of existence and face up to them. As we use a torch in the dark, we need the torch of *viveka* (distinguishing the real) while doing a *karma* or duty.

Realising all these factors and taking them into account we have to find out whether the *vṛtti* are sprouted from *manas, buddhi, ahaṁkāra, śarīra, tridoṣa, pañcaprāṇa* or *kleśa.* Then we try to restrain them *(vṛtti nirodha).* It is a tough job to restrain but through the process of *karma-śuddhi, vicāra-śuddhi, manaḥ-śuddhi, ahaṁkāra-śuddhi* and *citta-śuddhi* it is possible. The *aṣṭāṅga* of Patañjali's yoga are meant for these *śuddhi.* See what Patañjali says, *yogāṅgānuṣṭhānāt aśuddhikṣaye jñānadīptiḥ āvivekakhyāteḥ* (*Y.S.,* II.28). This *sūtra* indicates that we have to consider all aspects of yoga. I call them the eight petals of yoga. As the flower holds all the petals, we have to allow the flower of yoga to bloom along with the petals. You all talk about *cakra* and you know that *cakra* is considered to be having the petals. All the petals of *cakra* have to bloom to receive the energy and transform it into *ojas śakti* or spiritual splendour.

The yogic petals are *yama, niyama, āsana, prāṇāyāma, pratyāhāra, dhāraṇā, dhyāna* and *samādhi.* All these petals, when followed correctly, advertently, thoroughly, accurately, religiously and devotedly, it take us towards the ultimate. Patañjali explains in the *sūtra* the termination or the diminution of impurities *(aśuddhikṣaya)* takes place progressively and the knowledge shines until the *viveka jñāna* reaches its summit. Patañjali uses the term *sarvathā vivekakhyāti.*[1] When the *sādhaka* is totally free from the seed of all *kleśa saṁskāra,* including fissures in the consciousness *(chidra citta), buddhi* is untouched by the tinge of desires. Then this pure *buddhi* leads us to *dharmamegha samādhi* where all *(sarvathā)* aims of life cease.

Patañjali has not denied the body. He has not used the word *śarīra* or *deha* but *kāya.* He uses the word *aṅga.* Read *sūtra* II.40 and 43. *Śaucāt svāṅgajugupsā paraiḥ asaṁsargaḥ* (*Y.S.,* II.40) – Cleanliness of body and mind develops disinterest in contact with others for self-gratification. And, *kāya indriya siddhiḥ aśuddhikṣayāt tapasaḥ* (*Y.S.,* II.43) – Self-discipline *(tapas)* burns away impurities and kindles the sparks of divinity.

On one hand he says that *śauca* (cleanliness) terminates in *svāṅga jugupsā* – the abhorrence towards one's own body (*Y.S.,* II.39). On the other hand he says, *kāya siddhi* and *indriya siddhi.* The *tapas* burns the impurities of *kāya* – body, and *indriya* – organs of action and senses of perception, and these are accomplished (*Y.S.,* II.43). In the third chapter he says, *nābhicakre kāyavyūhajñānam* (*Y.S.,* III.30). If the body has to be neglected, why this *kāyavyūhajñānam?* The *vyūha* is orderly formation and arrangement. The military or police arrange their forces in an orderly manner when they have to attack and conquer the enemies. In our own body we find all our energies scattered and disarranged. Patañjali refers to it as *aṅgamejayatva* (*Y.S.,* I.31). We need to have a proper formation or arrangement of energy. We

---

[1] *prasaṁkhyāne api akusīdasya sarvathā vivekakhyāteḥ dharmameghaḥ samādhiḥ* (*Y.S.,* IV.29). The yogi who has no interest even in this highest state of evolution, and maintains supreme attentive, discriminative awareness, attains *dharmamegha samādhi:* he contemplates the fragrance of virtue and justice.

have to use proper strategy for it. The *vyūha* is especially used in battle. There has to be a formation and strategy which is kept secret from enemies. Our body is much complicated and affected with *vṛtti*, depression *(daurmanasya)* and *abhiniveśa:* take anger. It upsets the digestive system and even damages the nervous system disturbing the balance of *pañcavāyu* and the body gets affected with disease *(vyādhi)*. The source or centre of energy being the navel region, by controlling the area of the navel we acquire the knowledge of body *(kāya-vyūha)*. *Sūtra* from *Vibhūti Pāda, tataḥ aṇimādi prādurbhāvaḥ kāyasaṁpat taddharma anabhighātaḥ ca* (*Y.S.*, III.46).[1] conveys that it can achieve *aṣṭa-siddhi*, namely: *aṇimā, mahimā, laghimā, garimā, prāpti, prākāmya, Īśatva and vaśitva*[2] and *kāya* (body) will be unaffected by *bhūta-vṛtti, tridoṣa-vṛtti, mano-vṛtti* or *prāṇa-vṛtti*. Patañjali says, *prakāśa kriyā sthiti śīlaṁ bhūtendriyātmakaṁ bhogāpavargārtham dṛśyam* (*Y.S.*, II.18). It means the *triguṇa, bhūta*, mind, senses and organs exist eternally to serve the seer for enjoyment or emancipation. Though *bhoga-vṛtti* and *yoga-vṛtti* exist in us, it is only *yoga-vṛtti* which brings *kāya-vyūha jñāna* and *aṣṭa-siddhi* surface.

Apavarga (spiritual) and *bhoga* (sensual) *vṛtti*

The natural instinct in us draws our mind to sensual enjoyments *(bhoga)* though there is a possibility of switching over thoughts towards yoga which stands for spiritual endeavour. *Triguṇa* play a great role in this *apavarga* and *bhoga-pravṛtti*. *Pravṛtti* means processing with the way of thinking. If you are basically having interest for *bhoga-pravṛtti*, your mind and life gravitate towards sensual enjoyments. *Bhoga* being indulgence in the sensual objects of the world, one who indulges in it gravitates towards these enjoyments. But *apavarga-pravṛtti* pulls one to gravitate towards enlightenment, emancipation and liberation from *kleśa karma*.

One who depends upon these *bhoga* and *apavarga* tendencies, the *vṛtti* of *citta* get formed into *kliṣṭa* or *akliṣṭa* – painful or non-painful state of consciousness. The painful ones leave one in a tormented and perplexed state binding one into *bhoga-vṛtti*. If our thoughts are in *apavarga-vṛtti* we live in a non-painful *(akliṣṭa)* state. Thus, it makes us act in a smooth way without being caught in distress. Then it becomes *yoga-vṛtti*. In short, the *bhoga-vṛtti* and *yoga-vṛtti* depend upon one's inclination which is mostly dependent on the planes of *prakṛti*.

---

[1] From that arises perfection of the body, the ability to resist the play of the elements, and powers such as minuteness. (*Y.S.*, III.46)

[2] *aṇimā* = to become as minute as an atom, *mahimā* = to wax in magnitude, *laghimā* = to become light, *garimā* = to become heavy, *prāpti* = the power to dominate and obtain what one wants, *prākāmya* = the freedom of will and attainment of wishes, *Īśatva* = supremacy over all, *vaśitva* = the power to subjugate anyone or anything.

Therefore he needs to re-orient the component layers of *prakṛti* towards *yoga-vṛtti* or auspicious actions. No doubt the efforts are required for both. But for *yoga-vṛtti,* extraordinary efforts are required. Hence, it is not easy to transform one from *bhoga-vṛtti* to *yoga-vṛtti.* The *citta* may not be ripe to take the load of *yoga-vṛtti* divorcing from *bhoga-vṛtti.* If this transformation from *bhoga* to *apavarga* was easy we would have seen no conflicts at all in us.

Citta of each one has gradation according to the predominance of *sattva, raja* and *tamas* which are hidden in *kṣipta, mūḍha, vikṣipta, ekāgra* and *niruddha citta.* These five states of *citta* have their own ways of deliberation.

Pañcacitta bhūmikā-vṛtti

The *citta* along with its composites functions in five component layers according to its capacity. *Kṣipta citta,* with the predominance of *rajoguṇa* has the wandering nature without an aim. But the practice of *āsana* and *prāṇāyāma* curbs the fickleness in one.

The *mūḍha citta* is predominant in *tamas* and it remains in a state of nescience and inertia. Being irresponsible, one's practices interrupted, it takes a long time to change.

The *vikṣipta citta-bhūmi* is the oscillating one. Indecisiveness, distraction, unsteadiness is its basic nature. But sometimes the *vikṣiptā* person has the capacity to be attentive, decisive and steady. He shows his inclination to the *yogic sādhanā.* This state of *citta* is unlike *kṣipta* which is feeble. The person of *vikṣipta citta-bhūmi* has some rays of hope to go towards yoga. As we say that "Every black cloud has a silver lining", this will be his state. Such people are inclined more towards *rajas* and less for *sattva guṇa.* The moment such people discipline themselves, they realise their weaknesses and pursue their practice. If they practise for a long time uninterruptedly, they take a leap towards knowing higher aspects of life. As far as the people of *ekāgra* and *niruddha citta-bhūmi* are concerned, they are in a congenial state compared to those with *kṣipta, mūḍha* and *vikṣipta citta-bhūmi.*

Persons of *ekāgra citta-bhūmi* have strong aim in minds which do not waver at all. Their one-pointedness lifts them fast to subtler planes of consciousness but they need courage and vigour since their latest impressions *(saṁskāra)* hinder them. Those who belong to *niruddha citta-bhūmi* will be *tīvra saṁvegin* compared to those of *ekāgra* plane who are of *adhimātra saṁvegin.* The aspirants of the *vikṣipta* categories will be somewhere between *mṛdu* and *madhya,* whereas people belonging to *mūḍha* and *kṣipta citta-bhūmi* have to struggle a lot to start from the scratch in the *sādhanā.*

The ruffling and wavering will be found more in those of *kṣipta, mūḍha* and *vikṣipta citta.* They succumb easily to outer attractions, disturbances, enchantments and infatuations.

People of *pitta prakṛti* will be, *kṣaṇa cittam, kṣaṇa pittam* – moment-to-moment their haughty nature surfaces. People of *vāta prakṛti* are of *cale vāte calam cittam,* as the wind blows, their *citta* follows. People of *kapha prakṛti* will be slow in thinking. Their nature is like, "slow and steady will win the race". The people of *ekāgra* and *niruddha citta* are well balanced in thought, word and deed. The *yoga-vṛtti* in them overpowers *bhoga-vṛtti* and moves towards wisdom which dawns on them soon. Their journey is from *vṛtti nirodha* to *vṛtti-nāśa* (vanquishing of *vṛtti)* or from *pravṛtti* to *nivṛtti* or from *prakṛti* to *puruṣa* (final emancipation).

Vṛtti nirodha (kleśa tanukaraṇa)

The question arises that if yoga is *citta-vṛtti nirodha,* then why not arrest the thoughts straight away. It is easier said than done. It is not possible to jump towards the restraint of the consciousness, as we saw earlier how various things intervene, interfere and make it hard for *vṛtti nirodha.* Now the question is, as students of yoga, whether we handle first *vṛtti nirodha* or *kleśa-nivṛtti.* Patañjali himself gives the answer. He says, *tapaḥ svādhyāya Īśvarapraṇidhānāni kriyā yogaḥ* (*Y.S.,* II.1) and *samādhi bhāvanārthaḥ kleśa tanūkaraṇārthaśca* (*Y.S.,* II.2). These two *sūtra* are very important in connection with all I have explained earlier. I have not yet explained the *citta-vṛtti* though I explained *mano-vṛtti, buddhi-vṛtti, ahaṁkāra-vṛtti, kāya-vṛtti, pañcamahābhūta-vṛtti, pañcaprāṇa-vṛtti, pañcakleśa-vṛtti, bhoga-apavarga-vṛtti, pañcacittabhūmi-vṛtti* and the play of *tridoṣa.* The reason behind dealing with these *vṛtti* is that these *vṛtti* play a great role on *citta.* Their influence on *citta* is more than *pañca-vṛtti* which you will know soon.

The second *pāda* is called *Sādhana Pāda. Sādhana* conveys practice. Yet it covers the means or instruments available or needed for practice. When the mother asks the child to go and play, the child itself is a subject which is going to play, therefore child cannot be absent. Now the child needs objects to play with, such as friends instruments such as a ball, a playground or garden and a guide to coach him. If the child cannot catch exactly how to play, then the guide may change the play which is suitable for the child's level of understanding. Patañjali provides ways and means to practice *(sādhanā)*[1] that have to be adopted. In *Samādhi Pāda,*

---

[1] *prakāśa kriyā sthiti śīlaṁ bhūtendriyātmakaṁ bhogāpavargārtham dṛśyam* (*Y.S.,* II.18) Nature, its three qualities, *sattva, rajas* and *tamas,* and its evolutes, the elements, mind, senses of perception and organs of action, exist eternally to serve the seer, for enjoyment or emancipation.
viśeṣa aviśeṣa liṅgamātra aliṅgāni guṇaparvāṇi (*Y.S.,* II.19) The *guṇa* generate their characteristic divisions and energies in the seer. Their stages are distinguishable and non-distinguishable, differentiable and non-differentiable. (cont. page 260) .....

he explains *samādhi.* He touches the subject directly (knowing very well the capacity of *sādhaka)* to those who are *tīvra saṁvegin* (vehement *sādhaka).* The others belonging to the level of *mṛdu, madhya* and *adhimātra* will not be equal to *tīvra saṁvegin,* yet they are specified as eligible. He says that *bhakti* being the highest among *abhyāsa,* the *bhaktan* will reach the spiritual destination quicker than *tīvra saṁvegin.* Patañjali is a *parama bhaktan* or *Īśvara praṇidhānin.* This *bhaktan* will be having *paramaikāntika bhakti. Parama* means highest, *eka* means one and only one, *antika* means end. For such *parama-eka-antika bhaktan,* God is the only goal. He totally surrenders to God. His thoughts, devotion and dedication do not waver from God. He faces and removes all the obstacles which come in his way through *bhakti.* This type of *sādhaka* is completely different from other *sādhaka* – the aspirants.

Tapas, svādhyāya and *Īśvara praṇidhāna* which are bracketed as *kriyā* yoga, do not mean a special type of yoga. *Kriyā* means action, and action means practice to experience *samādhi bhāvanārtham* and *kleśa tanūkaraṇārtham.* We have two types of *citta* – *vyutthita* and *samāhita. Vyutthita citta* is outgoing *citta,* tending towards sensual joys *(bhoga-vṛtti).* People of *samāhita citta* have inclination toward emancipation *(apavarga-vṛtti).* For *vyutthita cittan, vṛtti nirodha* appears impossible, un-reachable and unimaginable. Patañjali does not deny yoga to anyone. On the contrary he advises to adopt *tapas,* then *svādhyāya* and later *Īśvara praṇidhāna.* In the name of *kriyā yoga* he covers *aṣṭāṅga yoga* and brings *karma mārga* in the form of *tapas, jñāna mārga* in the form of *svādhyāya,* and *bhakti mārga* in the form of *Īśvara praṇidhāna.* He wants the *sādhaka* to know *samādhi bhāvanārtham* which means conception or the feel of it *(bhāvanā).* This develops *yoga vṛtti* and then *kleśa tanu karaṇārtham.* It means attenuation of afflictions. This attenuation helps one to be free from *bhoga-vṛtti.*

An average intellect or *vyutthita cittan* is caught in the web of mundane world. He does not even realise the movements or modifications of *citta.* He is on the plane of *kṣipta, mūḍha* and *vikṣipta* states. Hence, his *vṛtti* are far from the field of emancipation. As he indulges in *bhoga-vṛtti,* probably he is unaware of *yoga-vṛtti.* This is Cārvāka's philosophy.

Cārvāka's philosophy came into existence from this *bhoga-vṛtti* which is very common in everyone. Cārvāka does not believe in the concept of virtuous and sinful action as he does not believe in concepts like heaven, hell or emancipation. The concept of God is far from his thoughts as he says that thought is connected with what one sees. God is not perceivable. He recognises the elements *pṛthvī, āp, tej* and *vāyu* and their *tanmātra.* He considers enjoyment as the end aims

---

(. . . . from page 259) *yama niyama āsana prāṇāyāma pratyāhāra dhāraṇā dhyāna samādhayaḥ aṣṭau aṅgāni* (*Y.S.,* II.29) Moral injunctions *(yama),* fixed observances *(niyama),* posture *(āsana),* regulation of breath *(prāṇāyāma),* internalisation of the senses towards their source *(pratyāhāra),* concentration *(dhāraṇā),* meditation *(dhyāna)* and absorption of consciousness in the self *(samādhi),* are the eight constituents of yoga.

of life. He believes, *ṛṇam kṛtvā ghṛtam pibet*. He says, "borrow or steal, but drink ghee (clarified butter) and enjoy". In other words he wants all to enjoy the worldly pleasures at any cost without thinking of their consequences. He was sure that there are no past births and never will there be future births. He did not believe in any scripture or *veda*. He denies even the parents since he says that there is no proof that they are the parents because when we are born, we have no knowledge of who our parents are. To a great extent his philosophy was, 'might is right'.

Probably from the *bhogic* philosophy of Cārvāka, the sages of yore gave a thought for six *darśana* to sprout.

By instinct *citta-bhūmi* knows only *bhoga-vṛtti*. But they do not realise that *pañcakleśa* are based on *bhoga-vṛtti*. Therefore we have to get educated from the above explained components that exist in us. We as *sādhaka* have to practise yoga in order to be free completely or to reduce them to a minimum to feel the quality or the essence of *samādhi (samādhi bhāvanā)*. This is an indication that the practice of *aṣṭāṅga yoga* is the answer to get rid of *pañcakleśa*.

Now let me explain *pañca-vṛtti*.

Pañca-vṛtti

The *vṛtti* are five. These are *pramāṇa, viparyaya, vikalpa, nidrā* and *smṛti*. *Pramāṇa* means correct, valid knowledge. It is right perception. *Pramāṇa* is dependent on three aspects – direct perception, inference and traditional scripts. *Viparyaya* is wrong, perverse or contrary knowledge. *Vikalpa* is fanciful, imaginary, dreamy, indecisive knowledge. *Nidrā* is sleep and *smṛti* is memory. These *vṛtti* are either *kliṣṭa* – painful, difficult to understand, perplexing, and *akliṣṭa* – non-painful, smooth going or un-distressing.

When do we call them *kliṣṭa* or *akliṣṭa-vṛtti?* When the *vṛtti* oppose our achieving a state of restraint, they are *kliṣṭa* and when they are congenial for restraint they are *akliṣṭa*. *Kliṣṭatā* depends upon all those factors mentioned earlier and more upon the afflictions. There is a close relationship between *vṛtti* and *kleśa*.

Let us start with *pramāṇa-vṛtti* – This has three aspects, namely, direct perception, inference and the authoritative sacred scriptures. Now, how many of us have this *pramāṇa-vṛtti?* If we have not exerted ourselves to know the thing correctly and not tried to verify the known or not tried to experience it, will there be the *pramāṇa-vṛtti?* The *pratyakṣa pramāṇa* is the direct experience from intuitive wisdom. Direct perception stands for inner journey towards the source, whereas senses of perception, with their characters of desire, infatuation, anger, greed, pride and envy cannot guide clearly. As they are imperfect, the afflictions remain in a fully activated state *(udāra)*, or interrupted or delicate and dormant state. *Kleśa* or afflictions cause *vṛtti* in the consciousness".

Anumāna is inference which needs a logical brain and earlier experiences. We can easily infer that a river is flooded because somewhere it has rained heavily. We can infer that the sky is clouded so it will rain. Similarly we may infer that whosoever is born will die. But for many this is not easy to accept. So Patañjali explains *abhiniveśa*, saying it is hard even for a wise man to accept death. The zigzag puzzle is, "Do *vṛtti* cause afflictions or afflictions cause *vṛtti?"*

That is why Patañjali wants us to weigh *vṛtti* and *kleśa* carefully and judiciously and in case of doubt, he advises to refer to sacred texts or experienced yogis before inferring.

Viparyaya vṛtti

When *pramāṇa-vṛtti* gets misdirected, the *viparyaya vṛtti* becomes strong. It is erroneous knowledge that has well set in us. *Anitya aśuci duḥkha anātmasu nitya śuci sukha ātma khyātiḥ avidyā* (*Y.S.*, II.5) – mistaking the transient for the permanent, the impure for the pure, pain for pleasure, and that which is not the Self for the Self; all this is called lack of higher knowledge. Lack of interest, lack of zeal, lack of courage and lack in verifying is *viparyaya.* Some don't even see in the right perspective *(tadrūpa)*, but without real understanding *(atadrūpa).* Some believe hearsay as *āpta-vacana*, but do not believe in *āgama-pramāṇa. Āpta* means the one who is close to us, related to us, but it does not mean that he has knowledge *(jñāna).* Even one who is close to us may distort which is nothing but *viparyaya jñāna*, which may further lead to *kleśa-vṛtti.* As such, one has to depend upon scriptures as *āgama-pramāṇa.*

Vikalpa vṛtti

This is another perplexing *vṛtti* like *viparyaya.* In *viparyaya* the object is mistaken whereas in *vikalpa* the object does not exist but depend on words. Hence *vikalpa* is fanciful imagination with no substance. It is like thinking of the objects which do not exist. *Vikalpa* is like daydreaming. Often *vikalpa* may lead to psychological problems as *kliṣṭa-vṛtti.* However it is very useful in the field of literature. Such imaginations do not take us towards spiritual endeavours.

If it is brought to the level of factual knowledge by means of trials and errors, then *vikalpa* could be an *akliṣṭa-vṛtti*, provided it leads towards the transformation that has to occur in the practitioners.

Nidrā-vṛtti

Nidrā is sleep. In sleep there is no thinking, no knowledge and no time. In sleep there is absence of everything around us including ourselves which is felt only after waking up. Sleep is conditioned by *triguṇa*. One who goes to sleep tossing side to side has *rājasic* sleep. Sleeping with tablets is *tāmasic*. Such a sleep makes one low, dull and drowsy. In *sāttvic* sleep, though we have the *abhāva pratyaya*, one feels freshness and joy after waking up.

Abhāva pratyaya in sleep is an important word which has to be thought of. *Abhāva* means absence, and *pratyaya* means device. In sleep, though all our belongings are around us, we lose the feeling of their existence. Only in a wakeful state do we know that they all belong to us *(parigraha)*. Suppose you like a dress or jewellery or a car, in sleep you dream of the same dress or jewellery or car. Then it is not *abhāva pratyaya*. Hiraṇyakashyapu, the demon king started dreaming of Lord Nārāyaṇa all the time since the Lord was his staunch enemy. A common man may worship Lord Nārāyaṇa, yet will not dream of Nārāyaṇa. That is why Patañjali says *citta-prasādana* to develop *sāttvic* nature even in dreams. A disturbed sleep may bring headache or fatigue. Then we search for painkillers. So sleep has its own special character of presenting *abhāva pratyaya* to simulate in the wakeful state.

There was a king who had a beautiful, soft bed. The servant of the king came at night to make the bed ready for the king. To feel the softness of the bed, he kept his head on a pillow and to sleep within a few seconds. The king arrived and woke him up. Now the servant began fearing the punishment the king might order. However the king laughed and the servant was surprised. Then the king asked him to bring a sword and tied it with a loose thread and asked the servant to sleep on that bed. He refused because he knew that the sharp sword could fall on his body at any moment. This story is the expression of one's real state.

Saint Tukārāma says, "Day and night we have to face the incident of battle. What is this battle? The six enemies of ours, desire, anger, greed, infatuation, pride and jealousy do not allow us to remain quiet and get good sleep".

What we experience in sleep, if it is simulated in wakeful state, it is *samādhi*.

Smṛti-vṛtti

Lastly, Patañjali refers to *smṛti-vṛtti* at the end. *Smṛti-vṛtti* is essential. Normally the unwanted memory surfaces quickly and useful memory vanishes. *Smṛti* or memory stores only those facts which have been read, seen, heard, inferred, perceived or experienced. Memory does not steal anything to store in it. Even if it is a verbal knowledge it remains in memory without any additional expressions. If we add something to memory then it is a manipulation of memory. *Smṛti* or memory stores the imprints of other *vṛtti* and acts as a fountain for other *vṛtti*. Therefore the *sādhaka* has to store *akliṣṭa-vṛtti* in *smṛti* and keep out *kliṣṭa-vṛtti* to make progression in *sādhanā*. *Kliṣṭa karma* or *vṛtti* becomes *kleśa saṁskāra* and one is born with these afflicted based actions.[1] That is why the *Sādhana Pāda* begins with *kleśa tanūkaraṇam* through *yogāṅgānuṣṭhānam* to experience *samādhi*. Practice of *aṣṭāṅga yoga* vigorously, carefully, consciously, uninterruptedly, continuously, zealously without questioning cleanses the *vṛtti* to reach *kleśa-karma-nivṛtti* and through that *citta-vṛtti nirodha* happens where the *mala* of *kliṣṭa – navrāntarāya* (nine obstacles) –[2] *vṛtti* are eradicated in totality.

Aṣṭāṅga yogāgni

You all know the eight aspects of yoga, *yama, niyama, āsana, prāṇāyāma, pratyāhāra, dhāraṇā, dhyāna* and *samādhi*. I am not going to deal in detail.[3] However, the eight aspects or petals are explained basically for the attenuation of *kleśa*. *Aṣṭāṅga yoga* brings good *saṁskāra* on *citta*. To be more precise the *aṣṭāṅga yoga* transforms the *saṁskāra* on all the components of man as we have gone through so far. By practising *āsana* regularly, one's circulation and digestion improve, the skin glows lustrously. These are external changes. But the internal and innermost changes are also there and they bring control from *bhūta* to *jīvātmā* (mortal self) leading to experience the Immortal Self.

Yama and *niyama* are meant to bring clarity in action and thinking. Though it is structured in the format of principles, these are not principles or ideologies, but they are meant to correct our behaviour and build up our character. They give us power to discriminate between *bhoga-vṛtti* and *yoga-vṛtti*. In order to get rid of *bhoga-vṛtti* the fire of yoga *(yogāgni)* has to be lit first through *yama* and *niyama*.

Actually, the aspects of yoga are like fire *(yogāgni)*. *Āsanāgni* burns out the dualities of body, mind, senses, *ahaṁkāra-vṛtti* and *buddhi-vṛtti*. *Prāṇāgni* cleanses the *pañcabhūta* and *pañcaprāṇa* by burning their impurities through *prāṇāyāma*. *Agni* of *pratyāhāra* burns the *bhoga-vṛtti* of senses and mind as well as *kliṣṭa-vṛtti*. Finally, *dhāraṇāgni, dhyānāgni* and *samādhyāgni*

---

[1] *kleśamūlaḥ karmāśayaḥ dṛṣta adṛṣta janma vedanīyaḥ* (*Y.S.*, II.12) – The accumulated imprints of past lives, rooted in afflictions, will be experienced in present and future lives.

[2] *vyādhi styāna saṁśaya pramāda ālasya avirati bhrāntidarśana alabdhabhūmikatva anavasthitatvāni cittavikṣepaḥ te antarāyāḥ* (*Y.S.*, I.30) – These obstacles are disease, inertia, doubt, heedlessness, laziness, indiscipline of the senses, erroneous views, lack of perseverance, and backsliding.
duḥkha daurmanasya aṅgame)jayatva śvāsapraśvāsāḥ vikṣepa sahabhuvaḥ (*Y.S.*, I.31) – Sorrow, despair, unsteadiness of the body and irregular breathing further distract the *citta*.

[3] See *Aṣṭadaḷa Yogamālā*, vol. 2.

burn out the impurities of *akliṣṭa-vṛtti* as Patañjali says that there are possibilities of *kliṣṭa-vṛtti* hiding in *akliṣṭa-vṛtti.* Often people are under the impression that *yogābhyāsa* is not to be found in *āsana* and *prāṇāyāma.* They think *dhyāna* is the true yoga. But unless *yama* and *niyama* are followed, the other aspects of yoga are of no value.

Here, I want to remind you all as *sādhaka,* that we are born with *śūdra tejas, vaiśya tejas, kṣātra tejas* and *brāhma-tejas.* These are called *varṇa. Varṇa* means colour. Colour itself is *tejas.* According to *tejas,* we have to ignite that fire to follow yoga as *anuṣṭhāna* (dedicated and devoted *sādhanā*). All of us have to start from *śūdra tejas* first. One has to laboriously practise with 100% perspiration. Then the *śūdra tejas* changes into *vaiśya tejas.* After labour work, sensitivity develops to bring balance between action (labour work) and sensitivity. This helps one to move towards *kṣātra tejas,* which shines lustrously. In the first three, the *tejas* get ignited gradually to burn the impurities *(aśuddhikṣaya)* and finally the knowledge of *brahma-tejas* shines *(jñānadīpti).* Undoubtedly, one has to start by striking a match to ignite fire. Then intensify the *sādhanā* as fuel for the fire in you to blaze to savour the *ātman.*

So our effort should be to practise the eight petals of yoga religiously on three tiers, three levels, namely, *tapas, svādhyāya* and *Īśvara praṇidhāna.* The word *kriyā* indicates laboured efforts or factual practice which is a journey from *śūdra tejas* to *brāhma-tejas.*

Tapas and *svādhyāya* lead us from *śūdra tejas* to *kṣātra-tejas* and finally with *Īśvara praṇidhāna* towards *brāhma-tejas.* This will lead one towards the attenuation of afflictions and to get the feel of *samādhi.* In *Samādhi pāda* he uses the word *samādhi prajñā.*[1] This is the step to *samādhi bhāvanā.* Again he says in the same *pāda* that through *Īśvara praṇidhāna* you get *samādhi siddhi.*[2]

Finally, in *dharmamegha samādhi* the *akliṣṭa-vṛtti* are also destroyed. The clouds of virtue pour like a rainfall and the disk of *citta* becomes clear.

Practice of the eight aspects of yoga removes all afflictions. When *kleśa-nivṛtti* (cessation of *kleśa)* comes to an end, then only *dharmamegha samādhi*[3] flashes like torrential rains.

---

1 *śraddhā vīrya smṛti samādhiprajñā pūrvakaḥ itareṣām* (*Y.S.,* I.20)

2 *samādhisiddhiḥ Īśvarapraṇidhānāt* (*Y.S.,* II.45)

3 *prasaṁkhyāne api akusīdasya sarvathā vivekakhyāteḥ dharmameghaḥ samādhiḥ* (*Y.S.,* IV.29) – the yogi who has no interest even in this highest state of evolution, and maintains supreme attentive, discriminative awareness, attains *dharmameghaḥ samādhi:* he contemplates the fragrance of virtue and justice.
tataḥ kleśa karma nivṛttiḥ (*Y.S.,* IV.30) – then comes the end of afflictions and of *karma.*

Thus *yoga sādhanā* begins from *kleśa tanūkaraṇa* and *vṛtti śodhana* (cleansing). Then *kliṣṭa-vṛtti* becomes *akliṣṭa-vṛtti*. Then *akliṣṭa-vṛtti* vanishes with *dharmamegha samādhi*. The *pratiprasava* of the *guṇa* takes place at this stage.

This elaborate explanation is meant for the purpose of cleansing *navāntarāya*, *pañcakleśa*, *pañca-vṛtti*, so that *citta* reaches a state untouched by all these obstacles for the spiritual journey to end the journey from *vṛtti nirodha* to *kleśa-karma-nivṛtti*.

When this journey ends, then there are no more *kleśa karma* and no more *kliṣṭa* and *akliṣṭa-vṛtti*.

Then *pañcabhūta* with *tanmātra*, organs of action, senses of perception, mind, intelligence and consciousness dissolve in *prakṛti* and *puruṣa* – the *citi* or the *ātman*, establishes itself in its own splendour and glory.

Thus the path of *aṣṭāṅga yoga* takes the *sādhaka* journeying from *citta-vṛtti* towards the end of the journey namely, *citi śakti*, or the power of the Soul.

KEYNOTE ADDRESS*

Dear friends, students and lovers of Yoga,

I am grateful to all of you who have gathered here to hear me. I am not a speaker but a *sādhaka*, and as a *sādhaka* I love to involve myself with your practices as you are *sādhaka*. As such I would like to share with you for the first time how my yogic journey progressively began from the periphery of the body to realise the distinction between the consciousness *(dṛśya)*, the seen, and the seer *(draṣṭā)*, kindling the spiritual light in my life. Hence I request you to listen patiently and I hope that my words will be of a great value in your practices for good.

I may repeat some of the things which I might have said on several occasions, as I have been in the public eye for more than seven decades. I request you to excuse and pardon me for any repetitions.

As a *sādhaka* I believe in practice and as a teacher I like to share my experiences with you all. Today, I am standing in front of you to inspire you to work as I worked with an inquisitive, enquiring mind to discover and rediscover this finite, yet immeasurable inner body through yoga. I request you, if possible, to proceed from my present search and discerning further to discover this mysterious body and its caretaker – the Self.

A religious devout disposition should be the prerequisite for a *sādhaka*. As a practitioner and a teacher, I have lived with precepts of yoga in my practice in totality. If I was a preacher I might preach with precepts but I may not follow as an obligation with dedication and devotion. As a teacher, I have to live as an ideal example by practising daily in front of you to see that I follow of what I say. This religiousness is needed by a pupil as well as by a teacher.

I have been living in yoga for more than seventy years and I say with a clear conscience that I never felt monotonous or bored even once in my practices. My practices alone acted as

---

* On the ocassion of the 10th Anniversary of Yoga Journal being held in Estes Park, Colorado,USA, September 2005.

a guiding star in educating me to find faults and then to re-charge each day with further intense efforts and these re-cultured and fresh efforts went on civilising my mind and intelligence to be in contact with the caretaker of my body, the Core of my Being. This reflective state of observation and re-valuation in my practices has not faded in me even to this day.

By the grace of yoga and God I keep my head, heart and self ever open to watch the various functional changes and subtle actions that happen in my *sādhanā*. Due to my attentive dedicated practice I began interchanging the functions, processes and gravitational changes in different *āsana* which made me grasp and absorb all the subtle changes in them which I combed all together to fit them into each and every *āsana*.

At the beginning of my *sādhanā*, my understanding moved at a snail's speed as I was not able to penetrate my mind due to want of understanding beyond my muscles and joints. After years of continuous *sādhanā*, I began to develop the sharpness in my observation to interpenetrate my mind by bringing the attention beyond the muscles and joints.

My first visit to the United States was in 1956, about fifty years back. At that time, very little was known about yoga and people were fond of enjoying the worldly pleasures through the three famous "Ws", - wealth, wine and women. With their materialistic richness, their approach to the disciplinary path of yogic life was not attractive to them.

During that visit to the States, I was taken aback to see the way of life here in contrast to that of my country. This made me think whether to come again or not. But destiny disposed and I came here again after a gap of seventeen years, that is, in 1973 when some members who came to my hometown to learn tempted me to re-visit to see the change.

No doubt I confess that I had to change my views as I saw much interest shown in yoga by a good number of members.

If I look back from 1973 to this day, I am delighted and proud to see that such a transformation in yoga has taken place in this country and I am happy to see the enthusiasm and will to delve into the depth of physical as well as spiritual values of yoga in your lives. It is for me a wonder of wonders that you have accepted this "yoga" as if it is in your genes.

This unbelievable love and affection to yoga that has taken place here, goes to your credit and merit though to some extent I may share these with you. Though I sowed the seed of yoga and nurtured it by my regular visits, I give all credit and merit of its popularity to you all who devotedly dedicated your time and energy to learn and transmit this yoga by going to the doorsteps of your brothers and sisters. Though this subject of yoga is becoming popular day by day, I want to advise you to keep an eagle eye on the new students and teachers so that they do not distort and give new colours to the subject. If the purity of the subject is divided with twists and turns, then it may get misguided and polluted and the future practitioners may lose the right essence of it to savour. No doubt, both of us made this yoga popular, but it is now your responsibility to see that you all maintain its pristine purity in the future also. Having said so much about the success and its popularity in your country, I express my heartfelt gratitude to all of you for your affection towards me.

Now I would like to take this opportunity in telling you of my early efforts in the field of yoga to understand the leap I made in this art, which may help you in cultivating and mastering the wisdom of yoga. No doubt, yoga was forced on me by destiny, as it was not my choice.

I was born in a remote backward village, in Bellur, about 60 kms. from Bangalore towards Chennai in Karnataka state, South India. I owe a lot to my parents who gave me birth and life as at that time my mother was afflicted by a worldwide Influenza epidemic and destiny made both of us survive.

Not only was I born with ill health but bouts of diseases one after the other like malaria, typhoid and tuberculosis sapped my life further and made me live a parasitic life. May be, these illnesses came to me as an unknown blessing to embrace yoga at the age of fourteen.

It is just a coincidence that my elder sister got married to Yogacharya Tirumalai Krishnamacharya in 1926. It took seven years for him to advise me to do yoga to gain health, though he knew that I was afflicted with bouts of diseases. Meanwhile he had initiated my younger sister and elder brother. My sister could not pursue as she got married and my elder brother left because of my brother-in-law's rigorous discipline imposed upon him. It was in 1934, the Maharaja of Mysore deputed my brother-in-law to propagate yoga in North Karnataka and to pay a visit to Kaivalyadhama at Lonavla, near Pune.

On his way from Mysore, he broke his journey at Bangalore and as it was summer holidays for schools, he asked me to be with my sister in these holidays till he returned from his tour.

The stay was meant for a few weeks. At once I agreed to proceed to Mysore as it was famous for palaces and lush gardens which was like a fantasy to me and my mind.

After his return from the tour I wanted to return to Bangalore. But he asked me to stay and join the school in Mysore to continue my studies and to learn *āsana* so that I might see the dawn of health in my life.

The word "health" charged me with enthusiasm and I stayed to learn the *āsana* as well as to pursue my studies.

On one auspicious day he called me and taught me to do a few *āsana*. When I bent forwards my middle fingers could not reach my knees. Probably this unbelievable stiffness made him indifferent towards me saying, "Do them daily". He left me alone to do what he had taught. As he initiated me into *āsana*, I considered him as my *guru* and as such he remains as my *guru* in my life.

Let me tell you of the turning point in my life to become a yoga practitioner. It so happened that one of his favourite pupils, Shri Keshavamurthy, who was staying as my companion with *Gurují* left the house without telling anyone, never to return. *Gurují* tried his best to trace him but he could not find him. This made him turn his attention on me and showed his seriousness in teaching me again.

My *guru* was known for his stern discipline. On account of this, gradually a fear complex grew in me. Having lost his best pupil, he took personal interest in me and forced me to do all the different and difficult *āsana* in a week's time and made me do them in public as his lectures were arranged every now and then.

Knowingly or unknowingly, this turned out to be a turning point for life.

In 1936, the Maharaja of Mysore deputed him again to visit Northern Karnataka to propagate yoga. As my studies came to an end, he took me with his senior pupils on tour. On this tour he gave me chances to conduct classes for women. Probably he wanted to sow the seed in me to become a teacher later on.

In 1937, on request by the authorities of the Deccan Gymkhana Club in Pune, my *Gurují* sent me to teach in the sports clubs and educational Institutions of Pune for a period of six months. But destiny made Pune my home.

This responsibility made me become more sincere in practice. So I began practising advertently for long hours each day to gain confidence in *āsana* for me to teach well. Actually I was practising ten hours a day independently as well as conducting classes explaining and showing first and then joining in with them.

In 1943, I got married to Ramāmaṇi. God blessed me with a true partner not only in my life but also to progress in my *sādhanā*. As I had no colleagues to see my shortcomings in my *āsana* practice, I began teaching *āsana* to my wife to give her the feel of the subject. Then I helped her through adjustments on her body in the *āsana* so that she got accustomed as to how, where, when and why to touch to learn and understand the flow of the skin and flesh in each *āsana*. Then I made her see my practices and showed her how to look at each part of the body in each *āsana* by guiding her ways as well as means of applying pressures and counter pressures to adjust my body wherever I needed corrections and rectifications.

My wife willingly began obliging me at any time I needed her help. Whenever I needed her help, she used to leave her household chores halfway to help me in my *āsana* practice which was not coming up to my expectations.

Her interest in me to master the art encouraged me to strive further and further to reach the needed alignment of the body with my mind, intelligence and consciousness. My guide lines for her to help me made me reach the state of stability and serenity in the *āsana* by right useage of pressures.

If I owed my life to my parents, my guru encouraged me to choose an aim in life, whereas my wife's involvement and encouragement made me reach a finer state of firmness in *āsana*.

As I was teaching I could notice the good and the bad points of the students which helped me with ideas not only to better myself but to impart new thoughts to my students in my teaching.

This observation of various bodies gave me time to understand the structure of the body, its function and constitution.

This way providence provided me with wonderful circumstances at the right time and helped me to mould and blend myself to penetrate the five layers of my being from *annamaya* to *prāṇamaya, manomaya, vijñānamaya* and *ānandamaya*. I perceptively inter-related with concrete ideas through intricacies of each *āsana* which transformed me to develop qualitative intelligence from a raw beginner to reach a ripe studentship and also made me become a conscientious teacher.

No doubt it was a mere chance that I became a follower of yoga; but I had to change the chance into choice in becoming a true pupil and a good teacher.

People who came to learn with different occupational hazards with different body structures awakened my intelligence and opened my eyes to look at them carefully and made me learn how to align their bones, muscles, joints, ligaments, fibres, tendons and so forth to bring uniformity in their frame of bodies in each *āsana*. As I came to know that the body is made of five elements of nature, earth, water, fire, air and ether, I had to understand their functions while I was practising on myself.

Lord Krishna's definition of yoga as "equanimity, harmony, balance, skilful adjustment" acted on my thoughts as a guiding star throughout my *sādhanā*. I began to introduce these qualities which came in my researches and began teaching which guided me to understand the needed anatomical adjustments and the physiological functioning of their bodies in each *āsana*.

This was the first progressive step that came to me in my *yoga sādhanā* as a teacher learner.

Though my *guru* was soft to his other students, he was strict with me at the time of his tutelage which made me follow him blindly without questioning him. I did ask him on occasions to guide me on the views of this great science but his answer was, "Do what I say and do not ask any further". Probably he must have thought that I was incapable of understanding this sophisticated philosophy or I may not have been up to his expectations.

Yet he sent me hundreds of kilometres away to teach. I began to read books on *āsana* to get some ideas on the subject. The word that attracted me was the meaning of yoga – 'union'. This word made a strong impression on my *sādhanā* to associate the organs of action and senses of perception together in order to connect them to the mind as these are cognisable to one and all.

The second progressive education began with this idea of connecting action and perception for the mind to conceive.

From this point, I worked to subordinate the action of *āsana* to the senses of perception as well as the mind.

Then I was lifted to the third state of progression to work on the subtle elements, namely, the intelligence and consciousness which remained dormant in me for years as my growth of intellect was far far below an average intellect.

In order to sublimate the senses of perception and mind, I had to understand what is intellect and what is intelligence and their transformations into wisdom. I learnt through watching that the intellect of the head fluctuates and oscillates while the intelligence of the inner heart, as wisdom, does not. I also had to watch these fluctuations to understand this in order to arrest the fluctuations of the intellect as well as to cultivate emotional stability, which is essentially needed in the *sādhanā*.

The *sūtra* I.17[1] and 33[2] helped me a lot in understanding the differences between intellect and intelligence and the relationship between the emotions of the heart and the intellect of the head.

Here I learnt how Patañjali divides the biological divisions according to the functioning of the four lobes of the brain into intellectual divisions – the seat of analysis, synthesis, contentment of bliss, and the seat of 'I'-ness, and the four chambers of the heart into emotional divisions like friendliness, compassion, gladness, and indifference towards effects. I had to think and act consciously and intentionally in associating the intellect of the head *(vitarka* – analysis, *vicāra* – synthesis, *ānanda* – bliss and *asmitā* – 'I'-ness), with the emotional intelligence of the heart, *(maitrī* – friendliness, *karuṇā* – compassion, *muditā* – gladness, and *upekṣā* – indifference towards the opposites of cold and heat, honour and dishonour, good and evil) to understand the values of yoga distinctly.

I realised in yogic *sādhanā* that the intellect of the head and the intelligence of the heart play a great role as they interfere both in thinking and acting. If the emotional upheavals are likely to influence cardiac diseases, the pressure on the brain leads to high blood pressure and so forth. In order to maintain the health in the intelligence of the heart, we need to follow *maitrī, karuṇā, muditā* and *upekṣā.* Similarly, in order to maintain health in the seat of the head, *vitarka, vicāra, ānanda* and *asmitā* have to co-ordinate and co-operate with each other. Then you as the practitioners progress intellectually and emotionally and balance these four petals of the head with the four petals of the heart for a balanced living. Actually, this association with co-ordination is the key to the majestic way in the art of living.

1 *vitarka vicāra ānanda asmitārūpa anugamāt saṁprajñātaḥ* (I.17) – practice and detachment develop four types of *samādhi*: self-analysis, synthesis, bliss and the experience of pure being.

2 *maitrī karuṇā muditā upekṣāṇāṁ sukha duḥkha puṇya apuṇya viṣayāṇāṁ bhāvanātaḥ cittaprasādanam* (I.33) – through cultivation of friendliness, compassion, joy and indifference to pleasure and pain, virtue and vice respectively, the consciousness becomes favourably disposed, serene and benevolent.

If the chambers of the brain represent the personal self, the chambers of the heart express the impersonal or universal Self.

From here, I was guided from within towards the fourth state of understanding the value of yoga.

I realised that the seed of all knowledge is the seer or the Self. This seed of knowledge sprouts and branches into two parts as consciousness and energy. If the movement of awareness is consciousness, the flow of life force is energy which the scientists call bio-energy.

After understanding the distinction between the intellect of the head and the intelligence of the heart, I thought of redefining my practices by bringing conjunction between the intellect and the intelligence. Hence, I began to do *āsana* using head and heart simultaneously in my practices.

Here, you may like to know the difference between the intellect of the head and the intelligence of the heart. Acquired knowledge is the intellect of the head and experiential knowledge is the intelligence of the heart. Experiential wisdom does not change but remains one *(eka)*. Head accumulates knowledge and heart filters that acquired and accumulated knowledge to experiment with pros and cons till one reaches a matured state of experience where a truth-bearing state of direct spiritual perception dawns *(ṛtaṁbharā tatra prajñā – Y.S.,* I.48). This way, I began to bring the intellect of the head to co-operate with the intelligence of the heart in my practice of *āsana* so that the head and the heart associate together and unite as single intelligence.

To bring this association and union, I had to study not only the elements of nature and their counterparts (sound, touch, form, taste and odour) but also energy with its divisional functions. Observing this close connection between the elements, awareness and energy, I began re-learning the *āsana* to bring unison between the elements, intellectual awareness and flow of energy. This opened my intellectual eye to feel the extension of intelligence through inner contact and expansion of consciousness with vibration in the body. This made me experience the revolving movement of energy and awareness while going into the *āsana*, staying, and coming out of it.

This attention of connecting awareness and energy helped me to learn each *āsana* in such a way that I could feel the reflection of each *āsana* on the mirrors of my senses of perception, mind, and intelligence re-reflecting on my body without any refraction. Similarly I made my body the mirror and intelligence as a reflector mirror for it to re-reflect on my core without distortions.

From here I moved towards self-education as the fifth step of the ladder of yogic knowledge and understanding.

We are made of five elements, namely, earth, water, fire, air and ether. To understand the function of the last two subtlest elements, I had to reintroduce the subtle form of practice for my intelligence to interweave in order to reach the remotest space in the body.

For this, I had to go back to study and understand health in its wholesomeness which needed total attention and awareness.

This thought of attention and awareness drew me to different dimensions of health, namely, physical health, moral health, mental health, energy health, intellectual health, conscientious health and divine health. If all these various dimensions of health have to work in unison and concord, it needed holistic attention and awareness of the intellect of the head and the intelligence of the inner or spiritual heart.

Actually health is nothing but awareness of life's force. As the river flows forward, life's energy too has only forward movements. As such the various facets of health follow the flow of life's energy. It is like a live wire. If one touches the live wire, one gets a shock or suffer burns. Similarly, the awareness of health at once has to prick the intelligence if something within the body gets disturbed. This disturbance in health means disturbance in consciousness.

In order to bring this unison between intelligence and consciousness, I began to remodel the techniques of *āsana* and *prāṇāyāma* to feel the attention and awareness concurrently moving with motion, action, observation, reflection and absorption in each *āsana* along with the breath to grasp the functioning of the consciousness and energy in this human body. This human body has five sheaths which are interrelated as anatomical, physiological or organic, mental, intellectual and the immeasurable space within – space of cosmic bliss.

Consciousness being the gateway to enter the core of the Being (the capital SELF), I peeped into the states of consciousness.

Though consciousness is one, it has seven states of functioning. They are emerging consciousness, restraining consciousness, tranquil consciousness, indivisible attentive consciousness, *sāttvic* "I" consciousness, split consciousness and crystal pure consciousness.

Though Patañjali explains yoga as the restraint of consciousness, see how difficult it is to bring these various facets of consciousness under control.

For me consciousness is like a carry bag with different contents in different packets.

It carries five fluctuations, five afflictions which may be physical, moral, mental, intellectual and spiritual. It also carries disturbing and distracting problems like disease, lack of interest, indecision, overlooking things, idleness, incontinence, illusive notions, disappointments, inability to pursue, aggravating further with distress, dejection, laboured breathing and tremors of the body. These disturbing factors may be in dormant, attenuating, alternating or fully active states.

So far I gave you thoughts on destructive contents. Let me take you to the other side of the consciousness which carries components to uplift the practitioner from nescience or want of knowledge towards the crown of knowledge and wisdom to experience the eternal cosmic bliss. These constructive suggestions are to remain quiet after exhalation, contemplation on a luminous effulgent light, to live undisturbed either in dreamy, sleepy or wakeful states or to concentrate on a thing conducive to the heart.

Defining the bad parts and good parts of the consciousness, I had to go back to my earlier thoughts regarding the intellect of the head and intelligence of the heart.

I had to communicate the facets of the head, namely, analysis, insight, elation, experiencing state of existence with the facets of the heart, which are friendliness, compassion, gladness and selfless living. I had to connect and commune these various compartments of the head and the heart through trust, physical power, mental power, intellectual will and memory as a means to repose consciousness for it to move closer towards the Self and God.

As a river with its tributaries joins the sea, I would like to take your consciousness with its tributaries to mingle and unite with the sea of the Self.

Patañjali begins his teachings with the path of surrender - (*bhakti mārga*) through devotion on God (*Īśvara Praṇidhāna*).

Knowing that the *bhakti mārga* (the path of devotion) is not possible to each and everyone, he takes us and proceeds towards the path of action (*karma mārga*) through *yama* and *niyama*, path of knowledge (*jñāna mārga*) through *āsana*, *prāṇāyāma*, *pratyāhāra* and *dhāraṇā* and ends up in *bhakti* in the form of *dhyāna*. From this, one can conclude that *aṣṭāṅga yoga* or the eight petals of yoga cover action, knowledge and surrender of oneself to the supreme soul - God.

Thus, this *aṣṭāṅga* yoga develops the practitioners with perfect action mingled with mature intelligence which in turn brings humbleness in the practitioners to see all evenly and treat all equally.

For this, he takes us to know nature's power existing in each human being in the form of five elements and their atomic qualities, organs of action, senses of perception, mind, intelligence, consciousness, cosmic intelligence with the nature's qualities namely illumination, vibration, inertia and then the soul and God or cosmic force.

He guides us to use these components of nature in conjunction with the Self to understand nature and then pacify nature so that the *atman* or the Self rests and dwells in its own abode.

The Self is stainless and choiceless. The Self being the perceiver, *aṣṭāṅga yoga* as an instrument helps the practitioner, who as a seeker, reaches ripeness in practice and sights the seer – the Self which was daunting as an object.

The principle of yoga is meant to remove that letter 'K' which is like a thick intellectual cloud abiding in between the see'k'er and the seer. When this intellectual cloud 'K' is removed, then the see'k'er is transformed into a seer. This is how yoga practices took me towards the culminating end – the Light of the Self.

Patañjali terms *sva* as individual *śakti* or self engulfed within body, and *svāmi* the *(puruṣa)*, as the Lord of the body. Lord Krishna – the Lord of yoga (*yogeshvara*), concurs with the thoughts of Patañjali and says in the 13th chapter of the *Bhagavad Gītā* that the Seer or the Self is the fielder or farmer (*kṣetrajña*) and body, the field (*kṣetra*). Sri Krishna explains the discrimination between the field – the body, and the knower of the body – the fielder as the Self, and shows how these two get wedded together through yoga.

As the fielder ploughs and removes weeds, sows the best of seeds and nourishes to get the best produce, Patañjali has given us the aspects of *āsana* to plough the field – the body to remove the unwanted desires like weeds which grow in it disturbing the tranquil state of consciousness. When the body is well ploughed, then the seer residing within this field – the body, yields the fruit of emancipation and eternal bliss.

God is *viśva cetana śakti* and cosmic energy is the *viśva caitanya śakti* or the universal source of life energy. Cosmic energy inspires the aspirations of nature as well as the seer.

Hence, I began to understand the importance of conjunction of energy with consciousness in my practice of *āsana* and *prāṇāyāma* which led me slowly towards the Light on Life.

This is the sixth progressive lead that yoga gave me.

Cosmic life force is the breath of all life. This cosmic breath divides and subdivides into five main and five subordinate energies.

While practising *āsana* and *prāṇāyāma*, I have to co-ordinate these ten energies with various facets of body and consciousness as a meeting point so that gladness, harmony, balance and concord are maintained with parity between the body, mind and Self.

Many *Upaniṣad* express that energy and consciousness are wedded together and diminish together. If one fades, the other also fades. If fullness is maintained in one, then the other also remains full.

With these new impressions I was lifted to the seventh stage of knowledge.

This twinness of energy and consciousness made me study the characteristics of *āsana* and began characterising the *āsana* through refinement and reach the state of singleness between intelligence and consciousness in each *āsana*. For this I had to make successive sequential changes in my practices to observe the distinctive differences by arranging and re-arranging the *āsana* in conjunction with energy, intelligence and consciousness to get the single state of oneness between the field – body, and its fielder – the Self.

I mentioned seven stages that I underwent to progress in my *sādhanā*. Patañjali in *Yoga Sūtra* II.27[1] says that through uninterrupted flow of discriminative awareness, one gains perfect knowledge which is of seven states. I have earned and I have integrated these seven states of awareness which started from my body, the senses, the breath, the mind, the intellect, the intelligence, the consciousness to experience the last state, that is, the Self or the Soul.

I can tell you with joy that I began my practice perspiring from the body to align its muscles and joints. From this gross perspiring state, I gradually proceeded through intellectual sweating along with the inspiration of the consciousness to align energy flow with the intuitive eye of the Self embracing the remotest parts of its frontier – the body from the skin to the Self and from the Self to the skin as a single unit.

---

1 *tasya saptadhā prāntabhūmiḥ prajñā* (II.27) – Through this unbroken flow of discriminative awareness, one gains perfect knowledge which has seven spheres.

Now my practices are directly dictated by the core – the seed of knowledge and understanding and not through the mind, intelligence or consciousness as it used to be earlier.

This right understanding of conjunction took me to the gates of that illuminating timeless eternal power – the Self.

After hearing from me these various states of intellectual ascension that took place in me and in my practices, I hope you can rightly guess of what quality the *sādhaka* should be and what type of *sādhanā* is needed to reach this level.

Patañjali categorises the practitioners into vehement, ardent, moderate and mild classes. Svātmārāma too categorises as conative practitioners, cognitive practitioners, intimate and consuming practitioners. *Śiva Saṁhitā* also distinguishes the practitioners as feeble, moderate, keen and supremely enthusiastic.[1] By these various classifications in practitioners, you can calculate that the span of time varies according to the efforts to reach the ultimate goal. If one is highly intelligent, then practice of *āsana* influences the intelligence to be efficacious. I am again emphasising on the importance of *āsana* and *prāṇāyāma* as these two are the only means to plough, eradicate desires, and irrigate the body to make it fertile to taste the effect of the efforts in integrating the consciousness and energy with the sea of the soul.

Similarly, you have to recharge the battery of energy to be of that high level through the practice of *prāṇāyāma* to receive that light of knowledge and wisdom that flashes at the ripe time as you ripen in memory and intelligence. These flashes of wisdom may come through sight or through vibrational feelings in the form of sound.

Thus my practice of yoga began from the grossest level and moved further in penetrating the finest infinitesimally small cells of the body for the Self to feel its presence before their birth and death. *Paramāṇu paramamahattvāntaḥ asya vaśīkāraḥ* (*Y.S.,* I.40). It means by the best practice of *āsana* and *prāṇāyāma,* the *sādhaka* can extend his intelligence from the grossest parts of the body to reach the finest of the finest particles, i.e., in today's knowledge – the cellular system. This helped me in harmonising the body mechanism and led me to pacify the power of nature.

From this I learnt the reason why so many *āsana* were invented and discovered for the yoga practitioners to practise so that each ingredient of the body lives in the stream of virtuous

---

[1] "Know that aspirants are of four orders: feeble *(mṛdu),* moderate *(madhyama),* ardent *(adhimātra)* and the most ardent *(adhimātratma)*" (*Śiva Saṁhitā,* V.10)

wisdom devoid of desires and ambitions; devoid of qualities of nature in order to live and lead a radiant life with freedom, beatitude and benevolence. This is the true essence of the Light of Yoga on Life's Light.

I devoted all my time on *āsana* for one reason as we have examples of great people of the past who reached the pinnacle of life by following one of the yogic principles like non-violence, truthfulness and so forth. Yogi Yājñyavalkya reached the zenith through *prāṇāyāma*. I used my energy and intelligence to find out the greatness of each *āsana*.

I took the clue from Patañjali wherein he says "one may attain an exalted state of consciousness by becoming totally engrossed, with dedication and devotion in his object of interest" (*Y.S.*, I.35). *Āsana* being my subject as well as object of interest, this aphorism stuck to my heart and I practised them uninterruptedly to reach parity in body, intelligence and Self.

Often the practitioners practise within the frame of their minds. But I went beyond this frame of mind. I interpenetrated in interweaving the life force with the body to the Self. As I had to give hundreds and hundreds of lectures / demonstrations (solo), I had to cultivate extroversion and the skill of exhibitionism and explicitness which might have been the reason for my yogic colleagues to misunderstand and misread my *sādhanā* and measure it on the physical level.

When I am in my practice – doing alone – I am not only totally an introvert but keep myself in the *sāttvic* state. Also I cannot practise *āsana* and *prāṇāyāma* with totality, without the other components of yoga being implicitly involved in my *āsana* and *prāṇāyāma sādhanā*. Without conjoining all the components of yoga, it is impossible to do *āsana* independently and distinctly as a unit of its own. *Āsana* is an integral part of the whole of yogic discipline. It only acted as an avenue for me directing me in the journey of yoga to experience the wholesomeness and glory of it.

Probably my *Gurujī* might have specifically initiated me to *āsana* to find out the subtlest of the subtle effects in them. I worked to find out the ultimate points in each *āsana* as far as my intellectual capacity carried and I am happy to say that I have fulfilled his dream by reaching the end of my journey in *āsana* with spiritual contentment wherein I differentiated between consciousness and the core of the being and now I do the *āsana* from the intelligence of the Self and not with the intelligence of the consciousness.

The see'k'er in me has disappeared long ago and only the seer in me dissects my practices.

As I practise *āsana* daily with a religious sense, many are under the illusion that I am still a see'k'er. Please note that I practise them daily because *āsana* uplifted me to this level and if I stop them, my conscience pricks me. Secondly, if I say that I have savoured the flavour of yoga, you may brand me as an arrogant yogi and in humility, if I say no, then my critics will be jubilant to say that I am still at the physical level, but my conscience knows the truth. Therefore, I follow the dictum of "silence". Hence let me advise you to practise without arrogance but with innocence in your head and heart.

As you all need to have information on the subject to begin practice, I have explained the ways of searching, removing the errors by discretion and to feel repose and tranquillity so that you live in the lustre of brilliance of that real Self as I live now.

I thank you all once again for your patience in listening to my harsh and rough voice and ask for your forgiveness.

Please take note of the best part of my address and unlock the yogic lock and dress it devotedly with discernment by the key of yogic wisdom so that the energy and wisdom flow perennially in each cell of your body, mind and intelligence and lead you to live blissfully as I am living in the spiritual empire.

May Patañjali's blessings be upon you all and once again I thank you.

ŚRĪ YOGA VIDYĀ YANTRA

WHAT IS A *YANTRA?*

YANTRA

Yantra means an instrument for holding, restraining or fastening anything in a specific way, a prop to function properly. *Yantra* is also a sort of plate or birch leaf on which the names of certain deities are written, worshipped and tied to the upper arm for the removal of demonic influences. It is like an ornament, a charm and a diagram of mystical nature or astrological character and then used as an amulet. It is a *digbandha,* which means binding or fettering the points of the compass by *mantra* to keep off all evils. Hence, *yantra* is treated as a secret *(guhya)* and sacred symbol. A machine is also called a *yantra.* It corresponds quite well to the multiple meanings of the English word device, which can be an instrument, a means, or a heraldic device bearing a symbolic diagram.

TANTRA

Tantra means a thread, a string, a leading principal action of a ceremony. It also means regular characteristic order of ceremonies, rites, a rule, a system and formalities. A *tantra* has a technical methodology for removing the problems or obstacles which come in one's way. Each machine has a technical method of functioning. For instance, take the bicycle. You peddle the cycle. The chain connecting the two wheels accelerates the wheels to move and the bicycle moves. The technique for the bicycle is peddling and holding the handles of it to cycle and reach the determined place. The cyclist keeps control over the brakes, handle, balance and speed so that he does not lose his balance. He applies the brakes when required, avoids the obstacles such as a heap of sand or rocks on the road. This way a cycle or any machine for that matter is a type of *tantra.*

MANTRA

Mantra is an instrument of thought or a *vaidika* verse or text of prayer or adoration addressed to a deity or deities. A format dedicated to a deity like *aṣṭākṣari (auṁ namō nārāyaṇāya)* or *pañcākṣari (auṁ namaḥ śivāya). Mantra* is a magical formula, an incantation, a charm or a spell. It is a secret council or plan or advice. *Mantra* and *tantra* means spells and devices, thinking or deliberating or counselling which leads towards a definite formula. It is a process of praising, invoking or consecrating with incantation.

The *mantra* initiates a technique *(tantra)* to formulate a *yantra.* The power of formulated *mantra* is transferred to *yantra* through *tantra.*

Lokmanya Tilak and Mahatma Gandhi gave the *mantra* of independence. Both uttered the *mantra* of *swarājya* as their birth right (Independent India). These two great men accredited the *mantra* of *swarājya.* This *mantra* of Gandhi brought oneness of people from the Kaśmir in the north to Kanyākumāri in the south, and from Peśāvar in the west to the eastern states of the seven sisters as one person. This is the power of that *mantra* of *swarājya.*

Once such a similar thing happened at the time of Rāmānujāchārya about 900 A.D. and after a thousand years it happened again at the time of Mahatma Gandhi. Rāmānujāchārya got the *aṣṭākṣari-mantra* from his *guru* and he at once invited people of all communities to gather to utter the *aṣṭākṣari-mantra* which would free them from worldly desires and take them towards *mokṣa.* That *aṣṭākṣari* was nothing but *auṁ namō nārāyaṇāya.* In the history of India it is Rāmānujāchārya who brought all of India as one man through the *aṣṭākṣari-mantra* and Gandhi through the *mantra* the *swarājya or Rāmarājya.*

If *tantra* is a methodology or appliance or a systematic way in channelling human force to achieve a goal in life, *yantra's* purpose is to find the mind to reach the goal that one has in mind.

The *mantra* is designed by *tantra* and concealed in the *yantra* with a mystical formation. For instance, when we have to perform a *pujā* or religious ceremonies or festivals, *raṅgavali* (a design) is drawn with rice paste on the ground before the function as a sacred diagram. The *maṅgala-kalaśa* or *maṅgala ghaṭa* is kept signifying the commencement of the auspicious worship like *pujā, homa* or *yajña* (rituals and sacrifices) involving a series of actions performed according to the prescribed order. Before starting the rituals a banana leaf is kept as a base. The grains of rice or wheat are spread on the banana leaf. Then the auspicious signs such as *svastika* 卐 or Hexagon ✡ like a star or symbolic words such as ॐ *(auṁ)* or श्री *(śrī)* is written. Then in the middle of the leaf an earthen or copper or silver vessel is kept filled with water. The vessel is called *kuṁbha*. It acts as an enclosure around the place of sacrifice in order to make adequate preparations for future eventualities. If *auṁ* is a *bīja mantra, śrī* stands for auspiciousness, purity *(śreyas)*. They are painted or written on banana leaves as well as vessels. Ingredients such as milk, water, grains, flowers, sandal paste, turmeric and vermillion powder are kept by the side of the vessel before starting the auspicious ritual. The coconut is kept on the mouth of the vessel surrounded by mango leaves. This *maṅgala ghaṭa* is kept during every *pūjā* to indicate the auspiciousness of the function.

YANTRA

Yantra is a potent and dynamic sacred symbol which conceives the quintessence of deities, the cosmological principles, metaphysical concepts or psychic unity according to the principles of rituals. It is drawn with geometrical figures with rhythmic unity. The *yantra* is consecrated with ritual worship. It is amalgamated with three principles – the form, function and power.

The figure of the *yantra* has a shape or a form *(ākṛti* or *rūpa)*. Its principle function is action oriented *(kriyā rūpa)*. *Yantra* suggests the procedure to reach the aim and the power *(śakti rūpa)*. The encased power kept in a figurative design has its own potentiality. The same is expressed in modern terminology as *vāstuālekha* (a plan for a dwelling place) or a design to structure the house. Then this house plan becomes the *yantra (ākṛti)* of *vāstu śāstra* as a workable design *(kriyā)* in the construction of a house. This method of construction is the *yantra*. This *yantra* needs to be activated to run on heat, electricity, magnetic power or solar power and water force. In the same way, the priests draw certain diagrams in all auspicious functions, as power or *śakti*, to keep the evils away.

In *yoga yantra* the body is the deity, *tantra* is the method of worship and *mantra* is the soul of the deity.

The *yantra* that is initiated through the *mantra* covers huge, large, vast, expansive and extensive knowledge in the form of idea with the divine power to hold the *śakti* - power of the *mantra* in it.

The concept of the divine power of the *mantra* is planted and reserved in a plate as *yantra* by narrowing the entire idea of the *mantra* without allowing its holistic potentiality to lose its value. If we go back to the history of civilization, it appears that in every civilization there are cosmic sites or sacred places which indicate such spiritual significance in the form of a *yantra*.

For instance the idol in the temple indicates *yantra.* The caves – the sculptural structures are the examples and they serve vital points or centres of accumulated energy. Once it is consecrated it stands separate as a special and auspicious place from its surroundings.

The *yantra* are designed in several forms which are based on trigonometric figures containing points, lines, triangles, circles and so forth. These are not mere drawings of symbols. They are based on the *vaidika* knowledge with spiritual perspective.

Yantra creates a cosmicized circuit of force in which the powers are invoked through *mantra* on chosen deities. As our planet is in space distinguishing itself as a solid mass compared to other planets of the universe, it is the same in our own body. Each organ is placed with inter-space. Similarly, *yantra* too has distinct space separating the lines from each other, yet remaining in a circuit.

The empty space is in itself a primordial substance and shares in the nature of divinity. I have compared *ānandamaya kośa* with space in *Light On Life,*[1] which signifies divinity. The inner and outer space merge within the *yantra* with purity and divinity. In this whole universe, the primordial substance is *mūla prakṛti* – the abode. This may remain in a manifested or un-manifested form or remain in an absolute state of void. Similarly, the space within *yantra* is brought symbolically into a manifested form as 'existence' or 'presence' from the un-manifested formless state.

The *Bṛhadāraṇyaka Upaniṣad* gives the metaphor of the spider. The spider through its own body forms the net and goes straight to the centre of the web to sit there. Similarly, we have the *antaryāmin* (universal soul) within. Lord Krishna says in the *Bhagavad Gītā, Īśvaraḥ sarva bhūtānām hṛd-deśe arjuna tiṣṭhati* I *bhrāmayan sarva-bhūtāni yantrārūḍhāni māyayā* II *(B.G.,* XVIII.61)

God abides in the heart of all creatures, causing each and everything including human beings to revolve according to one's own *karma* by his *māyā* – the illusive power. The body is the vehicle of that *Iśvara.* He is in that machine *(yantra)* and the machine moves at His will and that is *māyā.* Further Lord Krishna says, *tvam eva śaraṇam gaccha sarvabhāvena bhārata* I *tatprasādātparam śāntim sthānaṁ prāpsyasi śāśvatam* II *(B.G.,* XVIII.62)

Take total shelter in *Īśvara* alone with all your feelings *(Sarvabhāvena).* By His mere grace you attain the supreme bliss, supreme peace, and eternal place (state).

---

[1] Rodale publishers, 2005.

Our inner journey from body to soul is a pilgrimage *(yoga-yātrā)*. The body is the centre of all sacred rituals. Apart from physiological functioning with *āsana*, it is consecrated and sanctified through *prāṇāyāma* and *dhyāna*. As the body is the *yantra* of the soul, this *yantra* becomes the deity as the divine soul is enclosed in the *yantra*.

Even the elements *(pañcabhūta)* are suggested in this *yantra*, and the spot *(bindu)* which is in the centre of the *yantra* signifies *ākāśa tattva*. The multi angles such as heptagon, octagon indicate *pṛthvī tattva*. The vertical angle of triangle is *tejas tattva*. The innermost circle (encasing the tri-angle) signifies the *vāyu tattva*. Though a circle is only two dimensional, here the circle is representing the circling or spiral like movement *(nirvṛtti)* inwards, towards the core as involution. Moving outwards *(pravṛtti)*[1] signifies evolution. The circles indicate the *āp tattva* and the outermost square of the *yantra* is considered as *Bhū-pura* or the city of the whole universe.

If *Viśva caitanya śakti* is cosmic energy, *viśva cetanā śakti* is God. It is the substratum in the receptacle and the base of the manifest world. The figure of the petals of the lotus represents the eight aspects of yoga indicating the path towards self realization. Often, I express in teaching that "Yoga is the journey from the skin to the soul and from the soul to the skin." The petals of the lotus may remind the practitioners of yoga about the eighth petal for this inner journey.

YOGA YANTRA

Though *yantra* is a sacred and secret symbol, yet I am presenting this *yoga yantra* for each *sādhaka* to understand how important yoga is to bring union of *prakṛti* with *puruṣa*. This body is the *yantra* of *yoga vidyā* and its Deity is *Īśvara*. Yogic practice is the *tantra* as guided by Patañjali. The *mantra* of this *tantra* and *yantra* is *auṁ* (ॐ). (See table n. 3 pages 287 & 288)

---

[1] See the article *Physiology and Cakra* in *Aṣṭadaḷa Yogamālā* volume 2, pp. 174 and see also table n. 5.

	Ā	*U*	*Ṁ*	ॕ
1	*jāgratāvasthā* (wakeful)	*svapnā avasthā* (dreamy)	*suṣuptyāvasthā* (sleepy)	*turyāvasthā* (beyond these three states)
2	*manas* (mind)	*vāk* (speech)	*kāya* (body)	self (silence)
3	*citta* (consciousness)	*sthitaprajña* (stable intelligence)	*jīvātmā* (individual self)	*paramātmā* (universal soul, supreme soul)
4	*niṣkāma-vṛtti* (desirelessness)	*abhaya-vṛtti* (fearless thoughts)	*akrodha-vṛtti* (anger-less state)	*sthitaprajña* (stable intelligence)
5	*straiṇa* (feminine)	*pauruṣa* (masculine)	*napuṁsaka* (neuter)	*nirmātā* (creator beyond gender)
6	*sattva* (luminosity)	*rajas* (vibrancy)	*tamas* (inertia)	*guṇātīta* (beyond guṇa)
7	*guru-mātā* (mother as first teacher)	*guru-pitā* (father as second teacher)	*guru* as *ācārya* (third teacher)	*Parama Guru* – God (teacher of all teachers)
8	Brahmā	Vishnu	Shiva	*Paramātmā Parameśvara Puruṣa viśeṣa*
9	*bhūta* (past)	*vartamāna* (present)	*bhaviṣya* (future)	*kālātīta* (beyond time, unbound by time)
10	*diśā* (direction)	*kāla* (time)	*ākāra* (shape)	*nirākāra* (beyond dimension)
11	*āsana*	*prāṇāyāma*	*dhyāna*	*samādhi*
12	*śarīra*	*manas*	*buddhi*	*ātmā*
13	*tridoṣa samatvam (vāta, pitta, kapha)* – even flow of *tri-dośa*	*sapta dhātu śuddhi: rasa, rakta, māṁsa, meda, asthi, majjā, śukra* (chyle, blood, flesh, fat, bone, marrow, semen)	*trimala śuddhi (mūtra, puriṣa, sweda* – urine, faeces, sweat)	*arogatā* (freedom from all obstacles)
14	*dhāraṇā*	*dhyāna*	*samādhi*	*saṁyama*
15	*manas*	*buddhi*	*ahaṁkāra*	*citta* (absolute consciousness)
16	*sarvajña* or *jñāna bīja*	*sarva-śakti* or *śakti-bīja*	*sarva-vyāpt sarva-vyāpī*	*Īśvara* or *Paramātmā*
17	*karmendriya*	*jñānendriya*	*manasendriya*	*dharmendriya*

Table n. 3 – Correspondances of the *yantra* of *āuṁ*

18	*sapta citta (vyutthāna, nirodha, praśānta, ekāgra, nirmāṇa, chidra, divya)* – outgoing, restraining, tranquill, one-pointed, egoistic, fissured and divine	*sapta prajñā (śarīra, prāṇa, manas, vijñāna, ānubhavika, rasātmaka, ātmā)* – knowledge of body, breath, mind, intelligence, experienced wisdom, essence of wisdom	*sapta-kośa (annamaya, prāṇamaya, manomaya, vijñānamaya, anandamaya, cittamaya, ātmamaya)* and *saptacakra (mūlādhāra, svādhiṣṭhāna, maṇipūraka, anāhata, viśuddhi, ājñā* and *sahasrāra)*	*kaivalyāvasthā*
19	*sabīja samādhi*	*dharma megha samādhi*	*nirbīja samādhi*	*mokṣāvasthā*
20	*citta*	*Jīvātmā*	*puruṣa*	*Paramātmā*
21	*śakti*	*yukti*	*bhakti*	*paramaikānti* or *śaraṇāgati*
22	*dharma*	*artha*	*kāma*	*mokṣa*
23	*pañca kleśa (avidyā, asmitā, rāga, dveṣa, abhiniveśa)*	*pañca vṛtti (pramāṇa, viparyaya, vikalpa, nidrā, smṛti)*	*trayodaśāntarāya (vyādhi, styāna, saṁśaya, pramāda, ālasya, avirati, bhrānti darśana, alabdha bhumikatva, anavasthitatva, duḥkha, daurmanasya, aṅgamejayatva, śvāsapraśvāsa)*	*kleśa nivṛtti* *vṛtti nirodha* *antarāya abhāva*
24	*sthūla śarīra* (gross body)	*sūkṣma śarīra* (subtle body)	*kāraṇa śarīra* (causal body)	*paramātmā (śarīra)* *śarīra bhāva* (body) ▼ body ▼ *jīvātma* ▼ *puruṣa* *śariri-bhāva* ▼ *jīvātma* ▼ *puruṣa* ▼ *paramātma* or *paramapuruṣa*
25	*iḍā*	*piṅgaḷā*	*suṣumṇā*	*nāḍi-jaya (nāḍi-śuddhi)*
26	*bahiraṅga sādhanā*	*antaraṅga sādhanā*	*antarātma sādhanā*	*sādhanātīta* or *sādhanatraya*
27	*prāṇi-mātra jaḍa-ajaḍa*	*mūla prakṛti*	*puruṣa*	*puruṣa-viśeṣa*
28	*buddhi*	*citta*	*antaḥkaraṇa*	*antarātma*

Table n. 3 cont ....

THE SYMBOL OF *ŚRĪ YOGA VIDYĀ YANTRA*

This *yantra* of yoga is a connecting instrument that unites *jīvātmā* with *Paramātmā.* Let us understand the design of the *yantra* which reveals the philosophy of yoga. Start reading the *yoga sūtra* to understand the *yantra* from the periphery to the centre point to learn and follow it. The space outside the *yantra* indicates macrocosm *(brahmāṇḍa)* or *parama puruṣa, puruṣottama,* universal soul, God, *paramātmā, puruṣa viśeṣa* and the symbol within the frame is microcosm *(piṇḍāṇḍa)* or the universe *(prakṛti).* [See *Y.S.,* I.24, 25, 26, 27, 28 and *Y.S.,* II.19 and *Y.S.,* III.45, 46, 47, 48, 49].

DIGBANDHA – The *yantra* begins with *digbandha* (fig. 1). *Digbandha* means binding. It is a restricted area of the campus by *mantra* to keep off evils. It shows eight directions *(diśā)* from the points of the compass. The compass is the dot representing *brahmāṇḍa* on *piṇḍāṇḍa* (God in the body). *Aṣṭa dik* is eight directions. East *(Pūrva),* south-east *(Āgneya),* south *(Dakṣiṇa),* south-west *(Nairṛtya),* west *(Paśchima),* north-west *(Vāyavya),* north *(Uttara),* north-east *(Īśānya)* is the *digbandha* of the *yantra.* The open space outside the *yantra* and the dot within the *yantra* represents the universe *(brahāṇḍa)* and beyond. The outer space and the dot *(bindu)* in the centre is *ākāśa,* north-east stands for *pṛthvī,* south-west for *āp,* south-east for *tejas* and north-west for *vāyu tattva.*

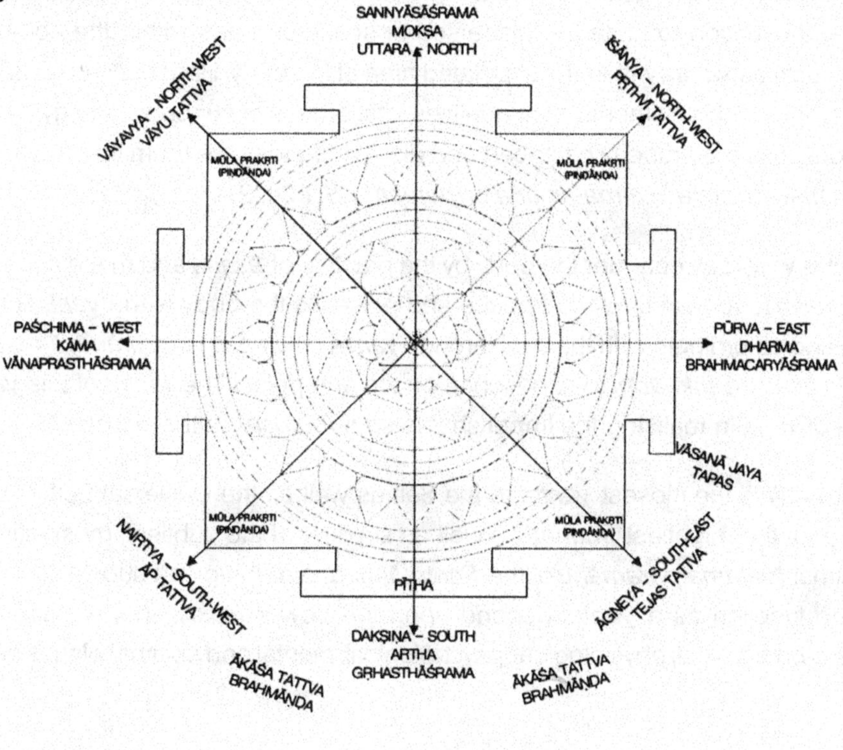

fig. 1

It has four basement plinths *(pīṭha).* Like the ray passing through the prism shows multiple colours, the *pīṭha* give different dimensions. They represent the four aims of life *(puruṣārtha)* and four steps *(āśrama)* in life. The *pīṭha* of the east represents right sense of duty *(dharma).* This primary plinth *(pīṭha)* is devoted to study *(brahmacaryāśrama).*

The *pīṭha* of the south represents a means to earn a living and economic stability *(artha).* This *pīṭha* stands for householder's life *(gṛhasthāśrama).*

The west *pīṭha* stands for offsprings or progeny *(kāma)* and then move towards the woods *(vānaprasthāśrama)* to learn non-attachment.

The *pīṭha* of the north stands for *mokṣa (sannyāsāśrama)* to live a detached life.

This *yantra* is structured for *yoga sādhaka* to reach *brahmāṇḍa* using the twentyfour evolutes of *piṇḍāṇḍa* through *aṣṭāṅga yoga sādhanā* using the body, organs of action, senses of perception, mind, five elements, their counterparts, five *prāṇa,* intelligence, consciousness and I-maker. All these suggest about the structure of nature in our body which has to be auspiciously sanctified and consecrated.

For example, each *āsana* and each *prāṇāyāma* is a *yantra* in itself as it has its own *digbandha* – a direction to unite the dispersed or scattered parts within the compass of the *āsana* which acts as *yantra* within the stipulated area of the body. Hence, *āsana* has to be done in such a way that all the elements, their qualities, vital organs of our body, energy, mind, senses and consciousness are properly balanced and disciplined to make them flow inwards towards the most enthralled circle – *ātma-sthāna* or *puruṣa* (*Y.S.,* II.20, 21).

That is why I say conquer the body by the practice of *āsana* and make it a fit vehicle for the soul *(puruṣa)* to remain in eternal peace and poise. As the body is the *yantra* of the soul it has to work and co-ordinate with the soul through *yama, niyama, āsana, prāṇāyāma, pratyāhāra, dhāraṇā, dhyāna* and *samādhi* to experience peace and poise. The *tantra* of this *yantra* is the culmination of yoga in realising the imperishable soul *(puruṣa)* as the *mantra.*

Our body is the closest *yantra* to the Self as well as the Universal Self. The Universal Self is mighty of the mightiest *(mahat)* as well as subtlest of the subtlest, most infinitesimal of the infinitesimal *(parama-paramāṇu* of the *Paramāṇu),* and nothing can substitute it. The body's structure and function as a *yantra* depend upon the power *(śakti),* shape *(ākṛti)* and action *(kriyā).* It works on physical, physiological, psychological, mental and spiritual planes and spreads beyond.

Our body is physical but its substratum is divinity. Each part of the body is a foundation or base *(pīṭha)* for God and Goddess. The body is the meeting of sacred rivers *(tīrthakṣetra)* or place of pilgrimage. The *nāḍī*, the *cakra* are connecting the body to the sacred place – the Self within and from Self to God. If the body is the *ghaṭa (kuṁbha)*, it is filled with energy *(prāṇa)* in order to live with attentive awareness *(prajñā)*, sanctity and purity of the body from *annamaya kośa* to *ānandamaya kośa*.

Our yogic journey is shown starting from the body to the soul. A pilgrimage is meant to reach the innermost part, that is God. As the *yantra* shows how *yoga sādhanā* consecrates and sanctifies all the sheaths of the body, the *yantra* becomes a Deity as the divinity is encased in the *yantra*.

Impressions as desires and memories exist in us from time immemorial. Emotional hunger like lust, anger, greed, infatuation, pride and malice (known as *ṣadripu* or six enemies) bind the self *(jīvātmā)* through cause and effect which are dependent upon the mixture of *guṇa* (*Y.S.*, I.30, 31; II.12, 13, 14; IV.10, 11). This cause and effect theory is well explained by Patañjali. He says that due to uncertain understanding of the REAL, it gives rise to nescience in the form of violence physically, morally, ethically, emotionally, intellectually and spiritually, making one to do directly or inducing one to act or abetting the act due to the influence of impressions and desires *(vāsanā)* in mild, moderate or to act in intense degree resulting in endless pain and ignorance (*Y.S.*, II.34).

All these are minimised, sublimated and if possible eradicated through the eight petals of *yoga sādhanā* (*Y.S.*, II.2).

THREE CIRCLES OF *TRIGUṆA (TAMAS, RAJAS* AND *SATTVA)* – The frame of the *yantra* represents root nature *(mūla prakṛti)* as a base for evolutory involution. Inside the frame there are three circles representing *guṇa*. The outer circle represents inexpressive *tamas*, *tamoraja* and *tamosattva* (inert state of being); the middle circle represents *rajotamas*, *rajoraja* and *rajosattva* (*rajas* – becoming to know the state of the inner being); while the inner circle stands for *sattva-tamas*, *sattva-rajas* and *sattvosattva* (*sattva* – consciously experiencing in the state of being).

***PRAKṚTI CATURVIMŚATI DAḶA* –** The twenty-four *tattva* of nature (fig. 2) are shown in the twenty-four petals of this lotus from the finest towards the grossest. Like a giant wheel, the wheels of *guṇa* revolve around the twenty-four principles *(tattva)* of nature in the body as the body is made of these *tattva*.

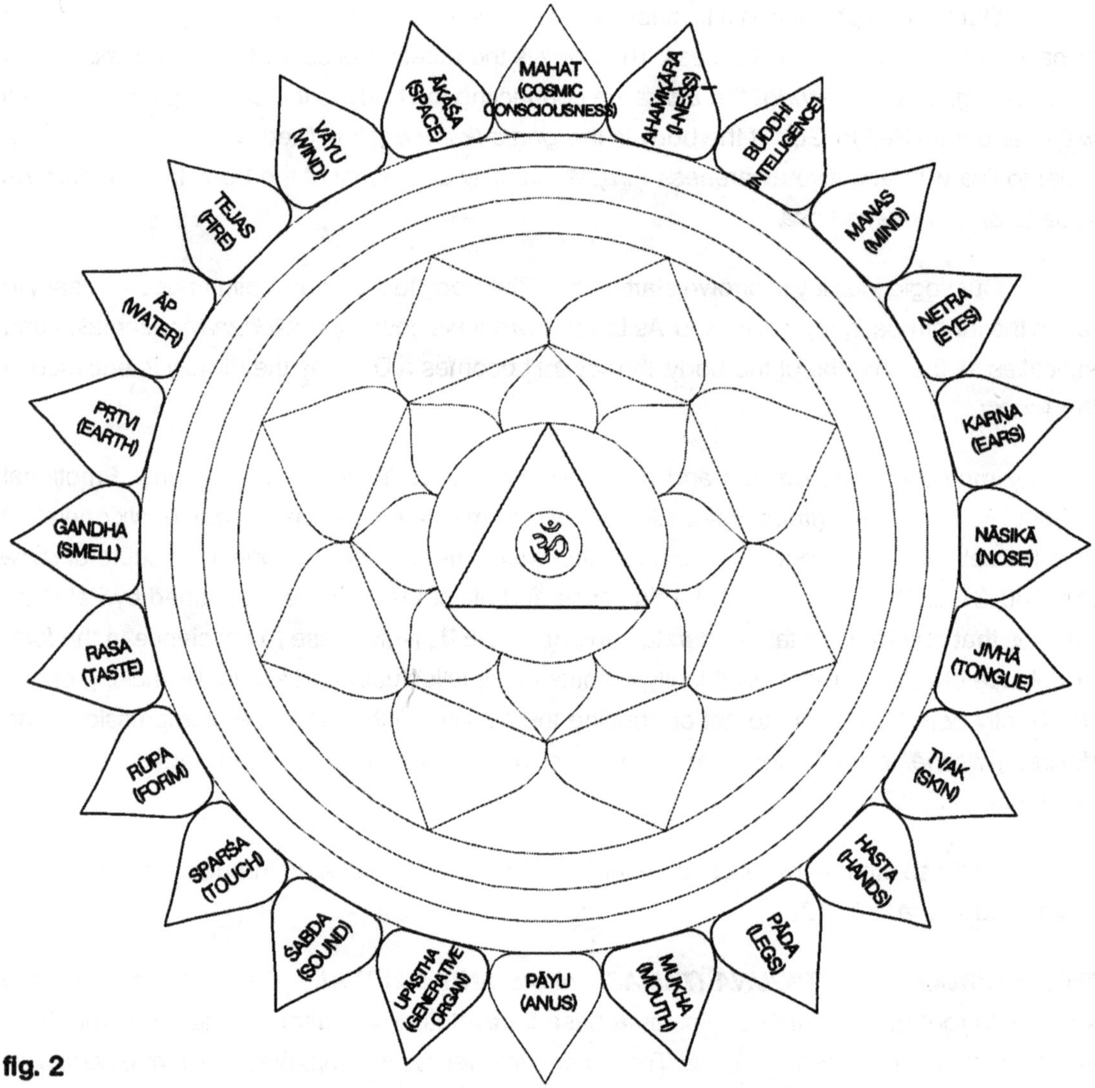

fig. 2

Quality of *sādhanā* (*Y.S.,* II.23, 25) as well as progress in one's effort are needed to evolve towards *Īśvara praṇidhāna* (*Y.S.,* I.23, II.1, 32) These three wheels act as a hub for a *yoga sādhaka* to progress from mild *(mṛdu)* to average *(madhyama)* and from average to keen *(adhimātra)* and then to reach the vehement *(tīvra)* state (*Y.S.,* I.21, 22).

It also signifies that the twentyfour *tattva* of *prakṛti* revolve around the movement of the wheels of *guṇa* to reach the centre point as maturity of intelligence and consciousness takes place.

When the *sādhaka* gets purified through the disciplines of yoga, (*Y.S.,* II.28) he reaches the *sāttvic* illuminative state to reach the centre point – the dot which stands for *antaryāmin, paramātmā* or God. The moment *sādhaka* reaches this state, the hub and the giant wheel stop revolving.

The twenty-four principles *(tattva)* of nature *(mūla prakṛti)* are cosmic consciousness *(mahat)* which becomes individual consciousness *(citta)* in the body. This *citta* branches into three parts as I-maker or I-ness *(ahaṁkāra),* intelligence *(buddhi)* and mind *(manas).* Then there are five *jñānendriya* (eyes, ears, nose, tongue, and skin), five *karmendriya* (hands, legs, mouth, excretory organ – anus, and generative organ), and then five elements (earth, water, fire, air or wind, ether or space) and their five infrastructures (smell, taste, form or shape, touch, sound; all these put together are the twenty-four principles of nature *(prakṛti)* (*Y.S.,* II.19).

THREE CIRCLES REPRESENT *SĀDHANĀ KRAMA* – These three circles (fig. 3) are the quest from the *annamaya kośa* to proceed towards *ānandamaya kośa* (*Y.S.,* I.12, 13, 14, 15, 16). The *sādhanā krama* of yoga is meant for purity *(prakṛti śuddhi)* (*Y.S.,* I.19; III.45, 46, 47, 48, 49, 50).

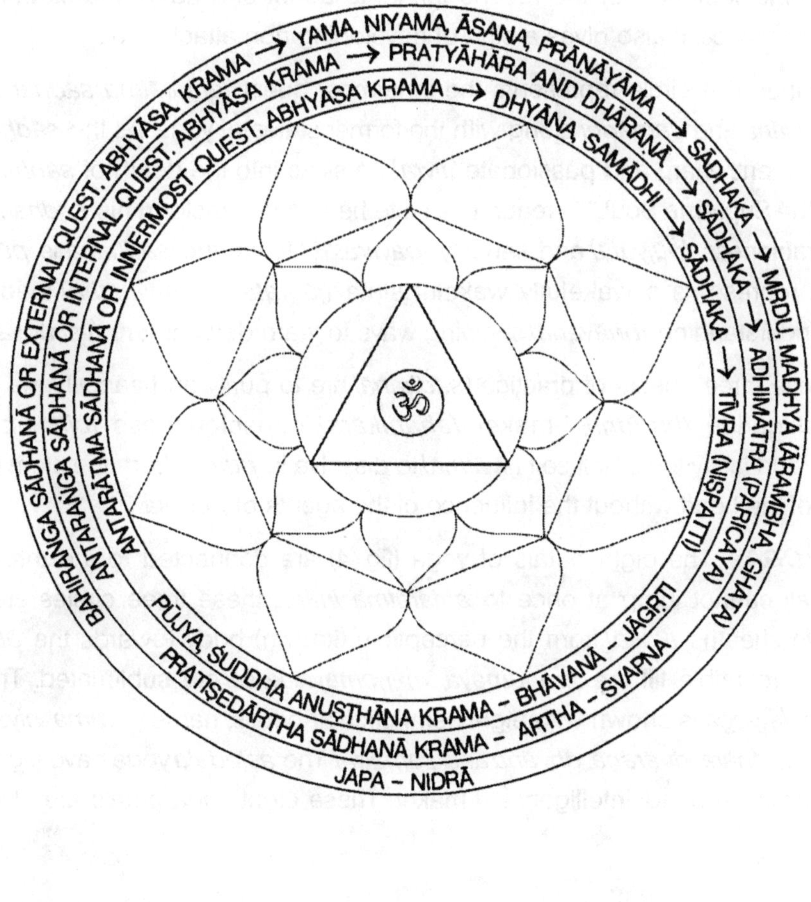

fig. 3

The outer circle represents the external quest *(bahiraṅga sādhanā)* of yoga. These are *yama, niyama, āsana* and *prāṇāyāma.* This circle represents repeated practice *(abhyāsa)* to get acquainted with the subject. Here the *sādhaka* is soft, mild, slow *(mṛdu)* or moderate *(madhyama)* and hence, he begins with a a specific way. It also expresses *japa.* As one utters the *japa-mantra* repeatedly and loudly, *abhyāsa* or practice reflects to do the same over and over again like *japa.* The practitioner being a beginner, he has .to start with the body *(ghaṭa)* and break slumbness, sloth, slackness, laziness and attachment or aversion *(rāga, dveśa)* (*Y.S.,* I.6; II.3) and dullness which are identical to the character of sleep *(nidrā).*

The middle circle represents the inner or internal quest *(antaraṅga sādhanā).* The *sādhanā* of yoga here is *pratyāhāra* and *dhāraṇā* along with the former four aspects of yoga as a means to encounter for preventing all the imbalances *(pratiṣedhārtha sādhanā)* to reach the state of purity *(śuddhatā* or *amiśritā)* in thoughts, words and deeds (*Y.S.,* I.32). As the *sādhaka* gains momentum, he has to infiltrate the inner sheaths with this intelligence in order to remove their disparities and co-ordinate them in perfect alignment. Intelligence progressively marinates the body towards its core of being. It represents dreamy state *(svapnāvasthā)* as one is hazy in thought and mind. It stands for the means *(artha)* to adopt and adapt the *sādhanā* towards progression in practice. It also gives a sign of developing non-attachment.

The innermost circle represents the innermost quest *(antarātma sādhanā).* Here the *sādhanā* is *dhyāna* and *samādhi* along with the former states of yoga. As the *sādhaka* by now becomes vehement, sharp and passionate *(tīvra),* he sinks into the depth of *sādhanā* to reach the soul and the Supreme Soul. To reach this state he has to transform his *sādhanā krama* for gaining venerableness *(pūjyatā)* and sanctity *(pavitratā).* Hence the *sādhanā* is *pūjya śuddha anuṣṭhāna.* It represents a wakefully wakeful state *(jāgrata-jāgratāvasthā)* leading toward experiential understanding *(bhāvanā)* showing ways to learn detachment *(vairāgya).*

All these three quests of practice (*sādhanā)* are to purify and sanctify tne body, mind *(manas),* intelligence *(buddhi),* I-maker *(ahaṁkāra),* consciousness *(citta),* conscience *(antaḥkaraṇa)* and lastly the small self *(jīvātmā)* to dissolve in *puruṣa* from the stem of the head to the centre of the heart without the influence of the agents of *puruṣa.*

AṢṬADAḶA YOGA - The eight petals of yoga (fig. 4) are connected to the three circles in *sādhanā.* As all cannot jump at once to *antarātma jñāna,* these three circles are shown to master the five sheaths *(kośa)* from the perceptible (known) body towards the *ātman* which remains non-perceptible till the *prāṇamaya, manomaya kośa* are sublimated. This *aṣṭāṅga yoga* or *aṣṭadaḷa yoga* is shown with eight semi-circular petals, namely, *yama, niyama, āsana, prāṇāyāma, pratyāhāra, dhāraṇā, dhyāna* and *samādhi.* The *aṣṭadaḷa* yoga have eight firm basis for gaining stability in mind, intelligence, I-maker. These eight yoga petals are also meant to cleanse the four petals of the brain *(vitarka, vicāra, ānanda* and *asmitā)* and four petals of the heart *(maitrī, karuṇā, muditā* and *upekṣā)* (*Y.S.,* I.17, 33).

For progress in *yoga sādhanā. Śraddhā, vīrya, smṛti, samādhi prajñā* are the pillars of yoga (*Y.S.,* I.20). *Śraddhā* acts as a pillar to *yama* and *niyama, vīrya* for *āsana* and *prāṇāyāma, smṛti* for *pratyāhāra* and *dhāraṇā* and *samādhi prajñā* for *dhyāna* and *samādhi.* By dedicated practice of yoga, the impurities are destroyed for mature wisdom to radiate in order to experience the glory of profoundness of the core of the being *(ātman).* Each *sādhaka* is caught in a perplexed dual state of mind. He is caught between the pleasures of the world *(bhoga)* or freedom from the worldly bondage *(apavarga).* The eight semi-circular petals of *aṣṭāṅga yoga* are meant to check, minimise or eradicate that which generates as well as causes the sea of grief and pain, namely uneasiness, unhappiness, sorrow, afflictions, distress, misery, agony, trouble, difficulty *(duḥkha).* They sanitize and nullify the happiness that causes attachment. (See *Y.S.,* II.23, 6, 7, 8, 9, 12, 13, 14, 15, 16, 18 and *Y.S.,* III.51 and *Y.S.,* IV.30).

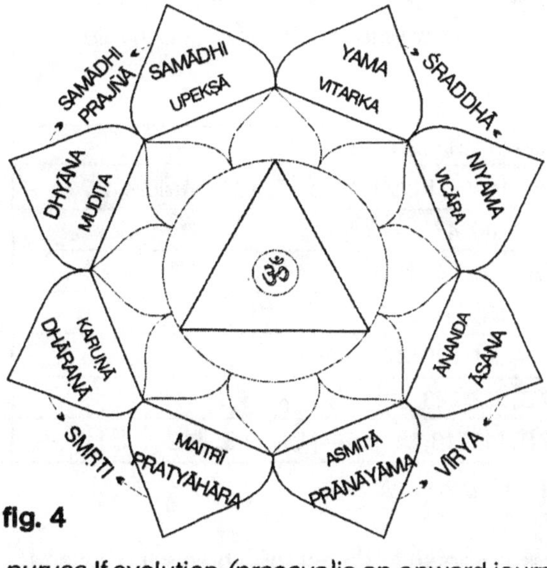

fig. 4

Patañjali says that the association and conjunction of the individual Self with nature is the cause of suffering. (*Y.S.,* I.4, *Y.S.,* II.17)

As the *Aṣṭadaḷa yoga* is exactly in the middle of *prakṛti* and *puruṣa,* the *yantra's* importance is great. It is shown in the middle for indicating the conjunction *(saṁyoga)* or association *(yuj)* of body *(prakṛti)* with soul *(puruṣa).* It is meant for the Self to discover its own true nature *(svarūpa upalabdhi)* (*Y.S.,* II.23). Secondly, yoga acts as a foundation for the evolution of the soul from *prakṛti* to understand its status and acts as a hub from *prakṛti* to *puruṣa.* If evolution *(prasava)* is an onward journey of *puruṣa* from *prakṛti,* involution is an inverse journey or return journey *(prati prasava)* where *prakṛti* returns to its abode for the *puruṣa,* illuminating *(sattva)* with his enriching qualities.

Aṣṭāṅga yoga acts as a bridge between *prakṛti* and *puruṣa.*

The mind, intelligence and consciousness are caught in between the object of enjoyment *(bhoga)* and illumination and emancipation *(mokṣa).*

This is the reason why yoga is termed as a physio-psychological and psycho-spiritual subject revolving cosmic *prāṇa* between *bhoga* and yoga (*Y.S.,* II.18). The outer three circles represent qualities *(guṇa)* of nature *(prakṛti).*

Though I have shown the five elements *(pṛthvī, āp, tej, vāyu, ākāśa)* in the *yantra,* I would like to bring to your attention the five elements that represent the body. The skeletal body as *pṛthvī tattva - annamaya,* vital body as *āp - prāṇamaya,* mind as *tejas - manomaya,* intelligence as *vāyu - vijñānamaya,* and Self *(puruṣa)* as *ākāśa* or *cidākāśa.*

If *viśva cetana śakti* is *paramātmā, Viśva caitanya śakti* is His cosmic energy. This cosmic energy multiplies in the body as *prāṇa, apāna, samāna, udāna* and *vyāna* (*Y.S.,* III.40, 41, 42, 43). Here please note that *apāna* represents *pṛthvī, prāṇa - āp, samāna - tejas, udāna - vāyu* and *vyāna - ākāśa.*

God is the substratum of the manifested world and hence yoga is a journey from the skin to the soul and from the soul to the skin expressing evolution of the soul and involution of the *prakṛti.*

1	The right first petal	*Yama*	Effects Y.S., II.30; II.35 to 39; I.33.
2	The right second petal	*Niyama*	Effects Y.S., II.32; II.40 to 45; II.33, 34; III.24, 25
3	The right third petal	*Āsana*	Y.S., II.46, 47
4	The bottom petal	*Prāṇāyāma*	Y.S., I.34; II.49 to 53
5	The left bottom petal	*Pratyāhāra*	Y.S., I.35; II.54, 55
6	The left bottom second petal	*Dhāraṇā*	Y.S., III.1; I.36, 37
7	The left third petal	*Dhyāna*	Y.S., III.2; I.23, 38, 39
8	The top petal	*Samādhi*	Y.S., I.17, 18; I.41 to 44; I.51; Y.S., II.12; III.3, 11

Table n. 4 - The eight petals and their related *sūtra*

***AṢṬADAḶA PADMA* OF *SAMĀDHI* (LOTUS)** - This is shown in an octagon below the *aṣṭadala yoga* (fig. 5) indicating the eight stages of *(aṣṭavidha) samādhi.* Though Patañjali defines *samādhi* as loss of the sense of self-being *(svarūpa śūnyatā)* (*Y.S.,* I.17, 18, 19, 41, 42, 43, 44, 45, 51; III.3; IV.29) he says that the yogi comes out from that state towards self establishment *(svarūpa pratiṣṭhā)* (*Y.S.,* IV.34) or *kaivalyāvasthā* (*Y.S.,* II.25; III.51, 56; IV.26, 34). These eight aspects of *samādhi* take the yogi close to *bhakti* or *Īśvara praṇidhāna* or *brahmāṇḍa* or the centre point *(bindu)* of the *yantra.*

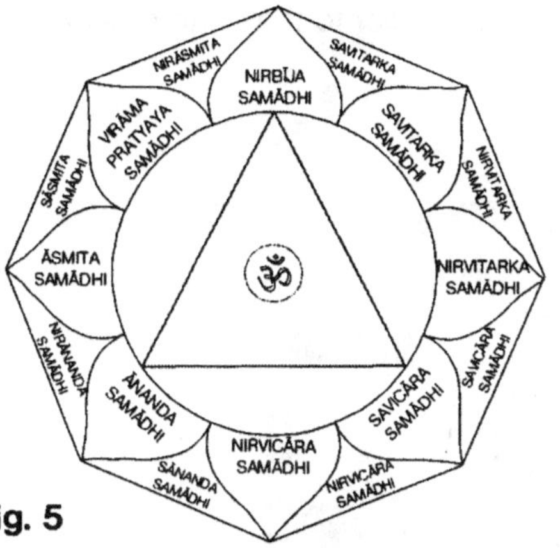

fig. 5

According to Patañjali the eight stages of *samādhi* lead us with involutary process where the journey is from the five elements, organs of action, senses of perception and mind which are distinguishable *(viśeṣa)* to the five *tanmātra* namely, sound, touch, form, taste, smell and the I-maker *(ahaṁkāra),* non-distiguishable *(aviśeṣa),* (*Y.S.,* II.19) and from there to *mahat* (first principle of *prakṛti)* as *liṅga* (mark). When all these dissolve in *mūla prakṛti* it is *aliṅga* (*Y.S.,* II.19). It is a noumenal state (*Y.S.,* I.19 and *Y.S.,* III.3).

The eight petals of the lotus indicate eight stages of *samādhi* to reach *puruṣa* or *ātman* to feel his pure state. Patañjali defines *samādhi* as one losing the sense of his self being *(svarūpa śūnyatā).* After experiencing the loss of self being, the yogi has to come out of that state towards Self establishment *(svarūpa pratiṣṭhā)* (*Y.S,* IV.34). This is *śri yoga vidyā yantra,* the ultimate in yoga as *kaivalyāvasthā* or *kevalāvasthā,* the compass or the *bindu.*

The eight petals of the inner lotus indicate eight stages of *samādhi* which are divided into two types as *sabīja* and *nirbīja samādhi. Sabīja samādhi* leads towards unalloyed and illuminative spiritual wisdom glowing with truth and reality – *ṛtaṁbharā prajñā. Ṛtaṁbharā tatra prajñā* (*Y.S,* I.48) – This state conveys the state of consciousness as matured wisdom or truth-bearing wisdom with intense insight. The consciousness then becomes aware of the self *(jīvātmā), puruṣa* (the real Self) and *antaryāmin (Īśvara),* the abode of the *puruṣa.* Water reflecting the visage on it seeing face to face, *puruṣa* sees *Īśvara* face to face. (*Y.S.,* I.3, 16, 47; II.20, 21, 47; III.3, 6, 56 and IV. 18, 25)

This wisdom is beyond the fountain of direct knowledge, informed or proven as factual (*Y.S.,* I.7). It is beyond the knowledge acquired through books, testimony or inference. (*Y.S.,* I.49)

This *ṛtaṁbharā prajñā* comes when the gates of the seven *cakra* and states of awareness *(sapta prajñā)* open. The seven *cakra* are; *mūlādhāra, svādhiṣṭhāna, maṇipūraka, anāhata, viśuddhi, ājñā* and *sahasrāra.* For example take *Cakrabandhāsana* The very name suggests how all the *cakra* get tied and united together. The spine is arched in this *āsana* in such a way that all the *cakra* act connected and co-related (*Y.S.,* III.27, 28, 29, 30, 31, 32, 33, 35). Take *Maṇḍalāsana.*[1] It suggests *ātma-pradakṣiṇā* – the body *(prakṛti)* going around the soul *(puruṣa).*

---

[1] See the author's *Light on Yoga,* Harper Collins, plate no. 525 to 535

It is the *parikramā* or *pradakṣiṇā* of the body around the soul, similar to the earth orbiting the sun.

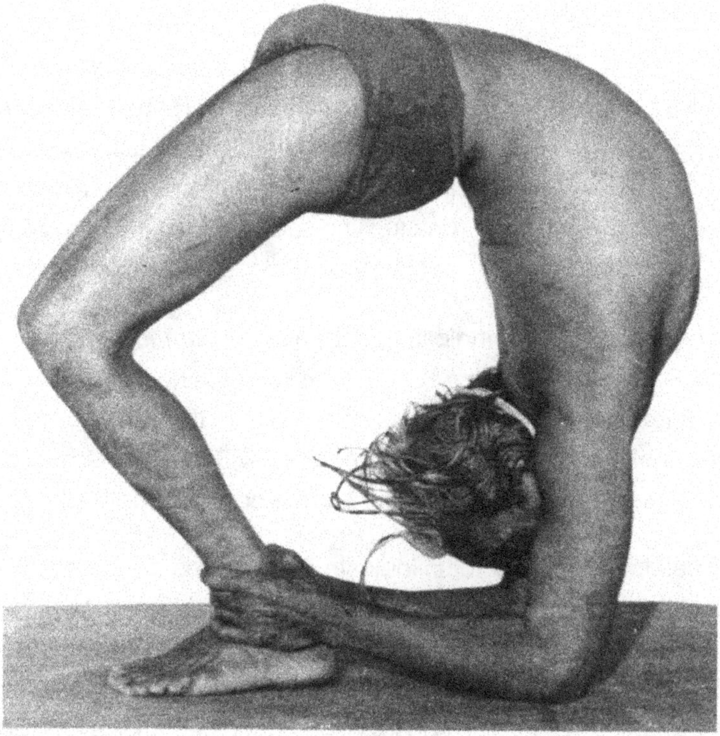

Plate n. 37 – *Cakrabandhāsana*

See Vyāsa's commentary. He enlists the *sapta prajñā* as follows – *1) parijñāta prajñā* – the knowable is known, 2) *heya kṣiṇa prajñā* – that which has to be discarded is discarded, 3) *prāpya prāpti prajñā* – the attainable is attained, 4) *kāryaśuddhi prajñā* – what must be done is done, 5) *caritādhikāra prajñā* – the aim to be reached is reached, 6) *guṇātīta prajñā* – untainted intelligence, 7) *svarūpa mātra jyoti prajñā* – Self illumed consciousness. All these seven states of *prajñā* are insights presented to a yogi who has gained matured wisdom accompanied with intense insight *(ṛtaṁbharā prajñā).*

From this new light of wisdom that comes from *sabīja samādhi* the yogi moves towards *nirbīja samādhi* where the *puruṣa* gets consecrated to live in its pure form (*Y.S.,* I.51). According to Patañjali, the eight petalled *samādhi* are: 1) *savitarka,* 2) *nirvitarka,* 3) *savicāra,* 4) *nirvicāra,* 5) *ānanda,* 6) *asmitā* (*Y.S.,* I.17), 7) *virāma pratyaya* as *asaṁprajñāta* (*Y.S.,* I.18) and 8) *dharma megha* or *nirbīja samādhi* (*Y.S.,* IV.29 and I.51). Some *Haṭhayoga* texts name *aṣṭa samādhi* as:

1) *savitarka,* 2) *nirvitarka,* 3) *savicāra,* 4) *nirvicāra,* 5) *sānanda,* 6) *nirānanda,* 7) *sāsmita* and 8) *nirāsmita.*

Though the word *samādhi* is yogic terminology, it stands for *bhakti.* Patañjali emphatically says that surrender to God brings perfection in *samādhi* or *samādhi* leads to *Īśvara praṇidhāna.* All the eight aspects of *samādhi* is a journey from *jñāna* to *vijñāna, vijñāna* to *prajñāna* and *prajñāna* to *bhakti.*

THE INNERMOST CIRCLE – This circle around the triangle (fig. 6) is the *puruṣa – ātman – draṣṭā – jīvātman* or *puruṣa-śakti.* As *puruṣa* has no shape, He is indicated with a circle showing no beginning and no end. The *Viśva caitanya śakti* moves spirally and widens or tightens around the axis – *viśva cetana śakti* or God. Hence, it is shown in the form of a circle. In *Light on Life,* I have compared the *vijñānamaya kośa* with *vāyu tattva.* Here it goes with the basic significance of *yantra.* Here the pinnacle of nature, the intelligence equals the intelligence and purity of the Self.[1]

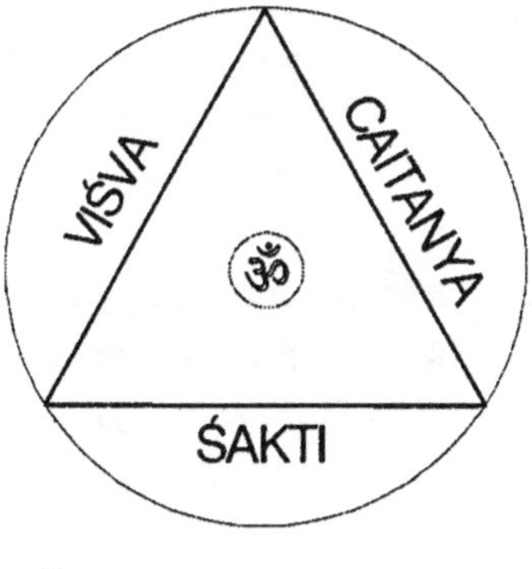

fig. 6

Puruṣa, draṣṭā / dṛṣṭru is pure. But he gets identified with thought waves *(vṛtti),* and gets tainted (*Y.S.,* I.4). Hence Patañjali explains, *yogaḥ cittavṛtti nirodhaḥ* (*Y.S.,* I.2). When *vṛtti* are restrained *draṣṭā* or *ātman* dwells in his original state (*Y.S.,* I.3). Hence, *Viśva caitanya śakti* becomes immobile *(stambha-vṛtti).* The steadiness of *viśva cetana śakti* and His *caitanya śakti* means knowledge and wisdom *(svarūpa prajñā).*

THE TRIANGLE – This triangle touching the circle (fig. 7) shows the conjunction of *puruṣa* with *paramātmā.* This triangle represents God in the form of ॐ or *akāra, ukāra, makāra.*

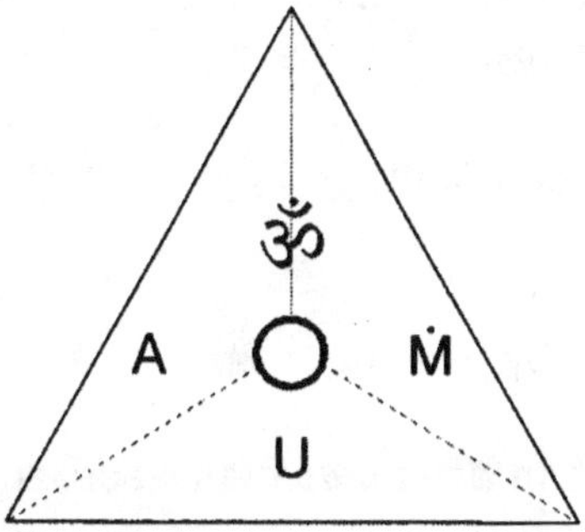

fig. 7

It also represents qualities of *Īśvara,* namely, omni-potent, omni-scient, omni-present, untouched by afflictions, actions and their results. God is the unsurpassed or unexcelled seed of all knowledge, He is said to be the first and foremost *Guru* of all *guru.* The space between the *bindu* and triangle

---

[1] *sattva puruṣayoḥ śuddhi sāmye kaivalyam* (Y.S., III.56) – when the purity of intelligence has reached the purity of the soul, the yogi has reached *kaivalya,* perfection in yoga.

indicates that God is untouched and untainted by any action, remaining eternally clean and clear. (See *Y.S.*, I.24, 25, 26, 27, 28)

The three points of the triangle touching the circle indicate the sign of evolutary process for *puruṣa (ātman)* to come in contact with *prakṛti's* attributes to test its highest state, the prowess of the soul *(citi śakti)*.

BINDU – Lastly, the dot *(bindu)* represents the seat of God which is reached through the achievement of *kaivalya*. It points out *Īśvara* which is recognised as *paramātman, puruṣa viśeṣa*, or God. He is represented by ॐ. The *yantra* indicates activity and mobility and movement in order to reach the *bindu, Paramātman,* who is ever in *jāgṛtāvasthā*. He keeps the world moving like a machine with His *yantramāyā*. *Bindu* as *Īśvara*, represents *ānandamaya kośa* and *ākāśa tattva*, the ultimate entity. When one reaches this ultimate entity, it is *kaivalya* (a state of aloneness). From this state of aloneness, the yogi realises freedom and beatitude *(kaivalya)*. From here he moves to *Īśvara praṇidhāna* with total surrender to God with devotion.

OUTSIDE THE *YANTRA* AND THE CENTRE OF THE *YANTRA*

Outside and inside the *yantra* suggest the immeasurable God or *puruṣa viśeṣa*. In *puruṣa sūkta*, *puruṣa viśeṣa* is said to have thousands of heads, thousands of eyes, thousands of legs engulfing not only the earth but the three worlds and extends and spreads further by ten fingers more.

auṁ

sahasra śīrṣā puruṣaḥ I sahasrākṣa sahasrapāt I sa bhūmim viśvatō vṛtvā I
atyatiṣṭaddaśāngulam I puruṣa eva idam sarvam I

This *yantra* suggests the ideology of yoga in bringing union of the Self *(puruṣa)* with God *(puruṣa viśeṣa)*.

The *yantra* indicates *adhyātma jñāna* through *yoga vidyā* by purifying *prakṛti*.

Samādhi takes us closer to experience *ātma darśana*. From *ātma-darśana* it leads us towards the *bindu – paramātma-darśana*. It is the journey from *prakṛti* to *puruṣa viśeṣa* and from *puruṣa viśeṣa* to *prakṛti*.

We have come to the world with the grace of God and go back to Him with His grace. Yoga is a process of *prasava* to *pratiprasava* evolution to involution and vice versa.

Prakṛti is the mother which helps us to get us purified through *bahiraṅga, antaraṅga* and *antarātma sādhanā* of yoga liberating us from the clutches of lust, greed, anger, infatuation, pride and envy to directly experience and live from the dictates of the *puruṣa.* Hence, in *Śri yoga vidyā yantra* we see the *puruṣa viśeṣa* in the outer space as well as in the centre *(bindu).* This reminds us of *Īśopaniṣad:*

pūrṇamadam pūrṇamidam pūrṇāt pūṇamudacyate I

pūrṇsya pūrṇamādāya pūrṇamevāvaśiṣyate II

So let me quote Swami Prabhupāda on *Iśopaniṣad* with reference to this *śloka.* He says, "He The personality of Godhead is perfect and complete and because He is completely perfect, all emanations from Him such as this phenomenal world are perfectly equipped as the complete whole. Whatever is produced of the complete whole is also complete in itself. Because He is complete and whole, and as such so many complete units emanate from Him, he remains the complete balance."

EPILOGUE

EDITING *AṢṬADAḶA YOGAMĀLĀ*

(LEARNING FROM THE MASTER)

The idea of these collected works started in 1991. Guruji was preparing *Light on the Yoga Sūtras of Patañjali* for publication. We were living in the Institute and had the privilege of being around Guruji when he was finalising the manuscript. We were noting, entering and retyping his corrections, trying to follow the unattainable flow of his new ideas and his very fast yet systematic way of reading, correcting and clarifying his own explanations.

Some moments were particularly vivid and they can give to the reader an idea of how that book was written. For example, we will never forget the time when Guruji was reediting his manuscript about the *sūtra* III.9 to III.13. His text was very beautiful, and it was ready to go to the final version when, very early one morning, he came to our room and took all his time to expose to us his new ideas on how to explain these *sūtra*. And the concept of the silent moments between the rising impressions and our attempt to restrain them came to be crystal clear for ever. But something else also was clear for both of us: this new and beautiful explanation was the fresh fruit of his own practice of pranayama that very morning!

And the same happened so many times. It was a marvel to witness that fountain of new explanations when Guruji was confronted by a *sūtra*, and was not very happy about the clarity or fluidity of his own ideas to explain it, and next morning, after his own practice, the sentences were flowing like a mountain stream, so powerful and so clear. We began to understand why he was not using for reference any book except two dictionaries. A few times, when we presented him ideas from traditional commentaries, he refused kindly to see them and told us, with a smile, that he would go through all of them once his own work was over. In deed, as with all his other writings, deeply anchored in tradition, he was proceeding like a thorough scientist, completely independent, using only his own experiential knowledge to present his invisible guru's text. It is said that a *sūtra* can be explained in an scholarly way or be used as a thread connecting the *sūtra* writer to the commentator, inspiring him to share his experiential knowledge, and we felt often that this was the case.

When *Light on Yoga Sūtras of Patañjali* was almost over, Guruji was always radiant, admitting with a great humility that his book was going to be a stepping stone for the future of the studies on Patañjali's text. We were so delighted with the experience we lived. In early seventies a great *pundit* from Benares, who had to his credit outstanding research works on *Sāṁkhya* and Pātañjala yoga, wrote about the difficulties of understanding the *Yoga Sūtras* declaring that they could be and they should be commented only by an accomplished yogi who himself experienced their intrinsic nature. And now, it was clear for us that nowhere could we find a study on Patañjali's *sūtras* where the interpretation was so deeply rooted in the personal experience of the author, and nowhere would be found an author with the unquestionable authority of a true yogi of the calibre of our Guruji.

That moment an idea struck the mind of Biria. He had already been collecting since the early eighties whatever material came to his hands, whether articles written by Guruji, or interviews given by him, question and answer sessions, even letters and aphorisms. A part of this collection became the raw material which gave birth to *The Tree of Yoga*.

We started wondering and imagining what could happen if all these articles, interviews and any other written or transcribed material from Guruji were collected, arranged systematically and edited under the beacon of his present day's experience. We dreamt about what could be the result if Guruji went again through all this material, as he did many times with his commentaries on the *Yoga Sūtras* of Patañjali. In one word our dream was that Guruji himself comments his own work. A *kārika*, a *bhāṣya* on his own experiences and theories. We thought that if this work sees the day, it would be a final reference about how Guruji himself lives his own experience, how he interprets his own teaching, and the ideas and concepts he wanted to convey through his teaching...

The beauty of this dream gave us enough courage to dare and to ask him one day : "Guruji, we will classify and type all your texts, everything which is scattered through-out the world, everything which is in the bottom of the lower shelves of your library, and we will put them in front of you. If you read them adding your rectifications, suggestions and commentaries, we will do all the manual work, from researching and editing till typing the entire text."

In fact, we were thinking: "Please, do with your own articles and interviews exactly what you did with the *Yoga Sūtras*. Infuse in them the light of your own present experience."

And he accepted. It took time to classify and enter everything in the computer. When two years later we came to Pune, we brought with us thirteen bound volumes of material and put them on his desk. His first reaction was, laughing: "How can it be that I wrote all this?" Then, to our great joy, he accepted to go through all this material.

This was the beginning of a great odyssey for both of us. Guruji not only took the entire task of reading, correcting, clarifying his writings, at the same time he was training us to be critical, to discuss with him and to argue about his new ideas. The library was transformed often into a laboratory of yoga science, where we pushed the chairs back and did the *āsana*, even *prāṇāyāma*, through which he conveyed to us the logic behind his ideas, making sure that they were well understood and received accurately. He taught us how the respect, love, learning, joy and even fun must go hand in hand in a healthy structure of research and study. The work sometimes was demanding, and he worked more than all of us, giving as ever a great example and creating tremendous courage and energy in us. He knew how to give us rest when we were tired, freshness when we were heavy, how to bring light when we were in the dark... He was always the first and the last reader of his own text. Not once there has been any excuse, like complexity of the subject, lack of time or fatigue, when he was involved in this process. Nothing could break that union between his soul and his work.

Though the material was arranged systematically, he couldn't withhold his unique quality of a great educator (the "emperor of yoga instructors", as he was called by his own *guru*), and composed his ideas and explanations in an evolutory way so that each text, being completely independent, could be also considered as a further evolution of preceding ones and an introduction for the following ones.

Geeta was reading and re-reading untiringly and with a great devotion the text along with us. She never limited her efforts when she thought that she could explain and clarify something still more to make the reader grasp Guruji's message better. Often, she took time to comment Guruji's ideas and made precious suggestions for inserting them in the text.

Prashant also, with his amazing knowledge of *yoga śāstra* and Hindu scriptures was always ready to help us whenever we were in difficulty to trace the precise and clear meaning of ideas, concepts and even the terminological references in the traditional sources.

Sometimes friends and colleagues were coming to the library and, to our surprise, they were telling us that we were working hard, that we should rest a little more... And we often smiled, as we realised that they were most probably not feeling what was going on. They did not know that when one is involved in an intense work with Guruji, one forgets time, effort, and even sometimes one's own existence, and has, in his own attitude, a glimpse of what yoga can be: living and doing without even the sense of 'I' in that a process which happens always under the magnificent umbrella of Guruji's presence. Sometimes, when asked, "But, are you not tired?" our answer was, "No, we are not tired, it is *Aṣṭadaḷa Yogamālā* that is going on." And Guruji saying, with his great smile, "This attitude is real yoga!"

Now that the work is coming to an end, only one word remains on our lips: Thank you, Guruji, for this most wonderful teaching class which went on for so many years and will enlighten our hearts and lives for ever.

Sricharan Faeq Biria

Patxi Lizardi

A LEGACY OF COURAGE AND SKILL

At the end of John Bunyan's religious masterpiece, *The Pilgrim's Progress*, (17th century), Mr Valiant-for-Truth, summoned to leave this life and cross over the final river, says these awkward yet lovely words of farewell: "I am going to my Father's, and though with great Difficulty I am got hither, yet now I do not repent me of all the Trouble I have been at to arrive where I am. My Sword, I give to him that shall succeed me in my Pilgrimage, and my Courage and Skill, to him that can get it".

The following reflections are on aspects of the great Difficulty that B.K.S. Iyengar has experienced in his long life and that have defined his pilgrimage to "arrive where he is". Like Mr Valiant-for-Truth, he is in a position to bequeath to us his legacy. Our inheritance, should we want it, is his Sword. What is his sword? Can it be other than the correct practice and knowledge of what yoga is, and of how to use these to progress towards a liberating truth? Mr Iyengar has spent a lifetime, and leaves us many volumes, on how to wield the "Sword", the practice and perfection of the techniques of yoga, without harming either ourselves or other people. That legacy is secure. The sword is ours, if we want to take the trouble to learn how to use it.

But what about the other part of the legacy, "my Courage and Skill, to him that can get it"? Mr Iyengar could claim that he found courage in his everyday life, in surviving the worst and being grateful for the best. In this way he bought time to acquire skill, and increasing skill helped him to unearth fresh courage.

It occurs to me that the template which helps us best to see clearly the young Iyengar in Pune, is that of the struggling young artist, a 19th century impressionist painter for example, a provincial dumped in the unfeeling yet exciting big city, half of him burning with his own inspiration, sense of purpose, opportunity, even destiny, - the other half a riot of self-doubt, youthful gawkiness, wounded sensibilities, and always the nag of empty pockets. After a few years, a companion arrives to relieve the loneliness, but soon that brings the complication of new young mouths to feed, and always there remains the sense of an unfair exclusion from society. That description would fit a dozen Paris artists whose names are now famous and whose work sells for tens of millions. It also fits the young Iyengar. He was passionate to explore and advance his art. His body was his living sculpture. Like other artists he accepted uncongenial tasks for the sake of putting food on the table. Like them, he wondered if success or even just a fair recognition would ever come, and if it did, would it come too late?

Artists had trouble with their parents and families. It was a madcap venture to wish to survive in the big city on art alone. In 1940's and 50's Pune, too, it was just as lunatic to aspire to live through yoga. As with art, people had a few clichéd pieties on the subject, but it was certainly no career. Confusingly families complained when you failed and complained even if you succeeded. When Mr Iyengar returned from his first trip to England, his uncle refused to let him in the house.

Such treatment, over time, takes its toll. Scars fade but they do not always disappear. Mr Iyengar learned how to counter even brutal criticism with indifference, cheerfulness and fortitude. Should we conclude that he was thick-skinned, or so charged with a sense of mission that arrows bounced off him? I only know that when the great painter, Edouard Manet, was in his final illness, by then recognized and acclaimed, he admitted what no one had ever guessed from the stoic courage of his life: that the callous taunts and rejection of the past had hurt him deeply, and that the hurt endured.

Make of these sketchy comparisons what you will. In the world of yoga and spiritual aspiration generally, the public are frequently so fixated on the final victory, the soul's realisation, which they have no hope of understanding anyway, that they ignore the dignity and triumph of the deeply human saga which preceded it. Is it not equally in the process of Becoming, of development, of evolution, that we should seek inspiration? Is it not there we should look for the Courage and Skill which Mr Valiant-for-Truth says he leaves us but which we still have to get for ourselves?

Another great artist described his work as "the one blessing which may be had for the asking". Mr Iyengar's philosophy is just that; his practice is a succour and a blessing. In good times or bad, it is always there. And he does not stop. Why? Is he like another artist who in his eighties and with failing sight, repainted the water lilies of his garden every day, saying that he "never quite managed to express everything he wanted to?" There is always a restless desire to discover and to say more, a sort of divine dissatisfaction. With that goes the feeling, expressed by many artists of every type and time, and on occasion by Mr Iyengar, that the public is missing the point. They would trade in some of the adoration if only people would understand their work better.

Part of what people want from yoga is for life to be more bearable and make a little more sense. Others have conquered adversity, they feel, how can I? Mr Iyengar could have marketed the bland certitudes of the holy man, the God merchant. In their place he chose to offer the fire of the artist, the heat of engagement, the struggle of battle.

Life is cluttered and real. Mr Iyengar could have become a sadhu. It is one way to leave behind many of life's troubles and complications. But in that direction he saw retreat and defeat. The stubborn, proud artist in him wanted to show the world that his "sculpture" was the best. And eventually he succeeded. Like other artists also, he hoped that one day his detractors would admit they had been wrong about him. Some did – others lacked the honesty.

Putting aside Iyengar the artist, let us look at how this untried young man related to the momentous political events and social changes of his time. Although that time brought "Trouble and great Difficulty" to most of the world, he at least was fortunate that in his country and in his century, there developed an unparalleled model for the evolution and emancipation of mankind. It was designed by a man whose life and struggles offered Mr Iyengar an inspiration which has motivated him ever since.

Mahatma Gandhi was the giant of the 20th century, a peaceful reformer, who, without demagoguery, led the subcontinent to freedom through a form of secular humanism which few had ever expected to succeed.

There are several ways in which we can see a young Iyengar, swiftly learning and benefiting from this extraordinary influence. Mr Iyengar learned at a practical level the yogic virtue of absorbing the best, wherever it was to be found, and of ignoring the worst. Gandhiji was without bitterness or rancour towards either the British who opposed him, or to those bigots and fanatics on both sides who undermined his work. Mr Iyengar chose to imitate this philosophy of inclusive tolerance.

When in 1938, aged 20, he moved to Pune, he found himself in a profoundly different environment to all he had known before. In his own words "I came from a difficult childhood of poverty and extreme (religious) orthodoxy, and to adjust to conditions in Pune was extremely difficult. Pune had a westernised lifestyle and what I took to be an intellectual arrogance, compared to my original place. It is yoga which took me through it". Yes, of course, yoga. But we should not imagine Mr Iyengar living in a vacuum, or a Himalayan cave. He spent his time on the streets, in private houses, schools and clubs, in cheap restaurants and cafés. India was soon engaged in both a world war and an independence struggle. It was in Pune that Gandhiji was imprisoned. Mr Iyengar was in no way impervious to all that was going on around him. And as if some form of enlightenment emanated from Gandhi's cell in the Aga Khan Palace, Mr Iyengar neither retreated to the limitations of ultra-orthodoxy nor did he succumb to a loss of identity or the temptations of freedom in novel surroundings. Instead, he "retrained myself, but maintained the dignity and nobility of the Indian way of living". In other words, it became second nature to him to preserve the best of the old and to adopt whatever had value in the new.

What did he learn from the new contacts he was making, and who were they?

In the years following World War II, art festivals sprang up all over Europe. One of these was the Gstaad Music Festival in Switzerland. Its leading light was the violinist, Yehudi Menuhin. There is a widespread myth that, from their first meeting in Bombay, Yehudi Menuhin waved a magic wand over a rustic Iyengar and transformed his life and career forever, rapidly bringing fame and riches. Mr Iyengar has never lost his gratitude for the opportunity that was presented and which he, by dint of merit alone, was able to take. But it is in no sense to diminish the genuine friendship between Menuhin and Iyengar, to look again at Mr Iyengar's relationship with an exclusive and talented international set.

There are no free rides with such people. Exclusive means keeping other people out. The barrier is lifted only insofar as they can make use of you. It is said that the rich pay late. Sometimes they do not pay at all. Temporary inclusion in the charmed circle does not equal acceptance.

In spite of the warmth Menuhin and one of his sisters felt for their new yoga teacher, boundaries of snobbery, of class, wealth and culture were firmly in place. Mr Iyengar, who, though still young, was already adept in yoga, gave full value to all those he taught. In return he took some things and, just as importantly, declined to take others. In reality there was not much money and only very limited renown. But the great gain was that he lost his provincialism, his awkwardness and above all, his fear. In childhood and youth Mr Iyengar had often been treated by those around him, and who should have known better, "like a slave, fit only for manual labour" (his words). This subjugation was doubled by the climate of colonialism in which all Indians belonged to a subject race and were even, by some, judged inferior. Independence did not banish these prejudices overnight. Especially a complex of inadequacy and inferiority was not easily eradicated from the Indian psyche. If Mr Iyengar has ever shown impatience with our fear in headstand, think what courage he needed to put an eighty year old queen on her head for the first time in her life.

People took advantage of him, sometimes even those with "spiritual" pretensions. But he lost his fear. He won confidence and self-reliance, social ease and courteous address. He learnt how to present his beloved art, not merely practise it. He saw Menuhin's beautiful, sensitive violinist's hands, looked at his own, rough as a workman's, and thought, "Mine should become like that". Today his hands would be the envy of any violinist. That is what he took from the rich. When he had learned what they knew, he moved on with gratitude for what he had received. What he deliberately avoided was their snobbery, an often unmerited sense of superiority, a tendency to look down on the vast majority of mankind. He remained true to the moral values of Gandhian socialism and equality. In so doing he remained true also to a much older tradition, one which touched the very roots of where he came from and who he was.

Ramanuja was the 11th century south Indian Brahmin saint and philosopher who both subjectively, through his own enlightenment, and objectively, through logic, refuted the taboos of the caste system. In particular, he said, the belief that the bodies of our inferiors are unholy was untenable. Pollution existed in the mind only. The body was sacred, and if one was, all were. Brahman did not pick and choose.

Nevertheless the orthodox society of the south in which Mr Iyengar was brought up, whilst proud of their Vaishnavite lineage stemming from Ramanuja, in practice lived within a narrow code. Perhaps because he was uprooted and treated as an outcast, perhaps because artists are notoriously brave enough to flout convention, this rich vein of spiritual liberalism surfaced in Mr Iyengar. There it found support from the generous and inclusive humanism of Gandhiji as he sought to redress the social, economic and political injustices of colonial domination. And it resonated too in the emergence and evolution of Mr Iyengar as an individual of talent, energy and perseverance making his way in the world.

Without the freedom of this broad enlightenment, his mission to put yoga in its rightful place before the world would have remained impossible. It enabled him to graft onto his strong traditional base an understanding of science, modern medicine, sickness, disease and the craft of teaching. The alchemical fusion of this knowledge, old and new, from near and far, was only possible within the cauldron of his own relentless practice. Already from this practice, a coherent philosophy was beginning to emerge.

William Blake, the 18th century mystic poet and artist, famously said, "A fool who persists in his folly will become wise". Mr Iyengar freely admits that in youth he was that fool: "I had no background of the culture of East or West. I was "foolishly" practising as I had no other channels to think. So I had to make up my mind to sink or swim in my line of choice".

The key words are Blake's "persists" and Mr Iyengar's "line". He persisted. He did not, like the true fool, jump from one thing to another. He held a "line", a direction. And he had a means. Both the line and the means were the practice of the art, science and philosophy of yoga.

Great artists are the first to admit that you are no artist unless you become a craftsman, unless you learn the science of your trade. Great scientists admit that, although method is paramount, breakthroughs happen through a sort of grace, on artistic intuition. Great philosophers are explorers of the physical and metaphysical universe, and of consciousness itself.

Mr Iyengar had no allegiance to the ideas of others. But he was insatiably curious and where he met intelligence it sparked his own. His inexhaustible reference library, in which he could sift true from false, gold from dross, was his own practice. With experience and over time, there accumulated a quantity of truth and gold.

Consequently he was increasingly able to compare his hoard of knowledge and maybe wisdom with that of others. Mr Iyengar reads. But he does not read to acquire second hand wisdom. He does it to check, to get his bearings, to compare and evaluate. The ultimate challenge that was always before him, was whether he could go far enough in his own practice to verify from experience the work of the master, the codifier and the father of yoga, sage Patanjali himself. Could Patanjali in effect become not "received" wisdom but "perceived" wisdom? By the time he achieved this, and illumined Patanjali's text from within, rather than from without, the least one might say, to return to Blake, is that this particular fool had come a very long way indeed.

A near contemporary of Patanjali was the Greek philosopher Socrates. Socrates suggested that the practice of philosophy permitted us to live "deliberately", by which he meant it offered an incremental progression, mindful of the pitfalls of cause and effect, towards where we wanted to go in life. His method was thought in action. Subject your questions, he said, to a form of logical inquiry. From this you will distil knowledge. An assimilated knowledge gives birth to wisdom. The result of all this, according to Socrates, is that we shall become "friendly with our own gods".

We have looked at Mr Iyengar as artist, as a man subject to the cultural, political and social currents of his time, and as a seeker of wisdom. Like Mr Valiant-for-Truth he only got to this point through Trouble and great Difficulty. He has led by example. That example exists not only in the present, in what he is today, but in a very human and loveable form, in the past.

Many try to glamorize themselves by association with Mr Iyengar, to promote themselves through his achievements. Those who wish only to teach may find that his example is of little benefit to them, except commercially. To those who wish to learn, he is, and will remain, available, accessible, a companion and a guide.

His present eminence is daunting. It creates a distance. He knows us, only too well perhaps, but we are no longer sure who, or where or what he is. One cure for that might be to imagine a strange, lonely, fiercely sensitive young man striding through the bustle of a Pune that is no more. Or think of him tramping the streets of London or the red dirt roads of Swaziland where, for lack of a bus fare, like Gandhi in those same places over forty years before him, he made his solitary way to his next appointment.

Intercept this young man. Stop him there. Make him your friend. He will inspire you.

If I could guess any one thing about Mr Iyengar, it would be that he is now, like Socrates, "friendly with his gods". And if we want to do something to thank and repay him for his life and work, for all his Trouble and great Difficulty, it is that one day we should be friendly with ours too. Who knows, they may even be the same gods?

JOHN J EVANS

INDEXES

OF

VOLUMES 1 TO 8

INDEXES
of the eight volumes of *Aṣṭadaḷa Yogamālā*

These indexes cover the eight volumes of *Aṣṭadaḷa Yogamālā*. Four indexes are presented to make easy for the reader to find the object of his/her search:

I – GENERAL INDEX

This is an encyclopedic presentation of the main terms, concepts, topics and ideas treated in the eight volumes, along with their interconections. When a theme has been treated in a very significant way, the corresponding page is marked in bold.

For the sake of easy search, the proper names are included in the General Index.

II – INDEX OF SANSKRIT WORDS

A complete list of all the Sanskrit words with all their appearances in the eight volumes. The names of *āsana*, *prāṇāyāma*, *bandha* and *mudrā* are not included in this index. The Sanskrit terms are classified according to latin alphabet, whether they are simple or compounds words

III – INDEX OF *ĀSANA*, *PRĀṆĀYĀMA*, *BANDHA* AND *MUDRĀ*

A complete list of all the names of *āsana*, *prāṇāyāma*, etc. with, in bold, the places where a particular entry has been treated in detail.

IV – INDEX OF QUOTATIONS

An exhaustive list of all the quotations of:

- *Yoga Sūtras* of Patañjali,
- *Bhagavad Gītā*,
- *Haṭhayoga Pradīpika*
- *Upaniṣads*

I – GENERAL INDEX

II – INDEX OF *SANSKṚT* WORDS

(The terms of this index are classified according to latin alphabet, whether they are simple or Compound words)

III – INDEX OF *ĀSANA*, *PRĀṆĀYĀMA*, *BANDHA* AND *MUDRĀ*

IV – INDEX OF QUOTATIONS

A) *YOGA SŪTRA*

Sūtra *Pages*

Samādhi Pāda

Sādhana Pāda

Vibhūti Pāda

Kaivalya Pāda

B) *BHAGAVAD GĪTĀ*

C) *HAṬHAYOGA PRADĪPIKĀ*

D) *UPANIṢAD*

Advayatāraka — I.213 (microcosm and macrocosm)

Bṛhadāraṇyaka — VI.61 (range of *Brahman*)
VIII.31 (from death to inmortality)
VIII.285 (metaphore of the spider)

Chāndogya — II.98 *(prāṇa)*
II.163 *(Brahmavidyā)*
II.274 *(vāyu* and *jñānendriya)*
II.276 *(prāṇa)*
III.32 *(ātman)*
III.220 (way of teaching)
IV.258 *(nāḍī)*
VII.162 (eyes and *prāṇa*)
VIII.45 (food as part of *manas*)
VIII.253 (Śvetaketu and Uddālaka)

Darśana — II.171 (spine)
II.322 (mastery of *āsana*)
VII.175 *(pratyāhāra)*

Haṁsa — VII.130 (sound of the breath)

Īśa — II.128 (fullness)
III.42 (fullness)
VIII.301 (fullness)

Īśāvāsya — III.308 (pervadeness of divinity)

Kaṭha — I.101 (body/soul as chariot/ charioteer)
I.120 (gates of the body)
I.135 (gates of the body)
I.195 (the present world scenario)
V.224 (body/soul as chariot/ charioteer)
V.289 (the spiritual path as a razor blade)
VII.73 (gates of the body)
VII.74 (gates of the body)

Kauśiṭaki — II.98 *(prāṇa)*
II.267 *(prāṇa)*

Kena — V.118 (related to the form in *āsana*)

Kṣurika — VII.175 (bring *citta* towards the inner body)

Maitrāyaṇi (or *Maitrāyaṇīya*) — VII.34 *(Aum)*
VII.128 (mind)

Māṇḍūkya — VI.313 *(Aum* is *Brahman)*

Muṇḍaka — I.164 (requirements for Self-realisation)
I.232 (two facets of consciousness)
II.45 (requirements for Self-realisation)
III.159 (requirements for Self-realisation)
IV.56 (requirements for Self-realisation)

Praśna — I.254-255 *(prāṇa* and *prajñā)*
II.163 *(prāṇa* and *prajñā)*
II.267 *(prāṇa)*

Śāṇḍilya — V.201 (mastery of *āsana*)

Śvetāśvatara — I.90 (God is one with different names)
I.120 (gates of the body)
I.135 (gates of the body)
III.160 (gates of the body)
VII.73 (gates of the body)
VII.74 (gates of the body)

Taittirīya — III.39 *(Brahma)*
VII.40 *(kośa)*

Triṣikhibrāhmaṇa — II.82 (mastery of *āsana*)
II.91 (mastery of *āsana*)
II.322 (mastery of *āsana*)
VII.175 (bring *citta* towards the inner body)

www.ingramcontent.com/pod-product-compliance
Lightning Source LLC
Chambersburg PA
CBHW081426270326
41932CB00019B/3114

* 9 7 8 8 1 8 4 2 4 3 9 1 8 *